SLEEP DISORDERS

Edited by **Chris Idzikowski**

Sleep Disorders
Edited by Chris Idzikowski

Published by InTech
Janeza Trdine 9, 51000 Rijeka, Croatia

Publishing Process Manager Mia Macek
Technical Editor Teodora Smiljanic
Cover Designer InTech Design Team

Additional hard copies can be obtained from orders@intechweb.org

Sleep Disorders, Edited by Chris Idzikowski
p. cm.
ISBN 978-953-51-0293-9

For EU product safety concerns :
IN TECH d . o . o . , Prolaz Marije Krucifikse Kozulić 3 , 51000 Rijeka , Croatia ,
info@intechopen . com or visit our website at intechopen . com .

Meet the editor

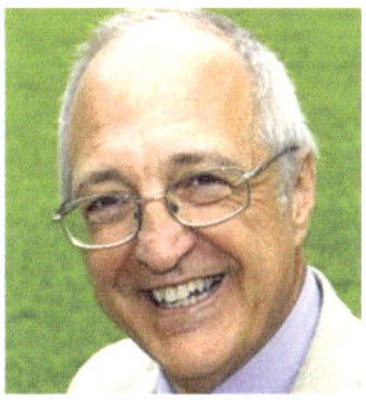

Dr Idzikowski's formal interest in sleep began in Edinburgh where he earned his PhD working with Emeritus Professor Ian Oswald, the UK's founding father of sleep research. He was Hon Treasurer of the British Sleep Society when it was first set up and subsequently became the founding Chairman of the Royal Society of Medicine Forum on sleep and its disorders and guided its transition to become the Sleep Medicine Section. He has held many honorary appointments, both health authority (Oxford) and University (e.g Queen's University of Belfast, Visiting Professor, Surrey University) and has also contributed to various sleep-related charitable organizations (e.g. Finland's Unettomat) as well as published numerous papers and books on sleep, including "Learn to sleep well" (Duncan Baird, 2000) and "Sleep" (HarperCollins, 2007). Currently he is the Director of Edinburgh Sleep Centre, a Consultant Psychologist at the London Sleep Centre and the Director of Sleep Assessment and Advisory Service in Belfast.

Contents

Preface

For progress to be maintained in a clinical field like sleep medicine, unimpeded, unrestricted access to data and the advances in clinical practice should be available. The reason this book is exciting is that it breaks down the barriers to dissemination of information. Researchers at the forefront of areas that have limited funding can find it difficult to get data from randomised, double-blind, (placebo-controlled), crossover or parallel group studies, etc., and so may be limited to the lowest level of scientific research, i.e. single case, or restricted observational series.

Nonetheless, data is data, and whilst the interpretation may be suspect (which can happen with even the best controlled studies), the data is the most valuable asset in a research paper. Of course insight that either consolidates or furthers our understanding is vital, but without data it can be nothing more than an armchair idea. Many journals require the highest levels of scientific rigour, which may make some research inaccessible - really a form of scientific censorship. Also established areas, or newly established areas can develop castes of mind that censor material by exclusion. Finally, access to scientific material can be very expensive. There are now numerous sleep journals but only larger departments are likely to be able to pay for these so a publisher that allows ready and free internet access has to be welcomed.

The chapters in this book reflect leading edge ideas, reflections and observations. Even though the modern era of sleep research evolved from Aserinksky's observations of rapid eye movements in the sleep of babies, most work is nonetheless done in adults. There is much less formal work done in youngsters and virtually none *in utero* and pregnancy itself is virtually unexplored. So, Dr Miller *et al*'s chapter reviewing sleep in pregnancy is particularly welcome as it incorporates current thinking in how disordered sleep impacts other adult pathological processes. Dr Tomoda and Dr Yamakazi's data-driven chapter on adolescents with sleep disturbance focuses on metabolic and endocrine data which sheds light on why gastrointestinal distress may arise in some children. Dr Silvestri and Dr Aricò's review examines the interrelationship of sleep disorders with the growing problem of Attention Deficit/Hyperactivity Disorder, a disorder which attracts considerable debate as to the role of sleep as a fundamental component or a state that exacerbates this complex condition.

Dr Kobal Grum and Dr Kobal's interesting work combines naturalistic observations in a quite unique observational setting found in Hg° mines. Armed with these occupational data, they consider the pathological mechanisms, given our current understanding of the neurobiology of sleep, that result in sleep disorders in these workers.

Sleep-related breathing disorders dominate sleep medicine so it is not surprising that there are several chapters in this area. The historical division in medicine of physicians and surgeons can be seen in this area or sleep disorders. It is dominated by respiratory physicians. However, surgeons also have a place, depending on the physical structures. Another curiosity in this area is that, whilst sleep apnoea demands treatment because of the adverse physical and social consequences if it is not treated, "snoring" is not regarded as such an urgent problem. However, there is evidence in terms of personal and social consequences as well as its symptomatic value, that highlight the need for more research in this area. Dr Kotecha's chapter is entirely pragmatic and practical, focussing on the evaluation of the upper airway so that the appropriate therapies can be applied.

Dr Del Campo *et al*'s timely chapter on Upper Airway Resistance Syndrome also highlights an area that is subject to discussion. As a diagnostic entity, it is not clear whether it is at one end of the obstructive sleep apnoea continuum or exists in its own right.

Dr Lovati *et al* take the book into another area, the possible bidirectional processes that can affect sleep and other disorders - in their case the two-way dynamics between sleep and migraine. From another perspective, Dr Rola examines the impact of stroke and neurological disorders on sleep disorders, bringing to the neurologists' attention the need to consider sleep a mediating factor in their nosological entities. Dr Büttner's broad ranging and comprehensive review goes beyond sleep apnoea and considers it and other disorders and their neuropsychiatric consequences on objective measures of performance.

Sleep disorders can be easily classified into three main areas: those that cause unwanted sleep or sleepiness, those that cause unwanted wakefulness and those that involve unwanted behaviours during sleep - the parasomnias. Dr Hizli Sayar and Dr Tarhan's review provides a helpful introduction into this area. Restless Legs Syndrome – a disorder which twenty years ago was 'treated' by a multitude of disparate therapies and which was only unified by its symptomatology. In recent years the mechanisms have become clearer and there is a degree of unification. Dr Taylor-Gjevre and Dr Gjevre's review brings the relevant clinical literature together in one location. The final chapter is extremely helpful in introducing methods of screening and evaluating REM Behaviour Disorder. This disorder is most easily confirmed using sleep laboratory methods (polysomnography and video), but these methods are expensive, so cheaper clinical methods are welcome and are discussed by Dr Miyamoto.

Chris Idzikowski
Director, Edinburgh Sleep Centre and
the Sleep Assessment and Advisory Service, Edinburgh,
UK

1

Sleep and Pregnancy: Sleep Deprivation, Sleep Disturbed Breathing and Sleep Disorders in Pregnancy

Michelle A. Miller, Manisha Ahuja
and Francesco P. Cappuccio
University of Warwick
UK

1. Introduction

There are many factors that can influence an individual's sleep pattern and quantity and quality of sleep. These factors can be cultural, social, psychological, behavioural, patho-physiological and environmental. Sleep patterns can also be influenced by society and by changes within society. In recent times we have seen the introduction of longer working hours, more shift-work and 24-7 availability of commodities. At the same time secular trends of curtailed duration of sleep to fewer hours per day across westernized populations (Akerstedt & Nilsson 2003) has led to increased reporting of fatigue, tiredness and excessive daytime sleepiness (Bliwise, 1996). It is of interest that whilst some studies indicate that women may have better sleep than men in general (Lindberg et al, 1997; Goel et al, 2005), they also report a larger difference in the estimated time of sleep that they believe they require and the actual sleep time they achieve than men. This might indicate that their sleep debt (amount of sleep deprivation) is higher in women than in men (Lindberg et al, 1997). There is now a wealth of evidence to support the epidemiological link between quantity of sleep (short and long duration) and quality of sleep (like difficulties in falling asleep or of maintaining sleep) and cardiovascular risk factors. These include hypertension (Cappuccio et al, 2007; Stranges et al, 2010), type-2 diabetes (Cappuccio et al, 2010a) and obesity (Cappuccio et al, 2008; Stranges et al, 2008; Cappuccio et al 2011a) as well as cardiovascular outcomes (Cappuccio et al, 2011b) and all-cause mortality (Ferrie et al, 2007; Cappuccio et al, 2010b). Additionally, there may be important gender differences in sleep and associated health outcomes (Miller, 2009 et al; Cappuccio et al, 2007). The deleterious effects of sleep deprivation can be seen on a variety of systems within the body, with detectable changes in metabolic (Knutson, et al. 2007; Spiegel, et al. 2009), endocrine (Spiegel, et al. 1999; Taheri, et al. 2004) and immune pathways (Miller & Cappuccio 2007; Miller et al, 2009).

The physiological and hormonal changes that occur in pregnancy increase the risk of developing Sleep Disordered Breathing (SDB). It has been estimated that 10-27% of pregnant women may suffer from habitual snoring (Pien & Schwab, 2004) and there is growing evidence to suggest that snoring and sleep apnoea during pregnancy are associated with an increased risk of gestational hypertension and pre-eclampsia. SDB and short sleep duration in pregnant women may also be associated with the risk of gestational diabetes.

This chapter will examine the evidence that suggests that short sleep duration and poor quality are associated with adverse maternal and foetal outcomes. Furthermore, it will examine the potential mechanisms which may underlie these associations including activation of the sympathetic nervous system, oxidation and inflammation and mechanisms leading to the development of insulin resistance (Izci-Balserak & Pien, 2010). It will also consider the prevalence of sleep disorders in pregnancy. The diagnosis, management and treatment of sleep disorders in pregnancy will be discussed along with implications for public health policy, etc.

2. Sleep and pregnancy

Pregnancy is associated with many maternal physiological and psychological changes both of which may have an effect on sleep. In the first trimester, hormonal changes may disrupt sleep and in the third trimester the large baby and the anxiety regarding delivery may have associated effects on sleep. Likewise post-partum, a newborn may disrupt sleep patterns. The review by Lee in 1998 demonstrated that there was a paucity of studies, which addressed the alterations of sleep in pregnant women, moreover many of these studies lacked sufficient power to allow consistent interpretation and replication of the results (Lee, 1998). Since then a number of studies have now been conducted but more research is still required to establish whether for example, a woman's pre-pregnancy sleep pattern can affect outcome and to determine whether there is any effect of parity on sleep related maternal and foetal outcomes. The changes in circadian rhythm of various hormones and the associated changes to sleep architecture that occur throughout pregnancy are discussed by Wolfson and Lee (2005) in 'The Principles and Practice of Sleep Medicine' (Kryger, Roth and Dement (Eds)).

2.1 Sleep deprivation: Adverse sleep changes in pregnancy quantity and quality

Due to the lack of good longitudinal studies there is still little information on what constitutes normal sleep quality and quantity both during pregnancy and in the period following delivery. In a recent study however Signal et al quantified the change and variability in sleep duration and quality across pregnancy and post-partum in 8 healthy nulliparous and 11 healthy multiparous women (Signal et al, 2007). The women wore an actigraph and completed a sleep diary for seven nights during the second trimester, one week prior to delivery, and at one and six weeks post-partum. They observed that compared to multiparous women, nulliparous women generally had less efficient sleep, spent more time in bed and had greater wake after sleep onset in the second trimester, and spent less time in bed and had fewer sleep episodes a day at one week post-partum. The largest change in sleep however occurred during the first week after delivery with the women obtaining 1.5h less sleep than during pregnancy. In a more recent and larger study sleep was assessed using the Pittsburgh Sleep Quality Index (PSQI) in 260 women during the second and third trimester of pregnancy (Naud et al, 2010). Of the 260 women, 192 (73.6%) had a term delivery without any adverse outcome. The investigators reported that there were no differences in sleep parameters between pregnancies with adverse outcome and without adverse outcome. The PSQI scores however indicted that sleep quality deteriorated from the second (5.26 +/- 3.16) to the third trimester (6.73 +/- 4.02; $P < 0.01$). This deterioration was displayed in five of seven sleep components ($P < 0.01$). Scores in the "poor sleeper" range were recorded by 36% of women in the second trimester and 56%, of women in the third ($P < 0.01$). "Poor sleep" in both trimesters was associated with low or high weight gain, low annual family income, and single motherhood ($P < 0.01$). A weak but not significant effect of season on sleep scores was recorded: The mean PSQI scores were 6.06 (+/-3.96) in winter, 5.21 (+/-3.21) in spring) 5.33 (+/-3.04) in summer and 5.53 (+/-2.41) in autumn); (P=0.076). In a similar study of 189 nulliparous women Facco et al demonstrated that compared with the baseline assessment (mean gestational age (13.8 (+/-3.8)) the mean sleep duration was significantly shorter at 30.0 (+/-2.2) weeks gestation ($p<0.01$). They also observed that in the third trimester the proportion of patients who reported frequent snoring (at least three nights per week) was significantly increased, and that there was an increase in those who met the diagnostic criteria for the recognised sleep disorder 'restless leg syndrome'. Furthermore, poor sleep quality, as defined by a Pittsburgh Sleep Quality Index score greater than 5, became significantly more common as pregnancy progressed (Facco et al, 2010).

In a separate study Wilson et al also found that sleep efficiency was decreased in late pregnancy and was associated with an increase in cortical arousals when compared to women in early pregnancy and non-pregnant women. Compared to a control group, they found that women in the third trimester of pregnancy had more awakenings and had had poorer sleep efficiency. They had less stage 4 sleep and more stage 1 sleep and spent less time in rapid eye movement (REM) sleep (Wilson et al, 2010).

Sleep quality also decreases as a woman approaches labour (Evans et al, 1995) but whilst little is known of the effect of sleep disturbance on labour or delivery outcome it has been common practice to administer morphine sulphate to women in either early or non-progressing latent phase labour to induce sleep. It has been observed that on awakening the contractions are more regular and active.

2.2 Sleep disorders in pregnancy

Sleep-Disordered breathing (SDB) is the term used to describe a group of disorders which are characterized by abnormalities of respiratory pattern (pauses in breathing) or the quantity of ventilation during sleep. A recent study evaluated the frequency of sleep disordered breathing in women with gestational hypertension compared to healthy women with uncomplicated pregnancies. They observed that women with gestational hypertension may have a significantly higher frequency of sleep disordered breathing than do healthy women with uncomplicated pregnancies of similar gestational age. The frequencies of sleep disordered breathing in the more obese gestational hypertension group and the healthy group were 53% and 12% ($p<0.001$) (Reid et al, 2011).

Obstructive sleep apnoea (OSA) is the most common of these sleep disorders and is characterized by the complete or partial collapse of the pharyngeal airway during sleep. To resume ventilation, feedback mechanisms arouse the individual, which leads to sleep disruption. OSA is associated with an increased CVD risk. Although, men are twice as likely to develop OSA as women, the risk is increased in women if they are overweight. Moreover, data from recent studies indicates that snoring and OSA increase during pregnancy. The prevalence of OSA is very low in normotensive women low-risk pregnancies but is increased among normotensive pregnant women with high risk pregnancies and, in those with gestational hypertension (pregnancy-induced hypertension (PIH)/pre-eclampsia) during pregnancy, the prevalence is even higher.

PIH is characterised by high blood pressure with a flat circadian rhythm and in particular does not have the normal nocturnal dip associated with sleep. Risk factors for PIH include first time pregnancy, long periods (>10years) between pregnancies, multiple pregnancies, women younger than 20 or older than 35 or women who are overweight, have a history or hypertension or kidney disease or diabetes. Recent studies indicate that OSA per se is an independent risk factor for gestational hypertension/pre-eclampsia and may contribute to other poor obstetrical outcomes. Good blood pressure control in pregnancy is important. Continuous Positive Airway Pressure (CPAP), which is used to treat OSA, may also have beneficial effects on blood pressure (Champagne et al, 2010). It may therefore be very useful in patients with PIH as this condition is associated with both increased blood pressure and a significantly narrowed upper airways and limited airflow during sleep (Izci et al, 2003). Continuation of treatment for OSA following the pregnancy may also be required.

Insomnia is a sleep disorder which is characterised by a difficulty in initiating or maintaining sleep in combination with adverse daytime consequences. The daytime effects may include excessive fatigue, impairment of performance or emotional changes. Data from self-reported questionnaires suggests that sleep complaints are more frequent in pregnancy and that sleep disturbances increases as the pregnancy progresses. In a recent study of 300 women (100 women in each trimester of pregnancy) it was observed that there was a significant increase in insomnia in the 2nd trimester, excessive daytime sleepiness (EDS) was also increased in pregnancy and the rate for specific awakenings increased by 63% in the first trimester, by 80% in the second trimester and by 84% in the third trimester ($p<0.001$) (Lopes et al, 2004).

Restless leg syndrome is a neurosensory sleep disorder which begins in the evening. The associated symptomatic leg movements can prevent a person from falling asleep and contribute to poor sleep quality. Pregnant women have at least two or three times higher risk of experiencing restless legs syndrome (RLS) than the general population and women affected by pre-existing RLS often complain of worsening symptoms during pregnancy. It is associated with iron deficiency anaemia. The women who are most at risk are those with low folate, ferritin or haemoglobin prior to conception. Data from the existing epidemiological studies suggests that the rates may be as high as 27% in the third trimester (Lee et al, 2001; Manconi et al, 2004). Whilst RLS is a reversible syndrome in pregnancy and is typically limited to the third trimester it has been associated with adverse pregnancy outcomes and therefore needs to be taken seriously. The standard medications for RLS that contain dopaminergics or opioids should be avoided but preventative measures to increase the amount of folate should be encouraged at the first prenatal visit.

Complaints of heartburn increase during pregnancy and if these progress to severe nocturnal oesophageal reflux may also contribute to sleep disruption.

2.3 Sleep disturbances and adverse maternal and foetal outcomes

In Western societies adverse pregnancy outcomes have been on the increase and in the United States over 1 million pregnancies are associated with adverse outcomes including increased maternal and infant morbidity. The current known risk factors however are insufficient for early detection of at risk individuals and attention has focused on sleep as an emerging new risk factor (Okun et al, 2009). A recent prospective cohort study of low-risk pregnant women suggested that there may be no differences in sleep parameters between pregnancies with adverse outcome and without adverse outcome (Naud et al, 2010). Other studies however have indicated that sleep deprivation in pregnancy may be associated with adverse maternal outcomes including gestational hypertension, pre-eclampsia and diabetes and difficulties with labour and delivery, depression and adverse effects on the foetus. Data suggests that women who snore or suffer from obstructive sleep apnea during pregnancy are more likely to suffer from gestational hypertension and pre-eclampsia. Data is also accumulating to suggest that both short sleep duration and sleep-disordered breathing may be associated with an increased risk of gestational diabetes (Izci-Balserak & Pien, 2010). A study of Taiwanese women compared sleep quality using the PSQI between 150 second-trimester and 150 third-trimester pregnant women and 300 non-pregnant women. (Ko et al, 2010). The study demonstrated that the prevalence of poor sleepers was increased in pregnant as compared to non-pregnant women and that sleep quality of pregnant women was related to stress and depression.

There is evidence to suggest that sleep deprivation during pregnancy increases the risk of preterm delivery and postpartum depression, and that systematic inflammation may be an important underlying mechanism in the association (Okun et al, 2009; Okun, et al 2011a, Chang et al, Okun et al, 2011b). Approximately 14.5% of women will experience an episode of post partum major depression (PPMD) and 25% will experience a recurrent episode (Wisner et al, 2006). Women with PPMD are also more likely to experience impaired relationships with their infant (Gavin et al, 2005). In a recent study 56 pregnant women with past history of PPMD but with no evidence of depression in their current pregnancy, had blood samples collected at 8 times during the first 17 weeks postpartum. The PSQI was also administered. Recurrence of depression was measured by two consecutive 21-item scores of $\geq$ 15 on the Hamilton Rating Scale for Depression (HRSD) and by clinical interview. The blood was analysed for estradiol, prolactin, cortisol and IL-6. The results indicated that in this study, self-reported poor sleep quality but not hormone or cytokine levels were associated with PPMD recurrence (Okun et al, 2011a).

Fatigue and sleep disturbance in late pregnancy are important determinants of both labour duration and delivery type. A prospective observational study of 131 women in their ninth month of pregnancy demonstrated that those women who slept less than 6 hours per night, as determined by 48-hour wrist actigraphy, sleep logs and questionnaires, had had longer labours and were 4.5 times more likely to have caesarean deliveries. Labours were also longer and were 5.2 times more likely end in caesarians in those women who had poor quality sleep (Lee & Gay, 2004).

Amongst pregnant women snoring is common and it may have adverse effects on the foetus. In particular, foetal hypoxia may occur leading to an increase in systemic inflammation and an elevation in the number of circulating nucleated red blood cells (nRBCs) with an associated decrease in foetal wellbeing (Tauman et al, 2011). A recent population-based case-control study investigated whether snoring, sleep position and other sleep practices in pregnant women were associated with risk of late still birth, i.e. $\geq$28 weeks' gestation)(Stacey et al, 2011). No relation was found between snoring or daytime sleepiness and risk of late stillbirth. However, women who slept on their back (O.R. 2.54, 95% C.I. 1.04 to 6.18) or on their right side (1.74, 0.98 to 3.01) on the night preceding the stillbirth or interview were more likely to experience a late stillbirth compared with women who slept on their left side. In addition women who got up to go to the toilet once or less on the last night (2.28, 1.40 to 3.71) and those who regularly slept during the day in the previous month (2.04, 1.26 to 3.27) were also more likely to experience a late stillbirth than the respective control counterpart. Possible mechanisms for the effect of sleeping position are: inhibition of venous return by compression and ensuing reduction in uterine blood flow (Milson & Forssman, 1984; Jeffreys et al., 2006), reduction in foetal oxygen saturation (Carbonne et al., 1996), reduced pulsatility index of the foetal middle cerebral artery (a surrogate for foetal hypoxia)(Khatib et al., 2011). An alternative explanation of these findings, however, could be of reverse causality, due to reduced foetal movement, one of the most common symptoms seen before stillbirth (Chappell & Smith, 2011).

The altered circadian patterns that accompany shift work are known to disrupt reproductive function in women. Female shift workers have more menstrual cycle irregularities than non-shift workers (Labyak et al, 2002) and some report more sleep disturbances. A link between adverse pregnancy outcomes and shift work has also been suggested (Kutson, 2003) although in a recent study no relationship was found between rotating shift work and adverse pregnancy outcomes but an increase in late abortions/still births was reported in women who were working fixed night shifts (Schlünssen et al, 2007).

The intense physical and psychological changes which women undergo during pregnancy may be associated with increased stress and reduced quantity and quality of sleep. These effects may in turn affect the mother-infant relationship either through pregnancy-related hormonal changes, changes in inflammatory markers, maternal fatigue or postpartum depression (Pires et al, 2010; Okun et al, 2011a).

2.4 Mechanisms

Sleep disturbances may affect maternal and foetal morbidity and mortality through a number of potential mechanisms. For example, increased nocturia (due to decreased bladder capacity and increased overnight sodium excretion) disrupts sleep. Gastro-oesophageal reflux also leads to awakening and disruption of sleep; first due to a relaxed lower oesophageal sphincter (progesterone working as a muscle relaxant); and then due to pressure on the stomach and reduced gastric emptying (Bourjeily & Rosene-Montella, 2009). Restless legs, leg cramps and increasing frequency of contractions all also contribute to disturbed sleep (Bourjeily & Rosene-Montella, 2009). Furthermore, sleep disordered breathing can be magnified or occur in pregnancy as a result of poor sleep and decreased functional reserve capacity, increased weight from gestation and pregnancy related nasopharyngeal oedema (Izci-Balserak, 2008; Pien & Schwab, 2004).

Sleep is not a passive state but is an active process in which memory consolidation, tissue restoration, metabolic and haemostatic processes occur (Adam,1980; Alvarez & Ayas, 2004; Ancoli-Israel, 2006; Benca & Quintas, 1997 as cited in Okun, 2011). Sleep disturbances are known to have effects on oxidation, glucose metabolism and the sympathetic nervous system and there is strong evidence to support an association with cardiovascular outcomes (Cappuccio et al, 2011b). Furthermore, the association between sleep deprivation and hypertension has been shown to be stronger in women than in men (Cappuccio et al, 2007). Cardiovascular disease is relevant to many adverse pregnancy outcomes including pre-eclampsia and intrauterine growth restriction (IUGR) both of which are also associated with a greater risk of developing cardiovascular disease in later life (Okun et al, 2009). Inflammatory processes have been shown to be important in the development of cardiovascular disease and emerging evidence has demonstrated an association between increased inflammation and medical morbidity, including various pregnancy complications. Some of the mechanisms by which sleep deprivation may lead to adverse maternal and foetal outcomes are discussed in more detail below.

2.4.1 Oxidation and inflammation

Increased oxidative stress, endothelial dysfunction and inflammation are important in the development of cardiovascular disease. In OSA, the associated sleep disordered breathing leads to episodes of hypoxia and then normoxia. This in turn leads to oxidative stress and a subsequent increase in inflammation. There is strong evidence that during pregnancy inflammation and oxidative stress is increased (Okun et al, 2009). There is also evidence that inflammatory markers and reactive species are present in a higher proportion of pregnant women who report sleep disturbances than those who do not.

Okun et al recently put forward a model for the possible role of sleep and inflammation in the pathogenesis of adverse pregnancy outcomes (Okun et al, 2009). They proposed that disturbed sleep has its major effects in the first 20 weeks of pregnancy. It is at this time that major physiological events occur, including the re-modelling of maternal blood vessels to the placenta so as to increase blood flow. This process is abnormal in pre-eclampsia and IUGR; in vitro studies indicate that this in part is due to excessive inflammation which inhibits trophoblastic invasion. It is postulated that is in non pregnant individuals disturbed sleep in pregnancy may contribute to this increased inflammatory state. Increased circulating cytokines through a positive feed forward process may in turn contribute to sleep disruption. In addition poor health behaviours including smoking, alcohol and obesity can also contribute to the increase in inflammation; thus having a profound effect on vascular re-modelling and hence leading to adverse pregnancy outcomes.

Interleukin 6 (IL-6) is a significant pro-inflammatory and anti-inflammatory agent. It is also released in several disease states, from muscles during exercise, from adipose tissue and blood vessel walls. In sleep, there is an increase in the availability of soluble IL-6-receptors during the late nocturnal period which enhances IL-6 signalling and was thought to have a positive effect on memory consolidation. The administration of intranasal IL-6 in a study in 2009 was shown to increase slow wave activity and the consolidation of only emotional memories during sleep in test subjects compared to a placebo (Benedict et al, 2009).

IL-6 is also increased in pregnancy as early as mid-gestation in women who report poor sleep duration and efficiency, poor sleep duration and sleep disordered breathing (SDB) (Okun et al, 2007a). In complicated pregnancies involving foetal hypoxia, there is evidence of foetal erythropoiesis shown by increased levels of circulating nucleated red blood cells (nRBCs). Levels of IL-6 and erythropoietin (EPO) mediate the production of nRBCs and, interestingly, a study on pregnant women who reported snoring (assessed using a sleep questionnaire) found high circulating levels of IL-6 and EPO in the umbilical cord blood shortly after birth (Tauman et al, 2011). In women suffering from pre-eclampsia compared with pregnant controls, levels of IL-6 are also markedly raised (Bernardi et al, 2008, Sharma et al, 2007). In addition they are shown to be more fatigued and suffer more from snoring and nasal airflow limitation (Bachour et al, 2008). This suggests that IL-6 could be a marker for foetal well-being raised in response to poor/disturbed sleep. It is also important because IL-6 is involved in the pathogenesis of insulin resistance and type 2 diabetes and gestational diabetes mellitus (Mohamed-Ali et al, 1997; Wolf et al, 2004).

Disordered sleep in the pregnant state has correlation with increased levels of IL-10 across all trimesters (Okun et al, 2007b). CRP is raised in both non-pregnant and pregnant states that report poor sleep. Studies on women with pre-eclampsia compared to normal control pregnancies offer differing results. One by Bernardi et al shows no change in IL-10 levels and others show decreased IL10 in pre-eclamptic women (Zusterzeel et al, 2001). This would suggest a non typical pattern of inflammation in these women as they do not have raised IL-10 or IL-1β (Bernardi et al, 2008). However, a major drawback of these studies is the measurement of IL-10 only once after diagnosis. Recent studies have suggested time dependent lipid peroxidation in pre-eclamptic patient which allows the use of plasma 8-isoPGF (2-alpha) as a marker for oxidative stress between 24-32 weeks but not 34-37 weeks of gestation. In a separate study whilst short sleep duration and poor sleep efficiency in both mid and late pregnancy were associated with higher stimulated levels of IL-6 there were no relationships were observed for TNF-α (Okun et al, 2007a).

Adiponectin has insulin sensitising and anti-inflammatory properties (Makino et al, 2006). Oxidative stress, TNF-α and IL-6 have been shown to reduce adiponectin, a hormone released by adipose tissue in people with SDB/OSA (Makino et al, 2006; Lain & Catalano, 2007). Insulin resistance increases in normal pregnancy, but is also associated with short sleep duration and SDB (Punjabi et al, 2004). Some studies have shown an increased risk of GDM in pregnant women who have lower levels of adiponectin and high levels of CRP (Willaims et al, 2004; Wolf et al, 2003; Qiu et al, 2004). Other studies have shown that pregnant women with GDM have lower levels of adiponectin TNF-α, IL-6 and IL-10 compared with controls (Ategbo et al, 2006).

One study has found that pregnant women with SDB have higher levels of malondialdehyde (MDA) than their non snoring controls. However this study found no comparable difference between any negative foetal outcomes after birth (Koken et al, 2007). Other studies conclude that SDB and the resulting hypoxia/re-oxygenation increase reactive oxygen species which can cause cellular damage (Jerath et al, 2009; Roberts & Hubel, 2004). This is hypothesised to contribute to pre-eclampsia and gestational diabetes in pregnant women (Roberts & Hubel, 2004).

2.4.1.1 Inflammation and maternal and foetal outcomes

Increased inflammation (higher levels of IL-6, TNF-α and CRP) is also associated with adverse pregnancy outcomes such as pre-eclampsia, Intra-Uterine Growth Retardation (IUGR) and preterm birth (Bartha et al, 2003, Romero et al, 2006 and Freeman et al, 2004). It is unclear if the increase in cytokines occurs as a result of increased stress or if sleep deprivation is a contributing factor. In a high proportion of these outcomes, studies have found a failure of re-modelling of spiral arteries, a process necessary for adequate placental perfusion following trophoblast invasion (Arias et al 1993). TNF-α was shown to interfere with trophoblast invasion in experimental studies (Fluhr et al, 2007 and Salamonsen, et al 2007).

Some studies have also linked the increase in inflammatory markers and maternal depression to pre term labour and babies with low birth weight. Groer & Morgan found that of the 200 women who were 4 - 6 weeks postpartum, those who were depressed, had significantly smaller babies and more negative life events. These women also had low levels of cortisol, suggesting an ineffective restrain on inflammation (Groer & Morgan, 2007). A study in Goa, India of 270 women also had similar results, and in addition positively correlated the severity of depression to the risk of low birth weight (Odds Ratio 2.5) (Patel & Prince, 2006).

Studies in the field of psychoneuroimmunology have shown that mothers suffering from postnatal depression have much higher levels of inflammatory markers than their non depressed controls. These markers include CRP, IL-6, interleukin-1β (IL-1β), TNF-α and IFN-γ (Miller et al, 2005). In the last trimester of pregnancy, raised markers are adaptive and prevent infection. However at abnormally large levels they increase the risk of depression (Maes et al, 2000). It was also shown that these women had lower levels of cortisol; however in response to an acute stressor, they produced much higher levels of IL-6 and TNF-α compared to the non-depressed controls. The authors from this study of 72 women concluded that they had "cortisol blunting" (Miller et al, 2005).

Author	Study Population	Maternal Effects	Foetal Effects	Inflammatory marker	Summary
Tauman et al (2011)	122 pregnant women recruited, of which 39% had SDB	Sleep Disordered Breathing	Increased Erythropoiesis	IL-6, EPO, nRBCs	In pregnant women who were habitual snorers, there was evidence of increased foetal erythropoiesis shown by increased umbilical cord levels of nRBCs, EPO and IL-6
Bachour et al 2008	15 pre-eclamptic women and 14 pregnant controls	Increased time with nasal flow limitations, generalised oedema, increased fatigue and poorer pregnancy outcomes		IL-6 , TNF-α, and CRP	Pre-eclamptic women presented with more snoring and had increased levels of IL-6 and TNF-α compared with controls. Overall their pregnancy outcomes were worse than controls.
Bernardi et al (2008)	35 pre-eclamptic women and 35 normotensive women	Pre-eclampsia		IL-6, IL-10, IL-1β TNF-α, protein carbonyls and plasma thiobarbituric acid	IL-6, TNF-α, protein carbonyls and plasma thiobarbituric acid were higher in pre-eclamptic patients. IL-6 and carbonyls had significant correlation with blood pressure as well as each other. No increase in IL-1β and IL-10 in pre-eclamptic patients. Effect of sleep disorders or complaints not investigated.

Author	Study Population	Maternal Effects	Foetal Effects	Inflammatory marker	Summary
Okun et al (2007a)	19 Women in mid – late pregnancy	Sleep complaints associated with increased inflammation.		IL-6	Short sleep and poor sleep efficiency in mid to late pregnancy is associated with higher stimulated and circulating levels of IL-6. Women having sleep problems as early as mid gestation could also have increased inflammation.
Okun & Coussons-Read (2007b)	35 pregnant women seen once a trimester. 43 non-pregnant women seen once.	Sleep complaints associated with increased inflammation.		IL-10, CRP and TNF-α	IL-10 and CRP were higher in pregnant women throughout the three trimesters. In women reporting sleep problems, TNF-α was significantly higher in pregnant women (across all trimesters) and CRP in non pregnant women.
Koken et al (2007)	40 snoring pregnant women and 43 non snoring pregnant women	Snoring		Glutathione peroxidase (GSH-Px), Malondialdehyde (MDA) and Myeloperoxidase (MPO)	Levels of GSH-Px were lower in the group that snored, and levels of MDA were much higher. Levels of MPO were comparable between the groups. There were no adverse outcomes associated with infants born to the mothers who snored.

Table 1. Sleep disturbances, pregnancy and inflammation

The table summarises the studies to date on the effect of sleep disruption on markers of inflammation and the possible association with maternal and foetal outcomes.

There is evidence to support the increase in inflammatory cytokines measured in amniotic fluids leads to preterm birth. A prospective cohort study of 681 women showed that depressed women were more than twice as likely to have preterm birth than their non depressed counterparts (9.7% vs. 4%; OR: 3.3). Prostaglandins in particular have a major role in uterine contractions and may be released early in response to increased pro-inflammatory cytokines in disturbed sleep. (Dayan et al, 2006). IL-6 and TNF-α have a role in ripening the cervix before birth; and in women who have preterm birth, these markers are raised in a study of 30 pregnant women. This suggests a link between inflammation and preterm birth, although in these women, stress was being assessed instead of sleep disturbances as a cause of raised cytokines. In a more recent study of 166 pregnant women, sleep was assessed by means of the PSQI. It was observed that for every one point increase in the PSQI score the odds of a preterm birth increased by 25% in early pregnancy and by 18% in late pregnancy (Okun et al, 2011b). Women who have SDB during pregnancy are also more likely to need an emergency caesarean (Leung et al, 2005).

2.4.2 Activation of neuroendocrine pathways

Activation of the sympathetic Nervous System (SNS) leads to the release of adrenal hormones (catecholamines), which can have an effect on sleep (Guggisberg, 2007). Furthermore, the production of catecholamines may stimulate the production of inflammatory cytokines. Inflammatory processes are modulated by numerous feedback and feed forward mechanisms. The Hypothalamic-pituitary-adrenal axis also regulates inflammatory processes via cortisol secretion, which is secreted in a diurnal manner following the sleep-wake cycle. Cortisol can suppress the production of pro-inflammatory cytokines and, as part of the negative feedback mechanism designed to prevent uncontrolled inflammation, pro-inflammatory cytokines stimulate the HPA axis to produce cortisol. However, as in the case of SDB and the resulting hypoxia, plasma cortisol is chronically raised (Meerlo et al, 2000). Prolonged cortisol secretion leads the glucocorticoid receptors becoming desensitised and results in a decrease in the protective effects of cortisol against inflammation (Sapolsky et al, 2000). Disrupted sleep can lead to mild stimulation of the HPA axis and increased inflammation, thus providing another mechanism whereby disrupted sleep in pregnancy may lead to dysregulation of normal homeostatic processes and potentially lead to adverse pregnancy outcomes (Okun et al, 2009).

2.4.3 Insulin resistance

Accumulating evidence suggests that both poor sleep quantity and quality are associated with impaired glucose tolerance and diabetes (Cappuccio et al, 2010a). Until recently little has been known about the effect of poor sleep during pregnancy on glucose tolerance and gestational diabetes. Qui et al interviewed a large cohort of 1,290 women during early pregnancy. They collected information regarding sleep duration and snoring during pregnancy. They obtained information on gestational diabetes mellitus (GDM) from the screening and test results in their medical records. They found that those women who slept 4 hours or less had a greater risk of GDM than those sleeping 9 hours per night. Furthermore they observed that whilst the increased relative risk was 3.23 (95% CI 0.34-

30.41) for lean women (<25 kg/m2) this was increased to 9.83 (95% CI 1.12-86.32) for overweight women (> or = 25 kg/m2). Snoring was also associated with a 1.86-fold increased risk of GDM and the risk of GDM was 6.9 xs higher in overweight than lean women (Qiu et al, 2010). These findings are consistent with data in non-pregnant women and warrant further investigation to determine the effect on pregnancy outcome.

2.4.4 Passive smoking

In Japan, two surveys were conducted to determine if passive smoking might have any effect on the sleep disturbances observed in pregnant women. 16,396 pregnant women were surveyed in 2002 and 19,386 in 2006. This is particularly important as 80% of passive environmental smoking comes from the spouse and in Japan there is a very high smoking rate amongst men (53%). The results indicated that passive smoking is independently associated with increased sleep disturbances during pregnancy. They observed that pregnant woman who were exposed to passive smoking were likely to suffer from difficulty in initiating sleep, short sleep, and snoring; those women who smoked suffered from the same disturbances and also reported early morning awakenings and excessive daytime sleepiness (Ohida et al, 2007). The authors suggest that some of the negative health outcomes observed in pregnant women may be mediated by the effect of active and passive smoking on sleep.

2.5 Diagnosis and management of sleep disorders in pregnancy

There are many different ways in which sleep data can be collected, the gold standard, however, is to measure sleep using polysomnography (PSG) as this provides an objective assessment of the sleep-wake cycle over the entire sleep period (Baker et al, 1999). Much of the data regarding sleep in pregnancy is limited to self-administered questionnaires and to diaries: very few recent studies have used PSG. However, it is recognised that undertaking multiple sleep studies at different time points during pregnancy is difficult. Despite this there is evidence to suggest that sleep disorders in pregnancy can in certain individuals have adverse outcomes for the mother or baby and therefore it would be useful to develop a screening tool that could be administered quickly by health professionals during routine pregnancy consultations. A simple and cost-effective alternative to PSG is to use actigraphy and sleep diaries. There are now many wrist-watch style actigraphs available. They are activated by movement and can differentiate when a person is awake or asleep, many also now have light monitors incorporated in them as well. They are useful in identifying night time awakenings and for determining their subsequent duration. When used in conjunction with self-recorded sleep diaries, actigraphs can help to establish a very detailed sleep pattern. Questionnaires administered to a bed partner can also help to establish a diagnosis of sleep disordered breathing. OSA is a common but often unrecognised condition in women of childbearing age. The likelihood is increased however in women with a past or current history of polycystic ovary syndrome, depression, hypertension, diabetes, hypothyroidism, metabolic syndrome, obesity (Champagne et al, 2010). The diagnostic test of choice would be a PSG, and referral to a sleep specialist to confirm and treat primary sleep disorders may be required. Further research is also required to establish if the management thresholds for treatment of OSA in non-pregnant women are applicable to pregnant women.

Pharmacological treatment of sleep disorders in pregnancy needs to be viewed with caution, given the potential for harm to the foetus. Similar caution needs to extend to women who are breastfeeding.

2.6 Implications for public health

In the general population sleep duration has been declining. Women now occupy an increasingly prominent position in the workplace but often they do so without any reduction in their home responsibilities. Consequently sleep needs are often of low priority. Preterm birth is a major public health priority and is a common adverse outcome in pregnancy. Sleep quantity and quality are not only important determinants of maternal and foetal health but are also important for general health and need to be particularly addressed in the post-partum period where sleep disruption is likely to be very common. There is also some evidence to suggest that the effects of sleep deprivation may be greater in women than in men. Despite this, the majority of studies undertaken are in men and there is now a clear need for more, large, multicentre, prospective studies to be performed in women.

There is also a paucity of studies evaluating sleep disturbances in the post-partum period and research is required to look at the effects of sleep deprivation on both maternal and paternal functioning and the effect on maternal-infant interaction. Factors such as the type of delivery, the type of infant feeding, return-to-work time and infant temperament may be important, along with the degree of support from the father or other family members. A recent randomised trial set out to investigate if modification to the bedroom environment could improve the sleep of new parents (Lee & Gay, 2011). They evaluated a modified sleep hygiene intervention for new parents (infant proximity, noise masking, and dim lighting) in anticipation of night-time infant care in two samples of new mothers of different socioeconomic status. They were randomized to the experimental intervention or attention control, and sleep was assessed in late pregnancy and first 3 months postpartum using actigraphy and the General Sleep Disturbance Scale. The investigators observed that whilst the sleep hygiene strategies evaluated did not benefit the more socioeconomically advantaged women or their partners they did improve postpartum sleep among the less advantaged women suggesting that simple inexpensive changes to the bedroom environment can improve sleep for new mothers.

Further studies are required fully to investigate the effects of smoking on sleep and associated adverse pregnancy outcomes but meanwhile educational programmes could be used to educate women on the possible harmful effects. Research to determine if other health behaviours could have beneficial effects on sleep in pregnant women is also required. For example, physical activity is recommended to pregnant women for health benefits but as yet there are insufficient studies to determine if this has any effect on improving sleep duration or quality.

3. Conclusion

A lack of sleep is known to affect both our physical and mental health. The few studies that have investigated sleep in pregnancy have found both an increase in total sleep time and an increase in daytime sleepiness in the first trimester whereas the third trimester appears to be associated with a decrease in sleep time and an increase in the number of awakenings. Sleep has an important impact on maternal and foetal health. It has been associated with an increased duration and pain perception in labour, with a higher rate of caesarean delivery and with preterm labour. Some pregnant women develop sleep disorders such as RLS or OSA or insomnia and others develop postpartum depression. Longitudinal studies are required to fully evaluate the effect of sleep deprivation on maternal and foetal outcome.

Better methods to measure sleep disturbances in pregnancy are required along with evaluation of the underlying cause so that appropriate and effect treatment can be administered. Particular attention needs to be given to women who develop leg complaints, who are overweight or become obese during pregnancy or develop conditions such as diabetes or PIH.

4. Acknowledgment

This work was in part funded by a University of Warwick Undergraduate Student Scholarship for Manisha Ahuja. We would like to thank Ms P McCabe for help in the preparation of the manuscript.

5. References

Akerstedt, T. & Nilsson, P. M. (2003). Sleep as restitution: an introduction. J Intern Med, Vol.254, No.1, pp. 6-12

Arias, F.; Rodriquez, L.; Rayne, SC.; Kraus, FT. (1993). Maternal placental vasculopathy and infection: two distinct subgroups among patients with preterm labor and preterm ruptured membranes. Am J Obstet Gynecol, Vol.168, pp. 585–591

Ategbo, J.M.; Grissa, O.; Yessoufou, A., Hichami, A,; Dramane, KL,; Moutairou, K,; Miled, A,; Grissa, A,; Jerbi, M,; Tabka, Z,; Khan, NA. (2006). Modulation of adipokines and cytokines in gestational diabetes and macrosomia. J Clin Endocrinol Metab, Vol.91, pp. 4137–4143

Bachour, A.; Teramo, K.; Hiilesmaa, V. & Maasilta, P. (2008). Increased plasma levels of inflammatory markers and upper airway resistance during sleep in pre-eclampsia. Sleep medicine, Vol.9, No.6, pp. 667-674

Baker, F.C.; Maloney, S. & Driver, H.S. (1999). A comparison of subjective estimates of sleep with objective polysomnographic data in healthy men and women. J Psychosom Res, Vol.47, No.4, pp. 335-341

Bartha, J.L.; Romero-Carmona, R. & Comino-Delgado, R. (2003). Inflammatory cytokines in intrauterine growth retardation. Acta Obstet Gynecol Scand, Vol.82, pp. 1099–1102

Benedict, C.; Scheller, J.; Rose-John, S.; Norn, J. & Marshall, L. (2009). Enhancing influence of intranasal interleukin-6 on slow-wave activity and memory consolidation during sleep. FASEB J, Vol.23, pp. 3629-3636

Bernardi, F.; Guolo, F.; Bortolin, T.; Petronilho, F. & Dal-Pizzol, F. (2008). Oxidative stress and inflammatory markers in normal pregnancy and preeclampsia. J Obstet Gynaecol Res, Vol.34, No.6, pp. 948-51

Bliwise, D. L. (1996). Historical change in the report of daytime fatigue. Sleep, Vol.19,,No.6, pp. 462-464

Bourjeily, G (Ed). & Rosene-Montella, K (Ed). (2009). Pulmonary Problems in Pregnancy. Pub Springer Verlag Gmbh

Cappuccio, F. P.; D'Elia, L.; Strazzullo, P. & Miller, M. A. (2010a). Quantity and quality of sleep and incidence of type 2 diabetes: a systematic review and meta-analysis. Diabetes Care, Vol.33, No.2, pp. 414-420.

Cappuccio, F. P.; D'Elia, L.; Strazzullo, P. & Miller, M. A. (2010b). Sleep duration and all-cause mortality: a systematic review and meta-analysis of prospective studies. Sleep Vol.33, No.5, pp. 585-592.

Cappuccio, F. P.; Stranges, S.; Kandala, N.-B.; Miller, M. A.; Taggart, F. M.; Kumari, M.; Ferrie, J. E.; Shipley, M. J.; Brunner, E. J., & Marmot, G. (2007). Gender-Specific Associations of Short Sleep Duration with Prevalent and Incident Hypertension. The Whitehall II Study. Hypertension, Vol.50, No.4, pp. 694-701

Cappuccio, F. P., Taggart, F. M., Kandala, N.-B., Currie, A., Peile, E., Stranges, S., & Miller, M. A. (2008). Meta-analysis of short sleep duration and obesity in children, adolescents and adults. Sleep, Vol.31, No.5, pp. 619-626

Cappuccio, F.P. & Miller, M.A. (2011a). Is prolonged lack of sleep associated with obesity? BMJ, Vol. 26, pp. 342:d3306. doi: 10.1136/bmj.d3306.

Cappuccio, F.P.; Cooper, D.; D'Elia, L.; Strazzullo, P. & Miller, M.A. (2011b). Sleep duration predicts cardiovascular outcomes: a systematic review and meta-analysis of prospective studies. Eur Heart J,Vol.32, No.12, pp.1484-1492.

Carbonne B., Benachi A., Leveque M.L., Cabrol D., Papiemik E. (1996). Maternal position during labor: effect on fetal oxygen saturation measured by pulse oximetry. Obstet Gynecol, Vol.88, pp. 797-800.

Champagne, K.A.; Kimoff, R.J.; Barriga, P.C. & Schwartzman, K. (2010). Sleep disordered breathing in women of childbearing age & during pregnancy. Indian J Med Res, Vol.131, pp. 285-301

Chang, J.J.; Pien, G.W.; Duntley, S.P. & Macones, G.A. (2010). Sleep deprivation during pregnancy and maternal and fetal outcomes: is there a relationship? Sleep Med Rev, Vol.14, No.2, pp. 107-14.

Chappel L.C., Smith G.C.S. (2011). Should pregnant women sleep on their left? BMJ, Vol.342, pp. d3649.

Dayan, J.; Creveuil, C.; Marks, M.N.; Conroy, S.; Herlicoviez, M.; Dreyfus, M. & Tordjman, S. (2006). Prenatal depression, prenatal anxiety, and spontaneous preterm birth: A prospective cohort study among women with early and regular care. Psychosom Med, Vol.68, pp. 938-946

Evans, M.L.; Dick, M.J. & Clark, A.S. (1995). Sleep during the week before labor: relationships to labor outcomes. Clin Nurs Res.,Vol.4, No.3, pp. 238-249

Facco, F.L.; Kramer, J.; Ho, K.H.; Zee, P.C. & Grobman, W.A. (2010). Sleep disturbances in pregnancy. Obstet Gynecol. Vol.115, No.1, pp. 77-83

Ferrie, J. E.; Shipley, M. J.; Cappuccio, F. P.; Brunner, E.; Miller, M. A.; Kumari, M. & Marmot, M. G. (2007). A prospective study of change in sleep duration: associations with mortality in the Whitehall II cohort. Sleep, Vol.30, No.12, pp. 1659-1666

Fluhr, H.; Krenzer, S.; Stein, G.M., et al. (2007). Interferon-gamma and tumor necrosis factor-alpha sensitize primarily resistant human endometrial stromal cells to Fas-mediated apoptosis. J Cell Sci,Vol.120, pp. 4126–4133

Freeman, D.J.; McManus, F.; Brown, E.A., et al. (2004). Short and long-term changes in plasma inflammatory markers associated with preeclampsia. Hypertension, Vol.44, pp. 708–714

Gavin, N.I.; Gaynes, B.N.; Lohr, K.N.; Meltzer-Brody, S.; Gartlehner, G. & Swinson, T. (2005). Perinatal depression: a systematic review of prevalence and incidence. Obstet Gynecol, Vol.106, No.5 Pt 1, pp. 1071-1083.

Goel, N.; Kim, H. & Lao, R.P. (2005). Gender differences in polysomnographic sleep in young healthy sleepers. Chronobiol Int, Vol.22, No.5, pp. 905-915

Groër, M.W. & Morgan, K. (2007). Immune, health and endocrine characteristics of depressed postpartum mothers. Psychoneuroendocrinology, Vol.32, No.2pp.133-9.

Guggisberg, A.G.; Hess, C.W. & Mathis, J. (2007). The significance of the sympathetic nervous system in the pathophysiology of periodic leg movements in sleep. Sleep, Vol.30, No.6, pp. 755-766

Holcberg, G.; Huleihel, M.; Sapir, O., et al. (2001). Increased production of tumor necrosis factor-alpha TNF-alpha by IUGR human placentae. Eur J Obstet Gynecol Reprod Biol,Vol.94, pp. 69–72

Izci, B.; Riha, R.L.; Martin, S.E.; Vennelle, M.; Liston, W.A.; Dundas, K.C.; Calder, A.A. & Douglas, N.J. (2003). The upper airway in pregnancy and pre-eclampsia. Am J Respir Crit Care Med, Vol.167, No.2, pp. 137-140.

Izci-Balserak, B. & Pien, G.W. (2010). Sleep-disordered breathing and pregnancy: potential mechanisms and evidence for maternal and fetal morbidity. Curr Opin Pulm Med,. Vol.16, No.6, pp. 574-582

Izci-Balserak, B. (2008). Sleep-disordered breathing in pregnancy. Int J Sleep Wakefulness, Vol.1, pp. 98–108.

Jeffreys R.M., Stepanchak W., Lopez B., Hardis J., Clapp J.F. 3rd (2006). Uterine blood flow during supine rest and exercise after 28 weeks of gestation. Br J Obstet Gynaecol, Vol.113, pp 1239-1247.

Jerath, R.; Barnes, V.A. & Fadel, H.E. (2009). Mechanism of development of preeclampsia linking breathing disorders to endothelial dysfunction. Med Hypotheses, Vol.73, pp. 163–166.

Khatib N., Haberman S., Belooseki R., Vitner D., Weiner Z., Thaler I. (2011) Maternal supine recumbency leads to brain auto-regulation in the fetus and elicits the brain sparing effect in low risk pregnancies. Am J Obstet Gynecol, Vol.204, pp. s278.

Knutson, K. L.; Spiegel, K.; Penev, P. & Van Cauter, E. (2007). The metabolic consequences of sleep deprivation. Sleep Med Rev, Vol.11, No.3, pp. 163-178

Knutsson, A. (2003). Health disorders of shift workers. Occup Med (Lond), Vol.53, No.2, pp. 103-108.

Köken, G.; Sahin, F. K.; Cosar, E.; Saylan, F.; Yilmaz, N.; Altuntas, I.; Fidan, F.; Unlu, M. & Yilmazer, M. (2007). Oxidative stress markers in pregnant women who snore and fetal outcome: a case control study. Acta Obstetricia et Gynecologica Scandinavica, Vol.86, No.11, pp. 1317-1321

Ko, S.H.; Chang, S.C. & Chen, C.H. (2010). A comparative study of sleep quality between pregnant and nonpregnant Taiwanese women. J Nurs Scholarsh, Vol.42, No.1, pp. 23-30.

Labyak, S.; Lava, S.; Turek, F. & Zee, P. (2002). Effects of shiftwork on sleep and menstrual function in nurses. Health Care Women Int., Vol.23, No.6-7, pp. 703-714

Lain, K.Y. & Catalano, P.M. (2007). Metabolic changes in pregnancy. Clin Obstet Gynecol, Vol.50, pp. 938–948

Lindberg, E.; Janson, C.; Gislason, T.; Björnsson, E.; Hetta, J. & Boman, G. (1997). Sleep disturbances in a young adult population: can gender differences be explained by differences in psychological status? Sleep, Vol.20, No.6, pp. 381-387

Lee, K.A. & Gay, C.L. (2004). Sleep in late pregnancy predicts length of labor and type of delivery. Am J Obstet Gynecol, Vol.191, No.6, pp. 2041-2046.

Lee, K.A. (1998). Alterations in sleep during pregnancy and postpartum: a review of 30 years of research. Sleep Med Rev, Vol.2, No.4, pp. 231-242

Lee, K.A. & Gay, C.L. (2011). Can modifications to the bedroom environment improve the sleep of new parents? Two randomized controlled trials. Res Nurs Health, Vol.34, No.1, pp. 7-19. doi: 10.1002/nur.20413.

Lee, K.A.; Zaffke, M.E. & Baratte-Beebe, K. (2001). Restless legs syndrome and sleep disturbance during pregnancy: the role of folate and iron. J Womens Health Gend Based Med, Vol.10, No.4, pp. 335-341

Leung, P.L.; Hui, D.S.; Leung, T.N, Yuen, PM,; Lau, TK. (2005). Sleep disturbances in Chinese pregnant women. BJOG, Vol.112, pp. 1568–1571

Lopes, E.A.; Carvalho, L.B.; Seguro, P.B.; Mattar, R.; Silva, A.B.; Prado, L.B. & Prado, G.F. (2004). Sleep disorders in pregnancy. Arq Neuropsiquiatr. June, Vol.62, No.2A, pp. 217-221.

Maes, M.; Lin, A-H.; Ombelet, W.; Stevens, K.; Kenis, G.; deJongh, R.; Cox, J. & Bosmans, E (2000). Immune activation in the early puerperium is related to postpartum anxiety and depression symptoms. Psychoneuroendocrinology, Vol.5, pp. 121-137

Makino, S.; Handa, H.; Suzukawa, K.; Fujiwara, M.; Nakamura, M.; Muraoka, S.; Takasago, I.; Tanaka, Y.; Hashimoto, K.; Sugimoto, T. (2006). Obstructive sleep apnoea syndrome, plasma adiponectin levels, and insulin resistance. Clin Endocrinol (Oxf), Vol.64, pp. 12–19.

Manconi, M.; Govoni, V. ; De Vito, A.; Economou, N.T.; Cesnik, E.; Mollica, G. & Granieri, E. (2004). Pregnancy as a risk factor for restless legs syndrome. Sleep Med, Vol.5, No.3, pp. 305-308. Review

Meerlo, P.; Sgoifo, A. & Suchecki, D. (2008). Restricted and disrupted sleep: effects on autonomic function, neuroendocrine stress systems and stress responsivity. Sleep Med Rev, Vol.12, pp. 197–210

Miller, M. A. & Cappuccio, F. P. (2007). Inflammation, sleep, obesity and cardiovascular disease. Current Vascular Pharmacology, Vol.5, pp. 93-102

Miller, M. A.; Kandala, N.-B.; Kivimaki, M.; Kumari, M.; Brunner, E. J.; Lowe, G. D. O.; Marmot, M. G. & Cappuccio, F. P. (2009). Gender differences in the cross-sectional relationships between sleep duration and markers of inflammation: Whitehall II study. Sleep, Vol.32, No.7, pp. 857-864

Miller, G.E.; Rohleder, N.; Stetler, C. & Kirschbaum, C. (2005). Clinical depression and regulation of the inflammatory response during acute stress. Psychosom Med, Vol.67, pp. 679-687.

Milsom I. & Forssman L. (1984) Factor influencing aortocaval compression in late pregnancy. Am J Obstet Gynecol, Vol.148,pp 764-771.

Mohamed-Ali, V.; Goodrick, S.; Rawesh, A., Katz, DR.; Miles, JM.; Yudkin, JS.; Klein, S.; Coppack, SW. (1997). Subcutaneous adipose tissue releases interleukin-6, but not tumor necrosis factor-alpha, in vivo. J Clin Endocrinol Metab., Vol.82, pp. 4196–4200

Naud, K.; Ouellet, A.; Brown, C.; Pasquier, J.C. & Moutquin, J.M. (2010). Is sleep disturbed in pregnancy? J Obstet Gynaecol Can, Vol.32, No.1, pp. 28-34

Ohida, T.; Kaneita, Y.; Osaki, Y.; Harano, S.; Tanihata, T.; Takemura, S.; Wada, K.; Kanda, H.; Hayashi, K. & Uchiyama, M. (2007). Is passive smoking associated with sleep disturbance among pregnant women? Sleep, Vol.30, No.9, pp. 1155-1161

Okun, M.L.; Roberts, J.M.; Marsland, A.L. & Hall, M. (2009). How disturbed sleep may be a risk factor for adverse pregnancy outcomes. Obstet Gynecol Surv, Vol.64, No.4, pp. 273-280

Okun, M.L.; Hall, M. & Coussons-Read, M.E. (2007a). Sleep Disturbances Increase Interleukin-6 Production During Pregnancy: Implications for Pregnancy Complications. Reproductive Sciences, Vol.14, pp. 560-567

Okun, M. L. & Coussons-Read, M.E. (2007b). Sleep disruption during pregnancy: How does it influence serum cytokines? Journal of reproductive immunology, Vol.73, No. 2, pp. 158-165

Okun, M.L.; Luther, J.; Prather, A.A.; Perel, J.M.; Wisniewski, S. & Wisner, K.L. (2011). Changes in sleep quality, but not hormones predict time to postpartum depression recurrence. J Affect Disord. Vol.130, No.3, pp. 378-384.

Okun, M.L.; Dunkel Schetter, C. & Glynn, L.M. (2011). Poor Sleep Quality is Associated with Preterm Birth. Sleep, (in press).

Okun, M.L. 2011) Biological consequences of disturbed sleep:Important mediators of health? Japanese Psychological Research, Vol 53, No. 2, pp 163–176

Patel. V. & Prince, M. (2006). Maternal psychological morbidity and low birth weight in India. Brit J Psychiatry, Vol.188, pp. 284-285

Pien, G.W. & Schwab, R.J. (2004). Sleep disorders during pregnancy. Sleep; 27:1405–1417

Pires, G.N.; Andersen, M.L.; Giovenardi, M. & Tufik, S. (2010). Sleep impairment during pregnancy: possible implications on mother-infant relationship. Med Hypotheses, Vol.75, No.6, pp. 578-582.

Punjabi, N.M.; Shahar, E.; Redline, S., et al. (2004). Sleep-disordered breathing, glucose intolerance, and insulin resistance: the Sleep Heart Health Study. Am J Epidemiol, Vol.160, pp. 521–530

Qiu, C.; Sorensen, T.K.; Luthy, D.A. & Williams, M.A. (2004). A prospective study of maternal serum C-reactive protein (CRP) concentrations and risk of gestational diabetes mellitus. Paediatr Perinat Epidemiol, Vol.18, pp. 377–384

Qiu. C.; Enquobahrie, D.; Frederick, I.O.; Abetew, D. & Williams, M.A. (2010). Glucose intolerance and gestational diabetes risk in relation to sleep duration and snoring during pregnancy: a pilot study. BMC Womens Health, Ma. Vol.10, p. 17

Reid, J., Skomro, R.; Cotton, D.; Ward,H.; Olatunbosun, F.; Gjevre, J.; Christian G, MD, (2011). Pregnant women with gestational hypertension may have a high frequency of sleep disordered breathing, Sleep in press

Roberts, J.M. & Hubel, C.A. (2004). Oxidative stress in preeclampsia. Am J Obstet Gynecol; Vol.190, pp. 1177–1178

Romero, R.; Espinoza, J.; Goncalves, L.F., et al. (2006). Inflammation in preterm and term labour and delivery. Seminin Fetal Neonatal Med.;Vol.11, pp. 317–326

Salamonsen, L.A.; Hannan, N.J. & Dimitriadis, E. (2007). Cytokines and chemokines during human embryo implantation: roles in implantation and early placentation. Seminin Reprod Med,Vol.25, pp. 437–444

Sapolsky, R.M.; Romero, L.M. & Munck, A.U. (2000). How do glucocorticoids influence stress responses? Integrating permissive, suppressive, stimulatory, and preparative actions. Endocr Rev, FVol.21, No.1, pp. 55-89.

Schlünssen, V.; Viskum, S.; Omland, Ø. & Bonde, J.P. (2007). [Does shift work cause spontaneous abortion, preterm birth or low birth weight?]. Ugeskr Laeger, Vol.169, No.10, pp. 893-900

Sharma, A.; Satyam, A. & Sharma, J.B. (2007). Leptin IL-10 and inflammatory markers (TNF-alpha, IL-6 and IL-8) in pre-eclamptic, normotensive pregnant and healthy non-pregnant women. Am J Reprod Immunol, Vol.58, pp. 21–30

Signal, T.L.; Gander, P.H.; Sangalli, M.R.; Travier, N.; Firestone, R.T.; Tuohy, J.F. (2007). Sleep duration and quality in healthy nulliparous and multiparous women across pregnancy and post-partum. Aust N Z J Obstet Gynaecol, Vol.47, No.1, pp. 16-22

Spiegel, K.; Leproult, R. & Van Cauter, E. (1999). Impact of sleep debt on metabolic and endocrine function. Lancet, Vol.354, No.9188, pp. 1435-1439

Spiegel, K.; Tasali, E.; Leproult, R. & Van Cauter, C. E. (2009). Effects of poor and short sleep on glucose metabolism and obesity risk. Nat.Rev.Endocrinol, Vol.5, No.5, pp. 253-261.

Stacey T., Thompson J.M.D., Mitchell E.A., Ekeroma A.J., Zuccollo J.M., McCowan L.M.E. (2011). Association between maternal sleep practices and risk of late stillbirth: a case-control study. BMJ, Vol.342, pp d3403.

Stranges, S.; Dorn, J. M.; Shipley, M. J.; Kandala, N. B.; Trevisan, M.; Miller, M. A.; Donahue, R. P.; Hovey, K. M.; Ferrie, J. E.; Marmot, M.G. & Cappuccio, F. P. (2008). Correlates of short and long sleep duration: a cross-cultural comparison between the United Kingdom and the United States: the Whitehall II Study and the Western New York Health Study. Am.J.Epidemiol, Vol.168, No.12, pp. 1353-1364

Stranges. S.; Dorn, J.M.; Cappuccio, F.P.; Donahue, R.P.; Rafalson, L.B.; Hovey, K.M.; Freudenheim, J.L.; Kandala, NB.; Miller, M.A. & Trevisan, M. (2010). A population-based study of reduced sleep duration and hypertension: the strongest association may be in premenopausal women. J Hypertens, Vol.28, No.5, pp. 896-902

Taheri, S.; Lin, L.; Austin, D.; Young, T. & Mignot, E. (2004). Short sleep duration is associated with reduced leptin, elevated ghrelin, and increased body mass index. PLoS.Med, Vol.1, No.3, p. e62

Tauman, R.; Many, A.; Deutsch, V.; Arvas, S.; Ascher-Landsberg, J.; Greenfeld, M. & Sivan, Y. (2011). Maternal snoring during pregnancy is associated with enhanced fetal erythropoiesis - a preliminary study. Sleep Med, May, Vol.12, No.5, pp. 518-522

Williams, M.A.; Qiu, C.; Muy-Rivera, M.; Vadachkoria, S.; Song, T.; Luthy, DA. (2004). Plasma adiponectin concentrations in early pregnancy and subsequent risk of gestational diabetes mellitus. J Clin Endocrinol Metab, Vol.89, pp. 2306–2311

Wilson, D.L.; Barnes, M.; Ellett, L.; Permezel, M.; Jackson, M. & Crowe, S.F. (2010). Decreased sleep efficiency, increased wake after sleep onset and increased cortical arousals in late pregnancy. Aust N Z J Obstet Gynaecol, Vol.51, No1, pp.38-46.

Wisner, K.L.; Chambers, C. & Sit, D.K. (2006). Postpartum depression: a major public health problem. JAMA. December 6, Vol.296, No.21, pp. 2616-2618

Wolf, M.; Sauk, J.; Shah, A.; Vossen Smirnakis, K'; Jimenez-Kimble, R.; Ecker, JL.; Thadhani, R. (2004). Inflammation and glucose intolerance: a prospective study of gestational diabetes mellitus. Diabetes Care, Vol.27, pp.21–27

Wolf, M.; Sandler, L.; Hsu, K.; Vossen-Smirnakis, K.; Ecker, JL.; Thadhani, R. (2003). First-trimester C-reactive protein and subsequent gestational diabetes. Diabetes Care, Vol.26, pp. 819–824

Wolfson, R.; Lee, KA (2005). Pregnancy and the Postpartum Period. In: The Principles and Practice of Sleep Medicine. Kryger, MH (Ed), Roth, T (Ed) & Dement, WC (Ed). pp.1278-1286. Elsevier.

Zusterzeel, P.L.; Rütten, H.; Roelofs, H.M.; Peters, W.H. & Steegers, E.A. (2001). Protein carbonyls in decidua and placenta of pre-eclamptic women as markers for oxidative stress. Placenta, Vol.22, pp. 213–219

2

Adolescents with Sleep Disturbance: Causes and Diagnosis

Akemi Tomoda and Mika Yamazaki
Child Development Research Center,
Graduate School of Medical Sciences,
University of Fukui
Japan

1. Introduction

In our previous study, circadian rhythm sleep disorders have been reported in pediatric and adolescent populations (Tomoda, Miike, Uezono, & Kawasaki, 1994). Pediatric practitioners now commonly encounter sleep disturbance in previously healthy children and adolescents (Boergers, Hart, Owens, Streisand, & Spirito, 2007; Giannotti, Cortesi, Sebastiani, & Ottaviano, 2002; Stein, Mendelsohn, Obermeyer, Amromin, & Benca, 2001). The characteristic clinical features are well known, but the specific causes remain unknown. New types of circadian rhythm sleep disorders, such as familial advanced sleep phase syndrome (ASPS) and delayed sleep phase syndrome (DSPS), non-24-h sleep-wake syndrome (non-24), and morningness-eveningness have been described during the last decade. Such disorders are probably caused by various disturbances of circadian expression of the clock gene (Archer et al., 2003; Ebisawa et al., 2001; Iwase et al., 2002; Pirovano et al., 2005; Takimoto et al., 2005; Toh et al., 2001; Wijnen, Boothroyd, Young, & Claridge-Chang, 2002). Polymorphisms in clock genes are known to induce circadian rhythm sleep disorders. For example, mutations in the period2 (Per2) gene (S662G) or casein kinase1 d (CK16) gene (T44A) cause familial ASPS; furthermore, missense polymorphisms in the Per3 (V647G) and CK1e (S408N) genes increase or decrease the risk of developing DSPS.
In our clinical practices, we recognized that the majority of our patients have a circadian rhythm disorder even though they usually do not mention or recognize this problem at the first interview. **We hypothesized that there could be certain relationship between biological rhythm disorders in these patients and their indefinite symptoms as well as their sleep disturbances.** This chapter introduces sleep patterns, circadian rhythms of core body temperature (CBT), glucose metabolism, and human clock gene profile in children and adolescents with sleep disturbance.

2. Methods

2.1 Protocol

This study included 22 unmedicated patients with sleep disturbances (Table 1). All patients satisfied diagnostic criteria for circadian rhythm sleep disorders of the Diagnostic and Statistical Manual of Mental Disorders, 4th Edition, Text Revision (DSM-IV-TR®). The

diagnosis was made by three raters using the Structured Clinical Interview. The severity of those symptoms was measured using self-reported ratings (performance status scores), as described previously {Kuratsune, 2002 #890;Tomoda, 2007 #925}. Their performance status scores on admission were higher than 5 (mean, 5.6; SD, 0.8).
For at least one month prior to the initial assessment, prophylactic drugs (e.g. tranquilizers) were not given. Patients who had just recently started treatment with antidepressants or hypotension drugs, or who were diagnosed as having neurological illness, migraine, obstructive sleep apnea, below average intelligence, or serious psychopathology were excluded from the study. Serious psychopathology was evaluated by referral to at least one psychiatrist if the patient presented with some indicative symptoms. No patient had a history of drug abuse. Table 1 presents physical characteristics of the present subjects. The protocol was approved by the Committee of Life Ethics, Graduate School of Medicine, Kumamoto University. All participants gave written informed consent.

	Patient (n = 22)	Control (n = 9)	p-value
Mesor (°C)	36.71±0.17	36.61±0.18	p>0.1
Double amplitude (°C)	0.85±0.36	1.51±0.37	p<0.005
Acrophase (clock time):			
In advanced patients (n=6)	15.10±1.02	17.44±1.34	p<0.005
In delayed patients (n=16)	20.02±1.18	17.44±1.34	p<0.005

p-value: significant difference in ANOVA.

Table 1. Circadian rhythm of core body temperature: Results of a cosinor analysis.

2.2 Recording of the sleep-wake rhythm

Each subject kept daily recordings (logs) of their time of sleeping and awaking for 4 or longer weeks. These logs were used to analyze their sleep pattern during a 24-hour period. According to the International Classification of Sleep Disorders (ICSD) revised by the Association of Sleep Disorders Center in North America in 1990 (Diagnostic Classification Committee, 1990), our patients were diagnosed as either delayed sleep phase syndrome (DSPS), non-24-hour sleep-wake syndrome (non-24), irregular sleep, or long sleeper. DSPS is characterized by difficulty in falling asleep at night and an inability to be easily aroused in the morning, and this diagnosis corresponds to DSM-III-R: Sleep-Wake Schedule Disorder. Non-24 presents sleep-wake cycles longer than 24 hours, and this corresponds also to DSM-III-R: 307.45. Irregular sleep is characterized with no recognizable circadian patterns of sleep onset or waking time, and this does not correspond a sleep disorder diagnosis in DSM-III-R. Long sleeper have sleep times longer than 9 hours although they do not have any organic abnormalities, and this correspond to DSM-III-R: 780.54.

2.3 Circadian rhythm of core body temperature

Continuous monitoring of CBT for 3 days and at every one minute was carried out by using a deep body temperature monitor (Terumo Corp., Tokyo, Japan).

Mean values of the 3 measurements at each time point during the 3 consecutive days were used in the examination. A chronograph was used to determine the circadian rhythm, and the single cosinor method, to analyze the CBT circadian variation for both groups (Halberg et al. 1977). A cosine curve with a period of 24 hours was fitted to the data by using the least squares method, and the following parameters were obtained: mesor (°C, rhythm-adjusted average), amplitude (difference between the highest and lowest temperature), and acrophase (time of the highest point in the rhythm defined by a fitted cosine curve). To obtain data in normal age-matched persons, we recruited 9 healthy school children as volunteers. They were 6 males and 3 females, aged 10-21 years (mean age, 17.3 years), and who had no mental retardation, physical problems, or psychiatric psychopathology.

In statistical analysis, ANOVA was used, and when the *p*-value was less than 0.05, the group difference was considered to be statistically significant.

2.4 Hormonal secretion profiles

Melatonin, cortisol, ß-endorphin and temperature circadian rhythms. 24-hour blood sampling was performed through an indwelling catheter in a forearm vein at 4-hour intervals. Each blood sample was immediately centrifuged at 4°C and stored at -80°C until melatonin, cortisol and ß-endorphin were assayed by radioimmuno assay (RIA). The lower limit of melatonin sensitivity was determined to be 3 pg/ml.

Comparative data concerning the timing of hormonal production were obtained for a group of six normally-sighted healthy male volunteers aged 20-22 years (mean age, 20.6 years) who had no mental retardation or serious psychopathology.

The recordings of the deep body temperature were carried out with a deep body temperature monitor (Terumo Co., Tokyo, Japan) below Lanz's point every 1 minute for three consecutive days for the patient and the control group.

Both a chronograph and the single cosinor method were used to examine the rhythmicity and to analyze the circadian variation.

A cosine curve with a period of 24 hours was fitted to the data using the least squares method, and the following parameters were established; mesor (rhythm-adjusted mean), amplitude (difference between mesor and nadir) and acrophase (lag of the crest time in the best fitted cosine curve in relation to a given reference time). When the p-value was less than 0.05, the rhythm was considered to be statistically significant.

2.5 Evaluation of carbohydrate metabolism

A 3-h oral glucose tolerance test was performed the morning after a subject had fasted overnight. After the fasting blood sample was drawn, a subject was given a solution containing a predetermined amount of glucose based on body weight (1.75 g/kg to a maximum of 75 g). After glucose ingestion, blood samples were drawn at 30, 60, 90, 120, 150, and 180 min to measure blood glucose (BG) levels and immunoreactive insulin (IRI) response. Serum BG level was determined using the glucose oxidase reaction method. Serum IRI response was measured using radioimmunoassay (Eiken Chemical Co. Ltd., Tokyo, Japan).

The BG levels, IRI response, cumulative BG (sigma BG), cumulative IRI (sigma IRI), insulin/glucose ratio (delta IRI/delta BG), and insulinogenic index (sigma IRI/sigma BG) were then compared to normal control data that had been reported previously for 8 subjects aged 12–16 years without a personal or family history of diabetes mellitus or any factor affecting glucose metabolism (Iwatani et al., 1997). The control subjects were within ±2.0 SD of standard height, and within ±20% of ideal body weight. All indices were calculated using the same methods as those reported previously (Iwatani et al., 1997).

2.6 Experimental procedure for human clock gene measurement

Subjects were exposed to natural and fluorescent lighting of the institution during the awake period. Lights were turned off during the sleeping period. An indwelling catheter was placed in the antecubital vein for a 24-h period. Blood samples were taken at 4-h intervals beginning at 10:00 a.m. on the second day of hospitalization and continued until 6:00 a.m. of the following day. Samples were obtained under dim light (less than 30 Lux) without waking the patients during the sleeping period. We previously reported that subjects 12 years of age and older show similar metabolic characteristics to those of an adult (Iwatani et al., 1997). Therefore, we recruited 10 men aged 20–41 years (mean age, 27.4 years; SD, 6.1 years) as normal subjects from whom data were obtained (Reppert & Weaver, 2002; Takimoto et al., 2005): none had below-average intelligence, physical problems, psychiatric psychopathology, or irregular sleep or meal schedules.

Blood was collected in blood RNA kit tubes (PAXgene; Qiagen K.K., Tokyo, Japan). The tubes were incubated at room temperature for 24 h; then the total ribonucleic acid (RNA) was isolated according to the manufacturer's instructions. For quality assessment of total RNA during protocol development, deoxyribonucleic acid (DNA) digestion of the samples was performed with the RNase-Free DNase Set (Qiagen K.K.). Synthesis of complementary DNA was conducted (ReverTra Ace-α-®; Toyobo Co. Ltd., Osaka, Japan) for use with the reverse-transcription polymerase chain reaction (RT-PCR) kit. Quantitative real-time RT-PCR (TaqMan®) was performed using a sequence detection system (ABI PRISM® 7900; Applied Biosystems, Foster City, CA) to determine the expression levels of *hPer1, hPer2, hPer3, hBmal1, hClock,* and housekeeping gene *hβ-actin* expression relative to *hβ-actin,* with the standard protocol described by the manufacturer. Relative expression of the clock gene was determined as the ratio of expression of the clock gene to that of the β-actin gene for each sample. Values were normalized so that the peak value equaled 100%. The TaqMan® *hβ-actin* control reagents and primer sets, Assays-on-Demand™ Gene Expression Product for *hPer1, hPer2, hPer3, hBmal1,* and *hClock* were purchased from Applied Biosystems for the following: *hPer1,* Hs00242988_m1; *hPer2,* Hs00256144_m1; *hPer3,* Hs00213466_m1; *hBmal1,* Hs00154147_m1; *hClock,* Hs00231857_m1. In addition, *hPer2* was selected as the daily expression of the clock gene for determination of the circadian profile (Takimoto et al., 2005).

3. Results

3.1 Sleep-awake rhythm disturbance

Based on the self-recorded sleep-wake logs, all patients were diagnosed as having one of the 4 sleep disturbances, i.e., DSPS, non-24, irregular, and long sleeper. Among patients in these 4 disease categories, there were no significant differences in the duration of sleep disturbance, ages when the symptom first started, and their current age.

More than 80% of our patients with sleep disorders showed a tendency of a day/night reversal life style, especially in the period right after termination of school social life. An overnight EEG study revealed a decrease in deep NREM sleep and delayed latency of the

REM sleep phase (unpublished data). Most of them need about 10 hours sleep to keep awake for the rest of the daytime. These data suggest a deteriorated quality of night sleep. Even though sleep disorders are considered to begin in childhood and adolescents, there have been no in depth reports on this problem.

3.2 Abnormal core body temperature rhythm

It has been known that the sleep-awake circadian rhythm and other circadian rhythms such as the CBT and hormonal secretion rhythms are closely related to each other. With this background we examined the circadian CBT rhythm in our cases using a special instrument for CBT measurement. The CBT rhythm has been considered to well-match the brain temperature rhythm, according to a basic study. The 41 subjects studied (24 males and 17 females), aged between 10 to 19 years (mean: 15.2 years), were referred to our clinic. To obtain data for normal age-matched controls, we recruited healthy school children as volunteers. The comprised 6 males and 3 females, aged 10-21 years (mean: 17.3 years) for CBT controls. The results are summarized in Table 1. In those patients, the mesor of the circadian CBT rhythm was significantly higher than that in the normal controls. In particular, it is noteworthy that the mean CBT at nighttime was obviously higher in the patients than in normal controls. In those patients, the nadir was also significantly higher than in the normal subjects. The nadir recorded on appearance was significantly delayed in the patients compared to in the normal subjects.

In those patients, the amplitude of circadian CBT rhythm was significantly lower (0.85 ± 0.36°C) than the normal subjects (1.51 ± 0.37°C) ($P < 0.005$). Acrophase in the control subjects was recorded on 17.44 ± 1.34 PM, whereas it was advanced in 6 patients to 15.10 ± 1.02 PM ($P < 0.005$), and delayed in 16 patients to 20.02 ± 1.18 PM ($P < 0.005$). Advance or delay was determined in comparison to the time defined in the control subjects. In our subjects, there were no rhythmical changes in their CBT.

3.3 Disturbed hormonal secretion profiles

We have studied the hormonal circadian secretion rhythm, such as for melatonin, cortisol and β-endorphin. Each of them showed abnormal behavior, that is, a delayed peak secretion time and a decrease in the secreted amount. As to cortisol secretion in the patients, the area under the curve (AUC) was significantly smaller than in normal controls. In addition, the cortisol peak secretion time was significantly delayed.

These data suggested that circadian rhythms are deranged in our patients, and clearly explain that the starting time of daily life is seriously delayed, because of delayed preparation for mental and physical activity supporting daily life. We would like to emphasize the reason why those patients showed a bad condition in the morning and a relatively good condition in the afternoon. The decreased total level of hormonal secretion may be the main cause of the inactivity, dullness and stagnant condition.

3.4 Disturbed carbohydrate metabolism

Glucose tolerance was significantly lower in the patients than in normal controls: the mean sigma blood glucose level was significantly higher ($P < 0.05$) and the insulinogenic index was significantly lower ($P < 0.05$) in the patient group than in controls (Miike, Tomoda, Jhodoi, Iwatani, & Mabe, 2004).

The mean blood glucose (BG) level was not significantly higher in the patient group than in the controls at any time interval following oral glucose ingestion, except at 30 and 120 min (both $P < 0.05$) (Tomoda, Kawatani, Joudoi, Hamada, & Miike, 2009). The mean plasma insulin concentration in the patient group was not significantly different from the controls at any time interval following oral glucose ingestion, except at 120 and 150 min ($P <0.001$ and $P <0.05$, respectively). However, individual patient insulin levels varied widely compared with the corresponding BG levels. The insulin level did not correlate with the BG level in some patients. The mean sigma BG level in the patient group was significantly higher than that of controls (910.3 ± 189.9 vs. 865.1 ± 60.5 mg/dl, $P = 0.027$). However, the mean sigma IRI was not significantly different (patients vs. controls = 431.6 ± 194.8 vs. 892.8 ± 440.5 μU/ml, $P = 0.103$). The insulin/glucose ratio, the initial insulin response 30 min after glucose ingestion, was not significantly different (patients vs. controls = 0.95 ± 0.63 vs. 2.43 ± 1.03, $P = 0.315$). However, a significant difference was found in the insulinogenic index (patients vs. controls = 0.48 ± 0.20 vs. 1.04 ± 0.50, $P = 0.044$). The results are summarized in Table 2.

3.5 Abnormal mammalian circadian clock

18 of 22 unmedicated patients were examined. The mRNA level of *hPer2* was significantly higher at 6:00 in the control subjects. In contrast, the mRNA level of *hPer2* was higher at 6:00 in only 3 patients, at 2:00 in 3, at 10:00 in 4, at 14:00 in 3, and at 18:00 in 5. The timing of the *hPer2* peak expression level was significantly later in the patients than in the control subjects ($P < 0.05$, Mann–Whitney's *U*-test). The most phase-advanced cases (cases 1, 2, 11) showed the *hPer2* peak at 2:00, although the most phase-delayed cases (cases 9, 10, 15–17) showed the *hPer2* peak at 18:00.

There were no significant differences in expression levels of *hPer1, hPer3, hBmal1, hClock.*

4. Discussion

Deranged circadian rhythms have been well recognized in jet lag. In this condition, one may have symptoms, and i.e. dysfunction of the autonomic nervous system, sleep awake rhythm, mental and physical activity. We presume that those patients with sleep disturbance suffered from an atypical but continuous jet lag condition in their daily life.

The international classification of sleep disorders (ICSD) was revised as a new sleep disorder nosology by the Association of Sleep Disorders Center in North America in 1990. Circadian rhythm sleep disorders, such as the delayed sleep phase syndrome (DSPS) and the non-24-hour sleep-wake syndrome, have been described as new types of sleep-wake disorders in the last decade. In this study, we presented children or adolescents who were evaluated as not having physical abnormalities, psychiatric disorders, or specific social problems, but they were suspected to have sleep disturbance because of their daily life pattern. They were healthy in terms of physical and psychiatric examinations, but unable to attend school because their overall conditions did not allow. Those patients who satisfied our inclusion criteria to this study accounted for 40% of the total school refusal cases whom we examined in a 2-year period. This portion is quite large, and indicates the difficulty to prescribe appropriate therapy for these patients.

In our study, all 22 patients were diagnosed as having sleep-wake rhythm disturbance based on their sleep log evaluation and CBT monitoring. Their body temperature rhythm was disturbed in the manner typically shown in adult sleep disorder patients. Among our 6 school refusal patients diagnosed as having non-24, 3 did not show clear rhythm of CBT. Because non-24 is considered most difficult to treat among the 4 categories of sleep disorder, this therapeutic difficulty could be attributable to the severely disturbed CBT rhythm.

Case	Type of Sleep	*hPer2* Acrophase	Cortisol Acrophase	CBT Nadir	Component analysis of the cardiographic R-R interval		Carbohydrate metabolism			
No.	Disturbance	(clock hour)	(clock hour)	(clock hour)	LFC	HFC	Σ BG (mg/dl)	Σ IRI (microU/ml)	Δ IRI/ Δ BG	Σ IRI/ Σ BG
1	DSPS	2:00	6:00	2:00	7.6	2.1	924.0	338.2	0.12	0.37
2	DSPS	2:00	6:00	3:00	9.2	7.1	1096.5	394.1	0.32	0.36
3	DSPS	6:00	6:00	2:00	4.5	10.2	953.2	616.8	0.65	0.65
4	DSPS	6:00	22:00	19:00	8.4	10.5	773.0	340.6	0.18	0.44
5	DSPS	10:00	10:00	5:00	8.1	25.2	1022.3	392.4	0.64	0.38
6	DSPS	14:00	6:00	6:00	9.1	8.2	1280.6	981.6	1.05	0.77
7	DSPS	14:00	10:00	9:00	10.1	4.5	705.5	230	1.03	0.33
8	DSPS	14:00	18:00	9:30	10.4	3.4	604.2	460.6	2.01	0.76
9	DSPS	18:00	6:00	13:00	10.9	15.3	939.0	381.9	0.81	0.41
10	DSPS	18:00	22:00	2:30	7.6	6.5	715.3	474.2	0.51	0.66
11	Non-24	2:00	6:00	1:30	10.1	3.3	839.8	163.5	0.25	0.19
12	Non-24	6:00	10:00	8:30	8.0	18.2	912.7	338.2	2.21	0.37
13	Non-24	10:00	6:00	6:30	9.4	6.8	1244.3	456.3	0.51	0.37
14	Non-24	10:00	6:00	8:30	15.2	11.4	692.5	532.4	1.81	0.77
15	Non-24	18:00	10:00	9:00	1.9	1.5	821.3	372.6	1.27	0.45
16	Hypersomnia	18:00	6:00	5:00	8.6	5.2	788.3	419.6	1.03	0.53
17	Hypersomnia	18:00	6:00	8:00	13.0	8.9	949.3	710	1.17	0.75
18	Irregular sleep	10:00	2:00	8:00	7.0	2.8	1123.2	166.6	1.62	0.15
Controls	-	6:00	6:00 ± 1:14	3:41 ± 0:57	13.2 ± 4.0	20.6 ± 7.6	865.1±60.5	892.8±440.5	2.43±1.03	1.04±0.50

Non-24, non-24-h sleep-wake syndrome; DSPS, delayed sleep phase syndrome; LFC, low-frequency components; HFC, high-frequency components.

Table 2. Type of sleep disturbance, and times of *hPer2* peak, cortisol peak, and lowest core body temperature (CBT) over 24 h, and results of component analysis of the cardiographic R–R interval and glucose tolerance test of each patient(Tomoda et al., 2009).

The 2 biological rhythms (sleep and CBT) are sometimes desynchronized with each other, e.g., when the person was completely isolated from time cues. Once the desynchronization occurred, psychosomatic symptoms, such as headache, gastrointestinal discomfort, or general fatigue. These symptoms could make the affected person unable to perform ordinary daily activities.

Furthermore, our findings obtained in this study suggest that physiological homeostasis might be seriously impaired by sleep deprivation and emotional distress, as reflected clearly by depressive symptoms in these patients. Easy fatigability and disturbed learning and memorization are among the primary characteristics of sleep disturbance and chronic fatigue in adolescents (Miike et al., 2004). Fatigue and gastrointestinal discomfort were quite severe in our patients. Another feature of this illness is the individuality of symptom patterns and the unpredictability of symptom severity.

It is particularly interesting that diurnal hypersecretion of glucocorticoids and altered regulation of the hypothalamo-pituitary-adrenocortical axis are known in patients with poorly controlled or uncontrolled diabetes (Archer et al., 2003; Chiodini et al., 2006; Roy, Roy, & Brown, 1998). We found no cortisol hypersecretion in the present patients, suggesting the absence of diabetic status. However, those patients with sleep disturbance had glucoregulatory dysfunction. Results of a previous study show that emotionally stressful events result in hyperglycemia in diabetic patients (Lustman, Carney, & Amado, 1981). On the other hand, sleep deficit has a harmful impact on carbohydrate metabolism and endocrine function, even in healthy subjects (Spiegel, Leproult, & Van Cauter, 1999). Abnormalities of the biological stress response (hypothalamic-pituitary-adrenal axis and autonomic nervous system) were also identified in a previous animal study, the results of which suggested that cortisol can act directly on the central nervous system (Sandoval, Ping, Neill, Morrey, & Davis, 2003). Multiple factors including autonomic nervous system dysfunction, derangement of neuropeptides in the hypothalamus, and hormonal imbalance might also affect the glucoregulatory metabolism.

The biological clock (circadian clock) in human beings is formed and regulated through interrelationships of various clock genes such as *Per1, Per2, Per3, Bmal1, Clock, Cry1, Cry2, Bmal, Rev-ervA, CK1 d/e,* and *glycogen synthase kinase 3-b (GSK3ß)* (Ebisawa et al., 2001; Gietzen & Virshup, 1999; Jones et al., 1999; Takano et al., 2004; Toh et al., 2001; Vanselow et al., 2006). Currently, the markers of circadian rhythms are considered to be the profiles of plasma melatonin, cortisol, and core body temperature (Tomoda, Miike, Yonamine, Adachi, & Shiraishi, 1997). However, even if these markers show normal rhythmic patterns, certain patients suffer from circadian rhythm sleep disorders and indeterminate symptoms, suggesting that these markers may not be reliable for the diagnosis of circadian rhythm sleep disorders.

Presumably, autonomic and metabolic dysfunction causing sleep disturbance may be related to the *hPer2* phase shift because of chronobiological abnormality. Results of a previous study indicate that such disturbances might be related closely to the desynchronization of biorhythms, particularly the circadian rhythm of body temperature and the sleep-wake rhythm (Tomoda, Jhodoi, & Miike, 2001; Tomoda et al., 2000). Previous and present results suggest that sleep deprivation may originate from a dysfunctional network of brain areas related to the circadian rhythm and peripheral nervous system involved in the autonomic nervous system including cardiac function and gastrointestinal digestion. However, dysregulation of the circadian rhythm is neither the only nor the dominant factor in the pathogenesis of such conditions. Immunological, autonomic, and neuroendocrine abnormalities might be mutually dependent and reinforcing factors. More studies must be done to elucidate this mechanism and to reveal the relation between clock gene expression in the suprachiasmatic nucleus and the peripheral blood cells. Furthermore, additional study of a larger series of cases will elucidate the usefulness of this technique.

5. References

[1] Tomoda A, Kawatani J, Joudoi T, Hamada A, Miike T. Metabolic dysfunction and circadian rhythm abnormalities in adolescents with sleep disturbance. *Neuroimage* 2009;47 Suppl 2:T21-6.

[2] Tomoda A, Miike T, Uezono K, Kawasaki T. A school refusal case with biological rhythm disturbance and melatonin therapy. *Brain Dev* 1994;16(1):71-6.

[3] Boergers J, Hart C, Owens JA, Streisand R, Spirito A. Child sleep disorders: associations with parental sleep duration and daytime sleepiness. *J Fam Psychol* 2007;21(1):88-94.

[4] Giannotti F, Cortesi F, Sebastiani T, Ottaviano S. Circadian preference, sleep and daytime behaviour in adolescence. *J Sleep Res* 2002;11(3):191-9.

[5] Stein MA, Mendelsohn J, Obermeyer WH, Amromin J, Benca R. Sleep and behavior problems in school-aged children. *Pediatrics* 2001;107(4):E60.

[6] Archer SN, Robilliard DL, Skene DJ, Smits M, Williams A, Arendt J, et al. A length polymorphism in the circadian clock gene Per3 is linked to delayed sleep phase syndrome and extreme diurnal preference. *Sleep* 2003;26(4):413-5.

[7] Ebisawa T, Uchiyama M, Kajimura N, Mishima K, Kamei Y, Katoh M, et al. Association of structural polymorphisms in the human period3 gene with delayed sleep phase syndrome. *EMBO Rep* 2001;2(4):342-6.

[8] Iwase T, Kajimura N, Uchiyama M, Ebisawa T, Yoshimura K, Kamei Y, et al. Mutation screening of the human Clock gene in circadian rhythm sleep disorders. *Psychiatry Res* 2002;109(2):121-8.

[9] Pirovano A, Lorenzi C, Serretti A, Ploia C, Landoni S, Catalano M, et al. Two new rare variants in the circadian "clock" gene may influence sleep pattern. *Genet Med* 2005;7(6):455-7.

[10] Takimoto M, Hamada A, Tomoda A, Ohdo S, Ohmura T, Sakato H, et al. Daily expression of clock genes in whole blood cells in healthy subjects and a patient with circadian rhythm sleep disorder. *Am J Physiol Regul Integr Comp Physiol* 2005;289(5):R1273-9.

[11] Toh KL, Jones CR, He Y, Eide EJ, Hinz WA, Virshup DM, et al. An hPer2 phosphorylation site mutation in familial advanced sleep phase syndrome. *Science* 2001;291(5506):1040-3.

[12] Wijnen H, Boothroyd C, Young MW, Claridge-Chang A. Molecular genetics of timing in intrinsic circadian rhythm sleep disorders. *Ann Med* 2002;34(5):386-93.

[13] Iwatani N, Miike T, Kai Y, Kodama M, Mabe H, Tomoda A, et al. Glucoregulatory disorders in school refusal students. *Clin Endocrinol (Oxf)* 1997;47(3):273-8.

[14] Reppert SM, Weaver DR. Coordination of circadian timing in mammals. *Nature* 2002;418(6901):935-41.

[15] Miike T, Tomoda A, Jhodoi T, Iwatani N, Mabe H. Learning and memorization impairment in childhood chronic fatigue syndrome manifesting as school phobia in Japan. *Brain Dev* 2004;26(7):442-7.

[16] Roy MS, Roy A, Brown S. Increased urinary-free cortisol outputs in diabetic patients. *J Diabetes Complications* 1998;12(1):24-7.

[17] Chiodini I, Di Lembo S, Morelli V, Epaminonda P, Coletti F, Masserini B, et al. Hypothalamic-pituitary-adrenal activity in type 2 diabetes mellitus: role of autonomic imbalance. *Metabolism* 2006;55(8):1135-40.

[18] Lustman P, Carney R, Amado H. Acute stress and metabolism in diabetes. *Diabetes Care* 1981;4(6):658-9.

[19] Spiegel K, Leproult R, Van Cauter E. Impact of sleep debt on metabolic and endocrine function. *Lancet* 1999;354(9188):1435-9.

[20] Sandoval DA, Ping L, Neill AR, Morrey S, Davis SN. Cortisol acts through central mechanisms to blunt counterregulatory responses to hypoglycemia in conscious rats. *Diabetes* 2003;52(9):2198-204.

[21] Hastings MH. Central clocking. *Trends Neurosci* 1997;20(10):459-64.

[22] Gietzen KF, Virshup DM. Identification of inhibitory autophosphorylation sites in casein kinase I epsilon. *J Biol Chem* 1999;274(45):32063-70.

[23] Jones CR, Campbell SS, Zone SE, Cooper F, DeSano A, Murphy PJ, et al. Familial advanced sleep-phase syndrome: A short-period circadian rhythm variant in humans. *Nat Med* 1999;5(9):1062-5.

[24] Takano A, Uchiyama M, Kajimura N, Mishima K, Inoue Y, Kamei Y, et al. A missense variation in human casein kinase I epsilon gene that induces functional alteration and shows an inverse association with circadian rhythm sleep disorders. *Neuropsychopharmacology* 2004;29(10):1901-9.

[25] Vanselow K, Vanselow JT, Westermark PO, Reischl S, Maier B, Korte T, et al. Differential effects of PER2 phosphorylation: molecular basis for the human familial advanced sleep phase syndrome (FASPS). *Genes Dev* 2006;20(19):2660-72.

[26] Tomoda A, Miike T, Yonamine K, Adachi K, Shiraishi S. Disturbed circadian core body temperature rhythm and sleep disturbance in school refusal children and adolescents. *Biol Psychiatry* 1997;41(7):810-3.

[27] Tomoda A, Miike T, Yamada E, Honda H, Moroi T, Ogawa M, et al. Chronic fatigue syndrome in childhood. *Brain Dev* 2000;22(1):60-4.

[28] Tomoda A, Jhodoi T, Miike T. Chronic fatigue and abnormal biological rhythms in school children. *J Chronic Fatigue Syndrome* 2001;60:607-12.

3

Sleep Disorders Diagnosis and Management in Children with Attention Deficit/Hyperactivity Disorder (ADHD)

Rosalia Silvestri and Irene Aricò
Messina Medical School, Department of Neurosciences, Italy

1. Introduction

ADHD is an increasingly prevalent developmental disorder, especially in the western world where prevalence rates are estimated around 12%.

According to both the DSM-IV and the ICD-10 it refers to three major problematic domains: attention, hyperactivity and impulsivity. Subtypes of ADHD have been coded accordingly as a predominantly hyperactive-impulsive type (H), predominantly inattentive (I) and a combined type (C).

Age is an important factor in the clinical/behavioral manifestations of ADHD. Symptoms, in fact, vary according to brain maturation. The hyperactive aspects, for instance, tend to subside with age, even if longitudinal research demonstrated that over 30% of children with ADHD grow up to be adults with significant ADHD related problems.

Gender also plays an important role in ADHD, with a 1:10 male prevalence in clinical samples (Cortese et al., 2006). It also appears to have a strong influence over behavioral symptoms and co-morbid disorders, which appear generally less disruptive in girls.

ADHD holds a high potential for psychiatric and cognitive co-morbidity (mood, anxiety, conduct disorder and learning disability), with a nearly 50% rate of oppositional defiant conduct in males.

2. ADHD and sleep

Sleep disturbance is by far one of the most reported problems (>80%) especially by parents and care-takers, who commonly recount restless, inadequate and often delayed and/or fragmented sleep in their children.

A clear distinction, however, needs to be drawn between subjective and objective sleep reports and, with respect to the latter, actigraphyc versus video-polysomnographic (vPSG) studies present a palpable difference in terms of method and quality of data accessed.

Several metanalytic reviews have been published within the last ten years, dealing with many confounding factors including gender, referral source, age range, co-morbid disorders, first versus follow-up visits, medications, number of studied nights with or without adaptation. (Owens, 2005; Cortese et al., 2006; Sadeh et al., 2006).

They all address, through various approaches, the multilevel/dimensional relationship among sleep alterations and neurobehavioral/neurocognitive functioning.

In particular, the interaction of sleep with attention/arousal mechanisms in children has been highlighted by most recent studies.

2.1 Subjective reports

Items more often referred to by subjective studies on sleep and alertness in ADHD include (Cortese et al., 2006): bedtime resistance, sleep onset insomnia, night awakening, sleep duration, restless sleep, parasomnias, problems with morning awakening, sleep disordered breathing (SDB) excessive daytime sleepiness (EDS).

No major differences between adolescents with ADHD and controls were detected (Mick et al., 2000) after excluding confounding factors such as medications and psychiatric comorbidity. As for ADHD children, significantly over reported by comparison with controls were EDS (Marcotte et al., 1998, Owens et al., 2000), whether or not sleep disordered breathing (SDB) related, movements during sleep (Corkum et al., 1999, Owens et al., 2000). Also a longer sleep duration with increased night awakenings and parasomnias were observed upon comparison with controls (Owens et al., 2000). Despite the fact that bedtime resistance and sleep onset insomnia did not come across as significantly different by comparison with control subjects, after controlling for psychiatric co-morbidity and medications, it cannot be ruled out that a subgroup of ADHD children may display significant difficulties with sleep onset. Endogenous circadian alterations have been postulated by several authors (Vander Heijden et al., 2005) along with forced ultradian cycling (Kirov et al., 2004), which would make these children more prone to a delayed sleep phase (DSP). In this respect, melatonin use before bedtime with different regimen schedules and dosing has been acknowledged by several clinicians (Hodgkins et al., 2011; Owens et al., 2010; Larzelere et al., 2010).

2.2 Objective studies

Only a few actigraphic studies (Wiggs et al., 2005; Dagan et al., 1997; Corkum et al., 2001) and few video PSG studies were obtained in ADHD children, probably due to objective constraints as imposed by health policies, children restless and oppositional behavior and parents' reticence to over-night hospitalization. Concerning actigraphic studies, measures of objective sleep patterns (sleep duration, activity mean, wake time and number of awakenings) resulted not predictive of ADHD symptom severity after regression analysis (Wiggs et al., 2005) and did not correspond to parents' reports except for waking time in the morning. In particular, bedtime for the IADHD children was usually grossly underestimated by their parents, probably because of less externalizing behaviors during daytime.

Correspondence between subjective and objective assessment has been usually inconsistent with a few exceptions (Acebo et al., 1999). In fact, despite an overall very high parental report of sleep disturbance, actigraphic data did not confirm parents' concerns. Of course, some of these results could rely on the inherent incapacity of actigraphy to confirm specific sleep disorders such as SDB or sleep fragmentation at a microstructural level. Nevertheless, these results may still prove of some utility in order to provide parental reassurance and correct some of their distorted beliefs.

3. Sleep architecture

Sleep architecture with phase distribution, wake time, arousal and sleep fragmentation could be seen at best only via PSG studies. A major issue in this context is the exclusion of confounding factors such as the effect of medications, co-morbid neurological and psychiatric conditions and, above all, primary sleep disorders. In fact, ADHD children could be generally subdivided in children without sleep disorders, probably less than 50% according to most estimates, and children with sleep disorders.

Many authors claim that in the absence of an abnormal apnea hypopnea index (AHI) or periodic leg movements (PLMs) index, sleep variables in ADHD children are not far from age normative values (Sangal et al., 2005). In a recent thorough metanalysis of polysomnographic (PSG) studies, Sadeh et al. (2006) examined other factors of variance, including age and gender. Age, in fact, reflects maturational changes of neurobehavioral and neurotransmitter systems, which may deeply influence sleep patterns.

Females with ADHD usually present less disruptive behaviors, which can also differentially influence sleep attitude and propensity.

Whether or not an adaptation night is performed, it may enable the exclusion of the effects of first night sleep deprivation and adaptation to the lab conditions.

All considered, total sleep time appears to be longer in comparison to controls in ADHD children who underwent an adaptation night. The same subjects also exhibited longer stage 2 than controls (Sadeh et al., 2006); there appears to be a gender-related effect also over time spent in stage 2, but the most consistent effect of TST and stage 1 time was age-related, with a shorter TST and longer stage 1 in younger children (<9 years) compared to older children (>9 years), as if to indicate a more severe sleep impact in the younger group, which is usually also more severely affected in terms of ADHD symptoms, especially as far as hyperactivity is concerned.

A critical review (Bullock & Schall, 2004) examining dyssomnia in ADHD children, reports an overall concordance between authors (O'Brien et al., 2003a; Miano et al., 2006; Silvestri et al., 2009) with respect to a decreased REM percentage and an increased REM latency in ADHD kids. Most reports from France, however, contradict these studies (Lecendreux et al., 2000, Konofal et al., 2001). Furthermore, these data are not confirmed in most studies on HADHD children with nighttime periodic limb movements (Crabtree et al., 2003), as if the REM effect were more consistent with the IADHD type.

Kirov et al. (2004), instead, noticed an increased duration of REM sleep and of the number of sleep cycles in ADHD children compared to controls. Also, REM latency resulted shorter in his subjects as already previously reported by Kahn (1982) and Greenhill (1983), as if a forced REM initiation may have produced a longer REM sleep duration along with an increased number of sleep cycles.

A decreased dopaminergic activity in ADHD may be responsible for cortical dysinhibition of the motor frontal cortices, which would in turn result in the forced ultradian cycle of ADHD with REM-increased propensity. Later on, the same group reported an increased REM drive with shorter REM latency in children with coexisting tick disorders and ADHD, ascribing this type of impact to hypermotor symptoms (Kirov et al., 2007), partially contradicting previous findings (Crabtree et al., 2003) on reduced REM sleep in ADHD children with periodic limb movements.

3.1 Microstructural aspects of sleep

What almost all authors agree about is an increase of sleep oscillations within the night that contribute to the overall daytime "hypoarousal" phenotype via a possible decrease of sleep efficiency (Gruber et al., 2007). However, while a few authors notice an increase of spontaneous or event-related arousals in their subjects' PSG (Silvestri et al., 2009; O'Brien et al., 2003a), arousals have mostly not been formally identified or reported in ADHD PSG studies. Rather, an increased number of phase shifts has been reported (Miano et al., 2006) with the same clinical significance.

The only dedicated paper in terms of a formal approach to explore the microstructural aspects of sleep in ADHD has been written by Miano et al. (2006) who analyzed the cyclic alternating pattern (CAP) in ADHD children without abnormal AHI or PLMs index. The authors reported an overall reduction of CAP rate, an index of sleep instability, in comparison to normal controls, with ongoing reduction of CAP sequences and A1 index, reflecting hypersynchronous delta waves with a protective effect on sleep continuity. This paper would then reconcile the increased fragmentation and low efficiency seen by other authors in ADHD sleep, with the relative compensatory increase of A2 and A3 subtypes, expressing sleep discontinuity.

A striking CAP similarity between ADHD and narcolepsy (Ferri et al., 2005) has been observed along with increased daytime somnolence on multiple sleep latency tests (MSLT). The latter observation is of seminal importance for the interpretation of ADHD as a primary disorder of vigilance (Weinberg & Brumback, 1990). A deficit of the arousal level fluctuations would underlie the concept and clinical considerations which tend to interpret ADHD as "a hypoarousal state" despite its contradictory daytime paradoxical hyperactivity. Further detailing of this theory and related studies are to follow in the sleep disorders section under "Narcolepsy".

4. Sleep disorders

4.1 Insomnia

Chronic sleep onset insomnia (SOI) is a frequent finding in ADHD children (Mick et al., 2000; Smedje et al., 2001; Corkum et al., 2001; Owens et al., 2000a; O'Brien et al., 2003a) with a prevalence rate of nearly 28% in unmedicated children (Corkum et al., 1999), almost double than the corresponding rate in the normal child population (Owens et al., 2000b; Meijer et al., 2000). Its daytime sequelae heavily impact the cognitive domain of children and, specific to this age group, also behavioral attitude and social conduct. Hyperactivity in fact, rather than overt EDS, is the general marker of insufficient sleep in most children, therefore aggravating the typical features of ADHD (Wiggs & Stores, 1999).

SOI in ADHD was demonstrated to co-occur with a delayed dim-light melatonin onset and sleep-wake circadian rhythm, whereas sleep continuity proved unaffected (Van der Heijden et al., 2005). These findings suggest a possible disturbance of the circadian pacemaker which, in turn, would be due to the alteration of clock genes (Archer et al., 2001), but no clear evidence has been found to confirm this assumption. Sleep hygiene habits of unmedicated ADHD children with SOI were later compared to those of ADHD subjects without insomnia, so as to ascertain whether poor sleep hygiene could at least partially explain insomnia in the affected group (Van der Heijden et al., 2006). The negative results of this study suggest that sleep hygiene practice is not related to sleep characteristics in ADHD children and does not differ significantly whether or not children complain of insomnia.

As early as 1991, Dahl et al. submitted a 10-year-old girl with ADHD and a long-standing SOI to chronotherapy, obtaining a significant improvement of the ADHD-related symptoms along with circadian sleep-phase advancement.

Subsequently, Ryback et al. (2006) confirmed these results in 29 ADHD adults with an open trial of bright-light therapy in the morning.

Interestingly, the reverse relationship does not appear to occur since ADHD symptoms are not commonly found in DSP. Therefore one might assume that SOI per se, as typical of DSP, is not enough to produce daytime feature of ADHD unless accompanied by nighttime hyperactivity/sleep fragmentation, as in most ADHD children (Walters et al., 2008).

As for sleep maintenance insomnia (SMI), several primary sleep disorders such as obstructive sleep apnea syndrome (OSAS), periodic leg movement disorder (PLMD), and restless legs syndrome (RLS) concur in increasing wakefulness after sleep onset (WASO) with night-time awakenings and lowering sleep efficiency with related detrimental effects on performance (Gruber et al., 2007).

These aspects will be developed later on in the course of this chapter, within their respective sections.

Early morning insomnia is not typical of children with ADHD, unless severely depressed and is described only in older groups of ADHD patients.

4.2 Excessive Daytime Sleepiness (EDS) and narcolepsy in ADHD

As previously reported in this chapter, the "hypoarousal state" theory regarding ADHD claims that there may be decreased sleep oscillations (CAP) in ADHD children without major co-occurring sleep disorders, and this might explain their daytime drowsiness as confirmed by MSLT data and, indirectly, by the Epworth Sleepiness Scale (ESS) results in ADHD adults (Oosterloo et al., 2006).

On a modified version of MSLT, ADHD children were found to be objectively more sleepy than controls, albeit a higher rate of OSAS in probands with respect to controls (50% vs. 22%) could represent a strong bias in this study (Golan et al., 2004).

Also, Lecendreux et al. (2000) found a shorter mean sleep latency in ADHD children compared to controls, with a significant correlation to hyperactivity impulsivity and inattentive-passivity indexes, as measured by Conners Parent and Teacher rating scales (CPRS & CTRS respectively).

Differences in nocturnal sleep could not account for any of these results. None of these authors, however, sought for the instrumental hallmark of narcolepsy (2 Sleep onset REMs) in their studies, nor reported on the clinical secondary features of narcolepsy (cataplexy, hypnagogic hallucinations and paralysis) in ADHD children.

The fact that reaction time values in these studies (Lecendreux et al., 2000) hold a negative correlation with the hyperactivity-impulsivity index of the CPRS indicates that a major distinction must be drawn between IADHD and HADHD. Generally, only a subgroup of ADHD children are found to be sleepier than most average ADHD subjects, thus suggesting an impaired control of their arousal system, which may induce them to switch rapidly from wakefulness to sleep when insufficiently externally stimulated during daytime (Ramos Platon et al., 1990).

A consequent implication of this theory would be an improved therapeutic option through the employment of noradrenergic α-1 agonists (Biederman & Spencer, 1999) such as modafinil, rather than the commonly used dopaminergic stimulants.

In a more recent study (Prihodova et al., 2010), SL on MSLT in unmedicated ADHD children exhibited significant time-related changes compared to the control group, but no inter-group differences were found regarding MSLT mean sleep latency when comparing the whole ADHD group with controls.

Likewise, no such differences were found when comparing different subgroups of ADHD with or without SDB/PLMs.
Again, a dysregulated arousal mechanism could be postulated in the absence of an overall objectively proven daytime sleepiness in ADHD.
Conversely, as for signs of ADHD in narcoleptic patients, memory, attention and executive functions were found to be affected in most, but not all, studies (Naumann & Daum, 2003). In particular, divided attention and complex cognitive tasks prove selectively sensitive to arousal fluctuations in narcolepsy (Hood & Bruck, 1996). However, automatic but not hyperactive behaviors have been reported or searched for in narcolepsy research in an attempt to allow a better clinical comparison between the two disorders.

4.3 Sleep apnea (OSAS)

Most of the recent attention to the ADHD co-morbidity with OSAS came from a paper reporting the impact of adenotonsillectomy on adverse events and behavioral problems in SDB children (Li et al., 2006). The authors described an overall improvement of all measures [AHI, tests of variable attention (TOVA), and child behavior check list (CBCL) scores] with no correlation, however, between AHI and TOVA values.
The correlation between OSAS and ADHD is difficult to explore, due to several confounding factors such as age, gender, recruitment sources and methodological approaches including the definition and the measurement of respiratory events in children (Sadeh et al., 2006).
Cortese et al. (2006) found and AHI 1/hour greater than controls in children with ADHD.
Race plays also an important role in the association between ADHD and OSAS. Hispanic children show a greater co-morbidity than Caucasian probands as far as learning problems, snoring and witnessed apneas (Goodwin et al., 2003).
Also, Huang et al. (2004), reported worse attention deficit and higher hyperactivity on the CBCL of ADHD with SDB compared to ADHD without SDB children, with an overall 57% of elevated AHI (>1) in their total group of ADHD subjects, against an AHI (>1) in only 4% of their control group. Both the cranio-facial predisposition to OSAS and the high prevalence of ADHD in Taiwan could, however, impede a generalization of these results. Adenotonsillectomy more than pharmacological treatment with stimulants lead to a favorable outcome in the same group (Huang et al., 2007).
Interestingly, most researchers agree on the association of only mildly severe OSAS to ADHD (O'Brien et al., 2003b; Sangal et al., 2005; Silvestri et al., 2009) suggesting that SDB leads to a mild mimic of ADHD, rather than a true form of it.
Possible mechanisms accounting for the association between ADHD and OSAS are intermittent hypoxia and sleep fragmentation which could both be responsible for neurochemical alterations of the pre-frontal cortex and their related effects including executive dysfunction with emotional liability and impulse control disorders (ICD).
Severe OSAS in the pediatric community is rare and usually linked to EDS rather than to hyperactivity, with a phenotypical change of behavior from mild to severe ADHD. It is unclear so far whether SDB may contribute only to mild ADHD mimics or really impact ADHD clinical expression and therapeutic management. While it is known that surgical treatment of OSAS may improve ADHD symptoms, no classic non-stimulant drugs (atomoxitin, clonidine, modafinil) used for the management of ADHD (Walters et al., 2008) induce a parallel improvement of OSAS.

4.4 Sleep related movement disorders

4.4.1 Periodic Leg Movements (PLMD) and RLS

Symptoms of ADHD have been found in 44% of children with PSG evidence of PLMs (Crabtree et al., 2003). Conversely, between 26% and 64% of ADHD children have a PLMs index >5/h of sleep (Picchietti et al., 1998; 1999). Furthermore, between 44% and 67% of the positive probands have a parental history of RLS, suggesting a possible genetic link between ADHD and RLS/PLMD.

When an additional co-morbidity with SDB was reported, the link between PLMs and ADHD appeared to be stronger, mediating the secondary SDB-ADHD association (Gaultney et al., 2005).

The reported prevalence of RLS in ADHD children ranges from 44% (Cortese et al., 2005) to no association at all (Gamaldo et al., 2007). Silvestri et al. (2009) reported that an RLS prevalence of 12% by interview and clinical criteria was increased to 25.4% after PSG evaluation, reflecting the frequent difficulties to elicit an appropriate history from children depending on their age-related verbal abilities.

PLM during wakefulness (PLMW) but not RLS itself were associated to lower ferritin values, unlike previous reports (Konofal et al., 2007, 2008; Oner et al., 2008). In particular, lower ferritin values in ADHD children, whether or not RLS+, were reported by Konofal et al. (2004), compatible with the ADHD dopaminergic dysfunction hypothesis. Iron, in fact, is a co-factor of the rate-limiting enzyme, tyrosine-hydroxylase, regulating dopamine synthesis.

Cerebrospinal fluid (CSF), Magnetic Resonance Imaging (MRI) and autoptic studies also proved reduced iron stores in the brain of RLS subjects.

Iron deficiency could therefore represent a link and an interpretation key to the dual pathology of RLS and ADHD related disorders (Cortese et al., 2008), D1 and D2 receptor density being also altered by an iron-deficient state (Walters et al., 2000; Konofal et al., 2008).

RLS was found to be significantly associated with H- and CADHD, rather than IADHD, with a strong impact on CPRS, CTRS and SNAP IV Teacher and Parent Rating Scale (Swanson, 1992) hyperactive and oppositional scores (Silvestri et al., 2009).

Preliminary data on dopaminergic treatment of ADHD-associated RLS suggested a dual improvement of RLS and ADHD symptoms (Walters et al., 2000). However, these results were not further replicated (England et al., 2011) since dopaminergic treatment of a larger number of ADHD-RLS+ children led to RLS improvement without any change in the ADHD-related symptoms and scores.

Iron supplementation (Konofal et al., 2008), or most recently levetiracetam (Gagliano et al., 2011) seem to hold promising results for the management of RLS in ADHD.

Even if it is not yet clear whether RLS and ADHD share a common genetic basis or have a distinct pathogenesis with one disorder (RLS) mimicking or leading to the other (ADHD), it is certainly important to look for RLS-related aggravation of ADHD symptoms to address separate or additional treatment of sleep related symptoms.

4.4.2 Rhythmic Movement Disorder (RMD)

RMD consists of head banging or body rocking behaviors primarily occurring in young children prior to sleep onset or during subsequent sleep.

The disorder often disappears with age over 18 months, but it is estimated to last sometimes in adolescents or adults with psychiatric problems or epilepsy (Simonds & Parraga, 1984; Mayer et al., 2007). Other PSG studies in pediatric populations disclosed RMD in 6/10 ADHD children, mostly with CADHD (Stepanova et al., 2005).

A percentage (21.8) similar to that of RLS (25.4) was reported in a group of 55 unmedicated ADHD children evaluated by means of PSG (Silvestri et al., 2009) co-occurring with other sleep related movement disoders, in particular PLMD and bruxism, but not SDB, at odds with previous records (Mayer et al., 2007).
A functional impairment of the pre-motor and striatal circuitry akin to that responsible for RLS could be hypothesized as a link between RMD and ADHD.

4.4.3 Bruxism

Highly co-occurring with other sleep related motor disorders such as PLMD, RLS and RMD, bruxism has also been described in ADHD reports, both subjectively and after PSG confirmation (Silvestri et al., 2009) up to 33% of the studied ADHD sample and with a gender distribution (female prevalence) confirming data in the general population (Hojo et al., 2007).
A dopaminergic dysfunction has already been accounted for this disorder (Lavigne & Montplaisir, 1994) and treated accordingly.

4.5 Parasomnias

Only few subjective studies report an overall increased number of parasomnias in ADHD children (Owens et al., 2000; Gau, 2006; Kraenz et al., 2004), whereas most studies (Corkum et al., 1999; Mick et al., 2000) notice no difference between ADHD children and controls after accounting for co-morbidity and pharmacotheraphy.
As far as objective studies are concerned, they mostly do not report about parasomnias with few exceptions (Miano et al., 2006), accounting for a maximum of 35% of generic parasomnias overall.
An increased prevalence of sleep talking (O'Brien et al., 2003b; Corkum et al., 1999) and enuresis is reported (O'Brien et al., 2003a; Kaplan et al., 1987; O'Brien et al., 2003c).
As far as REM-related parasomnias are concerned, an increased prevalence of nightmares in ADHD children was reported by three studies (Owens et al., 2000; O'Brien et al., 2003b; 2003c).
Disorders of arousal (DOA), which include sleep walking (SW), night terrors (NT) and confusional arousals (CA), albeit optimal candidates on the basis of familiar predisposition and SDB common association for a possible ADHD co-morbid occurrence have rarely been reported in ADHD subjects.
An early report (Ishii et al., 2003) found an overall low incidence (2.9%) of NT and SW in ADHD children, mean age 9.7 years. Most patients had mild ADHD, all being out-patients studied on the basis of subjective reports with an overall low co-morbidity load compared to Western countries.
On a broader sample of ADHD pediatric subjects, Gau et al. (2007) found an OR of 2.4 (95% CI 1.3-4.5) among subjects with definite ADHD, and 1.8 in probably ADHD probands (95% CI 1.4-2.3) between NT and inattention, with lower OR values between NT and hyperactivity. Similar results, not as strong, were reported for SW.
As a result of low CAP with decreased A1 sequences (Miano et al., 2006) suggested a possible disorder of arousal with a tendency to hypoarousability in their ADHD children who had otherwise no SDB nor other objectively identified sleep disorders.
On clinical interview Silvestri et al. (2009) found a 50% prevalence of DOA in a group of 55 ADHD children (28.5% CA, 47.6% SW, 38% NT), whereas on PSG, CA were recorded in 45.2% of their patients, SW in 2.3% and NT in 4.7%.

One patient reporting both dream enactment and SW episodes had a PSG evidence of CAs and REM without atonia, thus matching criteria for parasomnia overall disorder according to the International Classification of Sleep Disorders (ICSD-2).

Interictal epileptic discharges (IEDs), mostly on centro-temporal or frontal leads were seen in >50% of these unmedicated ADHD subjects and among them, in >40% of the DOA+ children, with nocturnal hypermotor seizures occurring in three children, none of which had ever presented evidence of diurnal paroxysmal disorders.

Complex behaviors during the DOA episodes were, however, easy to distinguish from nocturnal seizures in these children, even when co-occurring with IEDs.

Vulnerability of ADHD children to rolandinc seizures and foci is well known (Holtmann et al., 2003), along with an increased rate of DOA in patients with benign focal epilepsy of childhood.

A positive significant association of DOA with SDB in the form of snoring and with increased sleep instability was also described by the same authors (Silvestri et al., 2009), akin to previous reports emphasizing the same associations (Lopes & Guilleminault, 2006; Guilleminault et al., 2005).

A preferential impact on the cognitive domain rather than behavioral indicators is most typical of children with DOA and slow wave sleep (SWS) dysfunction, opposite to the effect of nocturnal hyperactivity which seems to preferentially influence daytime hyperactivity and oppositional behaviors.

Levitiracetam 750-1000 mg/day effectively controlled seizures and lead to total cessation of DOA with a >50% reduction of IEDs during a follow-up period of 24 months (Walters et al., 2008).

5. Therapeutic management and options to address co-morbid sleep disorders in ADHD

The effect of immediate (IR) or extended (ER) release stimulants in ADHD is well known and beyond the purpose of this review.

Stimulants still represent the first line of treatment of ADHD in pediatric populations across the world.

The majority of subjective report studies indicate increased parental complaints of sleep disturbance in medicated versus unmedicated ADHD children, irrespective of stimulant type or regimen (Cohen-Zion & Ancoli-Israel, 2004). However, objective studies, whether actigraphic or PSG, show overall conflicting results as far as sleep measures, continuity and architecture, major differences going in opposite directions with regard, in particular, to REM sleep (Chatoor et al., 1983; Greenhill et al., 1983); no influence, though, on specific sleep disorders such as SDB or PLMD.

A consistent co-morbidity with depression in many ADHD children could account for increased subjective and actigraphically confirmed sleep fragmentation in the most severe cases.

Besides stimulants (Smoot et al., 2007), nonstimulant drugs have been successfully employed for the treatment of ADHD including atomoxetine (Kemner et al., 2005), bupropion and now less commonly used, tri-cyclic antidepressants. Clonidine, Guanfacine and other adrenergic α-1 agonists along with modafinil might help IADHD children with the hypoarousal phenotype, whereas SSRIs and venlafaxine could be used to fight depression/anxiety-related sleep symptoms. Also, atypical anti-psychotic drugs such as risperidone (Reyes et al., 2006) might be employed to counteract conduct/behavior disorders as aforementioned several melatonin trials have addressed rhythmicity disorders and SOI, whereas levetiracetam, an anti-epileptic drug with antimyoclonic properties has been employed eihter in ADHD-RLS+ children or to treat DOA, seizures and related IEDs in ADHD children.

6. Conclusions

Sleep disorders comorbid to ADHD may aggravate cognitive and behavioral impairment in affected children.

They also severely affect parental negative attitudes and wellbeing.

Addressing and fostering a correct sleep diagnosis may add to the therapeutic benefit obtainable in ADHD children. In fact, a differential diagnosis according to subgroups of children in relation to their phenotypic sleep expression, allows to better characterize children and parental needs and to implement oriented therapeutic options. Future research needs to address better care and divulgate easy diagnostic means (Holter-PSG and self-administered questionnaires) for a home-based monitoring of children in their natural environment.

7. References

Acebo C, Sadeh A, Seifer R, Tzischinsky O, Wolfson AR, Hafer A & Carskadon MA. (1999). Estimating sleep patterns with activity monitoring in children and adolescents: how many nights are necessary for reliable measures? Sleep, Vol.22, No.1, (Feb 1999), pp.95-103

American Academy of Sleep Medicine. (2005). The International Classification of Sleep Disorders, diagnostic and coding manual (2nd ed.), American Academy of Sleep Medicine, Westchester, IL, USA

American Psychiatric Association. (1994). Diagnostic and statistical manual of mental disorders (4th ed.), American Psychiatric Association, Washington, DC, USA

Archer SN, Robilliard DL, Skene DJ, Smits M, Williams A, Arendt J & von Schantz M. (2003). A length polymorphism in the circadian clock gene Per3 is linked to delayed sleep phase syndrome and extreme diurnal preference. Sleep, Vol. 26, No.4, (June 2003), pp.413-5

Biederman J & Spencer T. (1999). Attention-deficit/hyperactivity disorder (ADHD) as a noradrenergic disorder. Biological Psychiatry, Vol.46, No.9, (Nov 1999), pp.1234-42

Bullock GL & Schall U. (2005). Dyssomnia in children diagnosed with attention deficit hyperactivity disorder: a critical review. Australian and New Zealand Journal of Psychiatry, Vol.39, No.5, (May 2005), pp.373-377

Chatoor I, Wells KC, Conners CK, Seidel WT & Shaw D. (1983). The effects of nocturnally administered stimulant medication on EEG sleep and behavior in hyperactive children. Journal of the American Academy of Child Psychiatry, Vol.22, No.4, (July 1983), pp.337-42

Cohen-Zion M & Ancoli-Israel S. (2004). Sleep in children with attention-deficit hyperactivity disorder (ADHD): a review of naturalistic and stimulant intervention studies. Sleep Medicine Reviews, Vol.8, No.5, (Oct 2004), pp.379-402

Corkum P, Moldofsky H, Hogg-Johnson S, Humphries T & Tannock R. (1999). Sleep problems in children with attention- deficit/hyperactivity disorder: impact of subtype, comorbidity, and stimulant medication. Journal of the American Academy of Child and Adolescent Psychiatry, Vol.38, No.10, (Oct 1999), pp.1285-93

Corkum P, Tannock R, Moldofsky H, Hogg-Johnson S & Humphries T. (2001). Actigraphy and parental ratings of sleep in children with attention-deficit/hyperactivity disorder (ADHD). Sleep, Vol.24, No.3, (May 2001), pp.303-12

Cortese S, Konofal E, Lecendreux M, Arnulf I, Mouren MC, Darra F & Dalla Bernardina B. (2005). Restless legs syndrome and attention-deficit/hyperactivity disorder: a review of the literature. Sleep, Vol. 28, No.8, (Aug 2005), pp. 1007- 13

Cortese S, Konofal E, Yateman N, Mouren MC & Lecendreux M. (2006). Sleep and alertness in children with attention- deficit/hyperactivity disorder: a systematic review of the literature. Sleep, Vol.29, No.4, (Apr 2006), pp.504-11

Cortese S, Lecendreux M, Bernardina BD, Mouren MC, Sbarbati A & Konofal E. (2008). Attention-deficit/hyperactivity disorder, Tourette's syndrome, and restless legs syndrome: the iron hypothesis. Medical Hypotheses, Vol. 70, No.6, pp.1128-32

Crabtree VM, Ivanenko A & Gozal D. (2003). Clinical and parental assessment of sleep in children with attention- deficit/hyperactivity disorder referred to a pediatric sleep medicine center. Clinical Pediatrics (Philadelphia), Vol.42, No.9, (Nov–Dec 2003), pp.807-13

Dagan Y, Zeevi-Luria S, Sever Y, Hallis D, Yovel I, Sadeh A & Dolev E. (1997). Sleep quality in children with attention deficit hyperactivity disorder: an actigraphic study. Psychiatry and Clinical Neurosciences, Vol.51, No.6, (Dec 1997), pp.383-6

Dahl RE, Pelham WE & Wierson M. (1991). The role of sleep disturbances in attention deficit disorder symptoms: a case study. Journal of Pediatric Psychology, Vol.16, No.2, (Apr 1991), pp.229-39

England SJ, Picchietti DL, Couvadelli BV, Fisher BC, Siddiqui F, Wagner ML, Hening WA, Lewin D, Winnie G, Cohen B & Walters AS. (2011). L-Dopa improves Restless Legs Syndrome and periodic limb movements in sleep but not Attention-Deficit-Hyperactivity Disorder in a double-blind trial in children. Sleep Medicine, Vol. 12, No.5, (May 2011), pp.471-7

Ferri R, Miano S, Bruni O, Vankova J, Nevsimalova S, Vandi S, Montagna P, Ferini-Strambi L & Plazzi G. (2005). NREM sleep alterations in narcolepsy/cataplexy. Clinical Neurophysiology, Vol.116, No.11, (Nov 2005), pp.2675-84

Gagliano A, Aricò I, Calarese T, Condurso R, Germanò E, Cedro C, Spina E & Silvestri R. (2011). Restless Leg Syndrome in ADHD children: levetiracetam as a reasonable therapeutic option. Brain & Development, Vol. 33, No.6, (Jun 2011), pp.480-6

Gamaldo CE, Benbrook AR, Allen RP, Scott JA, Henning WA & Earley CJ. (2007). Childhood and adult factors associated with restless legs syndrome (RLS) diagnosis. Sleep Medicine, Vol.8, No.7-8, (Nov 2007), pp.716-22

Gau SS, Kessler RC, Tseng WL, Wu YY, Chiu YN, Yeh CB & Hwu HG. (2007). Association between sleep problems and symptoms of attention-deficit/hyperactivity disorder in young adults. Sleep, Vol. 30, No.2, (Feb 2007), pp.195- 201

Gaultney JF, Terrell DF & Gingras JL. (2005). Parent-reported periodic limb movement, sleep disordered breathing, bedtime resistance behaviors, and ADHD. Behavioral Sleep Medicine, Vol. 3, No.1, pp.32-43

Golan N, Shahar E, Ravid S & Pillar G. (2004). Sleep disorders and daytime sleepiness in children with attention- deficit/hyperactive disorder. Sleep, Vol.27, No.2, (Mar 2004), pp.261-6

Goodwin JL, Babar SI, Kaemingk KL, Rosen GM, Morgan WJ, Sherrill DL & Quan SF. (2003). Symptoms related to sleep- disordered breathing in white and Hispanic children: the Tucson Children's Assessment of Sleep Apnea Study. Chest, Vol.124, No.1, (Jul 2003), pp.196-203

Greenhill L, Puig-Antich J, Goetz R, Hanlon C & Davies M. (1983). Sleep architecture and REM sleep measures in prepubertal children with attention deficit disorder with hyperactivity. Sleep, Vol.6, No.2, pp.91-101

Gruber R, Grizenko N, Schwartz G, Bellingham J, Guzman R & Joober R. (2007). Performance on the continuous performance test in children with ADHD is associated with sleep efficiency. Sleep,Vol.30, No.8, (Aug 2007), pp. 1003-9

Guilleminault C, Lee JH, Chan A, Lopes MC, Huang YS & da Rosa A. (2005). Non-REM-sleep instability in recurrent sleepwalking in pre-pubertal children. Sleep Medicine, Vol.6, No.6, (Nov 2005), pp.515-21

Hodgkins P, Sasané R & Meijer WM. (2011). Pharmacologic treatment of attention-deficit/hyperactivity disorder in children: incidence, prevalence, and treatment patterns in the Netherlands. Clinical Therapeutics, Vol.33, No.2, (Feb 2011), pp.188-203

Hojo A, Haketa T, Baba K & Igarashi Y. (2007). Association between the amount of alcohol intake and masseter muscle activity levels recorded during sleep in healthy young women. The International Journal of Prosthodontics, Vol.20, No.3, (May-Jun 2007), pp.251-5

Holtmann M, Becker K, Kentner-Figura B & Schmidt MH. (2003). Increased frequency of rolandic spikes in ADHD children. Epilepsia, Vol.44, No.9, (Sep 2003), pp. 1241-4

Hood B & Bruck D. (1996). Sleepiness and performance in narcolepsy. Journal of Sleep Research, Vol.5, No.2, (June 1996), pp.128-34

Huang YS, Chen NH, Li HY, Wu YY, Chao CC & Guilleminault C. (2004). Sleep disorders in Taiwanese children with attention deficit/hyperactivity disorder. Journal of Sleep Research, Vol.13, No.3, (Sep 2004), pp.269-77

Huang YS, Guilleminault C, Li HY, Yang CM, Wu YY & Chen NH. (2007). Attention-deficit/hyperactivity disorder with obstructive sleep apnea: a treatment outcome study. Sleep Medicine, Vol.8, No.1, (Jan 2007), pp.18-30

Ishii T, Takahashi O, Kawamura Y & Ohta T. (2003). Comorbidity in attention deficit-hyperactivity disorder. Psychiatry and Clinical Neurosciences, Vol. 57, No.5, (Oct 2003), pp.457-63

Kaplan BJ, McNicol J, Conte RA & Moghadam HK. (1987). Sleep disturbance in preschool-aged hyperactive and nonhyperactive children. Pediatrics, Vol. 80, No.6, (Dec 1987), pp.839-44

Kemner JE, Starr HL, Ciccone PE, Hooper-Wood CG & Crockett RS. (2007). Outcomes of OROS methylphenidate compared with atomoxetine in children with ADHD: a multicenter, randomized prospective study. Advances in Therapy, Vol.22, No.5, (Sep-Oct 2007), pp.498-512

Khan AU. (1982). Sleep REM latency in hyperkinetic boys. The American Journal of Psychiatry, Vol.139, No.10, (Oct 1982), pp.1358-60

Kirov R, Banaschewski T, Uebel H, Kinkelbur J & Rothenberger A. (2007). REM-sleep alterations in children with co- existence of tic disorders and attention-deficit/hyperactivity disorder: impact of hypermotor symptoms. European Child and Adolescent Psychiatry, Vol.16, Suppl.1, (Jun 2007), pp.45-50

Kirov R, Kinkelbur J, Heipke S, Kostanecka-Endress T, Westhoff M, Cohrs S, Ruther E, Hajak G, Banaschewski T & Rothenberger A. (2004). Is there a specific polysomnographic sleep pattern in children with attention deficit/hyperactivity disorder? Journal of Sleep Research, Vol.13, No.1, (Mar 2004), pp.87-93

Konofal E, Cortese S, Marchand M, Mouren MC, Arnulf I & Lecendreux M. (2007). Impact of restless legs syndrome and iron deficiency on attention-deficit/hyperactivity disorder in children. Sleep Medicine, Vol. 8, No.7-8, (Nov 2007), pp.711-5

Konofal E, Lecendreux M, Arnulf I & Mouren MC. (2004). Iron deficiency in children with attention-deficit/hyperactivity disorder. Archives of Pediatrics and Adolescent Medicine, Vol.158, No.12, (Dec. 2004), pp.1113-5

Konofal E, Lecendreux M, Bouvard MP & Mouren-Simeoni MC. (2001). High levels of nocturnal activity in children with attention-deficit hyperactivity disorder: a video analysis. Psychiatry and Clinical Neurosciences, Vol. 55, No.2, (Apr 2001), pp.97-103

Konofal E, Lecendreux M, Deron J, Marchand M, Cortese S, Zaïm M, Mouren MC & Arnulf I. (2008). Effects of iron supplementation on attention deficit hyperactivity disorder in children. Pediatric Neurology, Vol. 38, No.1, (Jan 2008), pp.20-6

Kraenz S, Fricke L, Wiater A, Mitschke A, Breuer U & Lehmkuhl G. (2004). Prevalence and stress factors of sleep disorders in children starting school. Prax Kinderpsychol Kinderpsychiatr, Vol. 53, No.1, (Jan 2004), pp.3-18

Larzelere MM, Campbell JS & Robertson M. (2010). Complementary and alternative medicine usage for behavioral health indications. Primary Care, Vol.37, No.2, (June 2010), pp.213-36

Lavigne GJ & Montplaisir JY. (1994). Restless legs syndrome and sleep bruxism: prevalence and association among Canadians. Sleep, Vol. 17, No.8, (Dec 1994), pp.739-43

Lecendreux M, Konofal E, Bouvard M, Falissard B & Mouren-Siméoni MC. (2000). Sleep and alertness in children with ADHD. Journal of Child Psychology and Psychiatry, and allied disciplines, Vol.41, No.6, (Sep 2000), pp.803-12

Li HY, Huang YS, Chen NH, Fang TJ & Lee LA. (2006). Impact of adenotonsillectomy on behavior in children with sleep- disordered breathing. Laryngoscope, Vol. 116, No.7, (Jul 2006), pp.1142-7

Lopes MC & Guilleminault C. (2006). Chronic snoring and sleep in children: a demonstration of sleep disruption. Pediatrics, Vol.118, No.3, (Sep 2006), pp.741-6

Marcotte AC, Thacher PV, Butters M, Bortz J, Acebo C & Carskadon MA. (1998). Parental report of sleep problems in children with attentional and learning disorders. Journal of Developmental and Behavioral Pediatrics, Vol.19, No.3, (Jun 1998), pp.178-86

Mayer G, Wilde-Frenz J & Kurella B. (2007). Sleep related rhythmic movement disorder revisited. Journal of Sleep Research, Vol. 6, No.1, (Mar 2007), pp.110-6

Meijer AM, Habekothé HT & Van Den Wittenboer GL. (2000). Time in bed, quality of sleep and school functioning of children. Journal of Sleep Research, Vol.9, No.2, (June 2000), pp.145-53

Miano S, Donfrancesco R, Bruni O, Ferri R, Galiffa S, Pagani J, Montemitro E, Kheirandish L, Gozal D & Pia Villa M. (2006). NREM sleep instability is reduced in children with attention-deficit/hyperactivity disorder. Sleep, Vol.29, No.6, (Jun 2006), pp.797-803

Mick E, Biederman J, Jetton J & Faraone SV. (2000). Sleep disturbances associated with attention deficit hyperactivity disorder: the impact of psychiatric comorbidity and pharmacotherapy. Journal of Child and Adolescent Psychopharmacology, Vol.10, No.3, pp.223-31

Naumann A & Daum I. (2003). Narcolepsy: pathophysiology and neuropsychological changes. Behavioral Neurology, Vol.14, No.3-4, pp.89-98

O'Brien LM, Holbrook CR, Mervis CB, Klaus CJ, Bruner JL, Raffield TJ, Rutherford J, Mehl RC, Wang M, Tuell A, Hume BC & Gozal D. (2003b). Sleep and neurobehavioral characteristics of 5- to 7-year-old children with parentally reported symptoms of attention-deficit/hyperactivity disorder. Pediatrics, Vol.111, No.3, (Mar 2003), pp.554-63

O'Brien LM, Ivanenko A, Crabtree VM, Holbrook CR, Bruner JL, Klaus CJ & Gozal D. (2003a). Sleep disturbances in children with attention deficit hyperactivity disorder. Pediatric Research, Vol.54, No.2, (Aug 2003), pp.237-43

O'Brien LM, Ivanenko A, Crabtree VM, Holbrook CR, Bruner JL, Klaus CJ & Gozal D. (2003c). The effect of stimulants on sleep characteristics in children with attention deficit/hyperactivity disorder. Sleep Medicine, Vol.4, No.4, (Jul 2003), pp.309-16

Oner O, Alkar OY & Oner P. (2008). Relation of ferritin levels with symptom ratings and cognitive performance in children with attention deficit-hyperactivity disorder. Pediatrics International, Vol.50, No.1, (Feb 2008), pp.40-4

Oosterloo M, Lammers GJ, Overeem S, de Noord I & Kooij JJ. (2006). Possible confusion between primary hypersomnia and adult attention-deficit/hyperactivity disorder. Psychiatry Research, Vol.143, No.2-3, (Aug 2006), pp.293-7

Owens JA, Maxim R, Nobile C, McGuinn M & Msall M. (2000a). Parental and self-report of sleep in children with attention-deficit/hyperactivity disorder. Archives of Pediatrics and Adolescent Medicine, Vol.154, No.6, (June 2000a), pp.549-55

Owens JA, Rosen CL, Mindell JA & Kirchner HL. (2010). Use of pharmacotherapy for insomnia in child psychiatry practice: A national survey. Sleep Medicine, Vol.11, No.7, (August 2010), pp.692-700

Owens JA, Spirito A, McGuinn M & Nobile C. (2000b). Sleep habits and sleep disturbance in elementary school-aged children. Journal of Developmental and Behavioral Pediatrics. Vol.21, No.1, (Feb 2000), pp.27-36

Owens JA. (2005). The ADHD and sleep conundrum: a review. Journal of Developmental and Behavioral Pediatrics, Vol.26, No.4, (Aug 2005), pp.312-22

Picchietti DL, England SJ, Walters AS, Willis K & Verrico T. (1998). Periodic limb movement disorder and restless legs syndrome in children with attention-deficit hyperactivity disorder. Journal of Child Neurology, Vol. 13, No. 12, (Dec 1998), pp.588-94

Picchietti DL, Underwood DJ, Farris WA, Walters AS, Shah MM, Dahl RE, Trubnick LJ, Bertocci MA, Wagner M & Hening WA. (1999). Further studies on periodic limb movement disorder and restless legs syndrome in children with attention-deficit hyperactivity disorder. Movement Disorders, Vol. 14, No.6, (Nov 1999), pp.1000-7

Platon, M. R., Bueno, A. V., Sierra, J. E., & Kales, S. (1990). Hypnopolygraphic alterations in attention deficit disorder (ADD) children. International Journal of Neuroscience, Vol.53, No.2-4, (Aug 1990), pp.87-101

Prihodova I, Paclt I, Kemlink D, Skibova J, Ptacek R & Nevsimalova S. (2010). Sleep disorders and daytime sleepiness in children with attention-deficit/hyperactivity disorder: a two-night polysomnographic study with a multiple sleep latency test. Sleep Medicine, Vol.11, No.9, (Oct 2010), pp.922-8

Reyes M, Croonenberghs J, Augustyns I & Eerdekens M. (2006). Long-term use of risperidone in children with disruptive behavior disorders and subaverage intelligence: efficacy, safety, and tolerability. Journal of Child and Adolescent Psychopharmacology, Vol.16, No.3, (Jun 2006), pp.260-72

Rybak YE, McNeely HE, Mackenzie BE, Jain UR & Levitan RD. (2006). An open trial of light therapy in adult attention- deficit/hyperactivity disorder. Journal of Clinical Psychiatry, Vol.67, No.10, (Oct 2006), pp.1527-35

Sadeh A, Pergamin L & Bar-Haim Y. (2006). Sleep children with attention-deficit hyperactivity disorder: A metanalysis of polysomnographic studies. Sleep Medicine Reviews, Vol.10, No.6, (Dec 2006), pp.381-398

Sangal RB, Owens JA & Sangal J. (2005). Patients with attention-deficit/hyperactivity disorder without observed apneic episodes in sleep or daytime sleepiness have normal sleep on polysomnography. Sleep, Vol.28, No.9, (Sep 2005), pp.1143-8

Shur-Fen Gau S. (2006). Prevalence of sleep problems and their association with inattention/hyperactivity among children aged 6-15 in Taiwan. Journal of Sleep Research, Vol. 15, No.4, (Dec 2006), pp.403-14

Silvestri R, Gagliano A, Aricò I, Calarese T, Cedro C, Bruni O, Condurso R, Germanò E, Gervasi G, Siracusano R, Vita G & Bramanti P. (2009). Sleep disorders in children with Attention-Deficit/Hyperactivity Disorder (ADHD) recorded overnight by video-polysomnography. Sleep Medicine, Vol.10, No.10, (Dec 2009), pp.1132-8

Simonds JF & Parraga H. (1984). Sleep behaviors and disorders in children and adolescents evaluated at psychiatric clinics. Journal of Developmental and Behavioral Pediatrics, Vol. 5, No.1, (Feb 1984), pp.6-10

Smedje H, Broman JE & Hetta J. (2001). Associations between disturbed sleep and behavioural difficulties in 635 children aged six to eight years: a study based on parents' perceptions. European Child and Adolescent Psychiatry, Vol.10, No.1, (Mar 2001), pp.1-9

Smoot LC, Boothby LA & Gillett RC. (2007). Clinical assessment and treatment of ADHD in children. International Journal of Clinical Practice, Vol. 6, No. 10, (Oct 2007), pp.1730-8

Stepanova I, Nevsimalova S & Hanusova J. (2005). Rhythmic movement disorder in sleep persisting into childhood and adulthood. Sleep, Vol. 28, No.7, (Jul 2005), pp.851-7

Swanson, J.M. (1992) School-based assessments and intervention for ADD students. K.C. Publishing, Irvine, CA, USA

Van der Heijden KB, Smits MG & Gunning WB. (2005). Sleep-related disorders in ADHD: a review. Clinical Pediatrics (Philadelphia),Vol.44, No.3, (Apr 2005), pp.201-10

Van der Heijden KB, Smits MG & Gunning WB. (2006). Sleep hygiene and actigraphically evaluated sleep characteristics in children with ADHD and chronic sleep onset insomnia. Journal of Sleep Research, Vol.15, No.1, (Mar 2006), pp.55-62

Van der Heijden KB, Smits MG, Van Someren EJ & Gunning WB. (2005). Idiopathic chronic sleep onset insomnia in attention-deficit/hyperactivity disorder: a circadian rhythm sleep disorder. Chronobiology International, Vol.22, No.3, pp.559-70

Walters AS, Mandelbaum DE, Lewin DS, Kugler S, England SJ & Miller M. (2000). Dopaminergic therapy in children with restless legs/periodic limb movements in sleep and ADHD. Dopaminergic Therapy Study Group. Pediatric Neurology, Vol.22, No.3, (Mar 2000), pp.182-6

Walters AS, Silvestri R, Zucconi M, Chandrashekariah R & Konofal E. (2008). Review of the possible relationship and hypothetical links between attention deficit hyperactivity disorder (ADHD) and the simple sleep related movement disorders, parasomnias, hypersomnias, and circadian rhythm disorders. Journal of Clinical Sleep Medicine,Vol.4, No.6, (Dec 2008), pp.591-600

Weinberg WA & Brumback RA. (1990). Primary disorder of vigilance: a novel explanation of inattentiveness, daydreaming, boredom, restlessness, and sleepiness. The Journal of Pediatrics, Vol.116, No.5, (May 1990), pp.720- 5

Wiggs L & Stores G. (1999). Behavioural treatment for sleep problems in children with severe learning disabilities and challenging daytime behaviour: effect on daytime behaviour. Journal of Child Psychology and Psychiatry, and allied disciplines, Vol.40, No.4, (May 1999), pp.627-35

Wiggs L, Montgomery P & Stores G. (2005). Actigraphic and parent reports of sleep patterns and sleep disorders in children with subtypes of attention-deficit hyperactivity disorder. Sleep, Vol.28, No.11, (Nov 1997), pp.1437-45

World Health Organization. (1992). International Statistical Classification of Diseases and Related Health Problems (10th ed.), World Health Organization, Geneva

4

Elemental Mercury Exposure and Sleep Disorder

Alfred Bogomir Kobal[1] and Darja Kobal Grum[2]
[1]*Department of Occupational Medicine, Idrija Mercury Mine, Idrija,*
[2]*Department of Psychology, Faculty of Arts, University of Ljubljana, Ljubljana, Slovenia*

1. Introduction

The sleep-wake rhythms cycle coincides with the solar 24-hour schedule. Most adult subjects in nontropical areas are comfortable with 6.5 to 8.0 hours of daily sleep, taken in a single period. It is known that normal sleep consists of four to six behaviourally and electrophysiologically (EEG) defined cycles. Sleep is divided in two main types: REM (rapid eye movements) sleep and non-REM sleep. In the general population, sleep disorders are common and usually associated with some illness, psychological and social disturbances. Insomnia as the most common sleep disorder is most often the consequence of psychological disturbances. It is characterized by the inability to fall asleep quickly. Sleepwalking, night terrors and nightmares are parasomnias which often reflect significant stress or physiopathology. Restless legs syndrome and periodic limb movements are a type of motor disorders. Restless legs usually occur before sleep onset, while periodic limb movements can fragment the sleep. Transient sleep disturbances are mostly associated with variety of factors including stress, life changes, shift work, jet lag, and some acute health disorders. The most popular drugs, such as alcohol, nicotine and caffeine, can adversely affect the quality and quantity of sleep (Hornyak et al., 2006; Lee & Douglass, 2010; Pinel, 2009; Vgontzas et al., 2010).

Occupational exposure to heavy metals, such as cadmium, lead, manganese and mercury, was very frequent in the 20th century. Many epidemiological studies show that these heavy metals can cause serious functional disability among exposed workers (World Health Organization [WHO], 1980). Inorganic lead, manganese and inorganic-elemental mercury (Hg°) exposure can, among others, cause neurotoxic effects with a typical, but different, clinical picture associated with sleep disorder.

Hg° a silvery-white liquid metal is quite attractive and very widespread which, despite being highly toxic, was used by humans as a medicine for thousands of years. We shall discuss its neurotoxic effects and the sleep disorders it can cause at increased occupational exposure. Hg° was first described by Aristotle in the 4th century A.D., and the alchemist's concept of Hg° leaned on his system of natural phenomena, which dominated all of science until the 17th century. For this reason Hg° was attributed with all those qualities of nature that accelerate development, growth and maturation. The famous Arabian physician Avicena, who was active in the 11th century, wrote that Hg° vapours cause paralysis, tremor and frequent limb spasms. In Columbus' time began to be used to treat syphilis. The use of its compounds was still widespread in the United States in the 19th century, and was among others also used to treat depression (Goldwater, 1972). The popularity of Hg at the time was considerable, for even President Abraham Lincoln found relief for his health problems in a pharmacy-prepared drug called "blue pills", which contained elementary Hg° (Hirschhorn et al., 2001). Various, mostly organic Hg compounds were still widely used in the 20th century, and even to a smaller extent today (Clarkson & Magos, 2006).

The Roman historian Pliny speaks of the first occupational Hg° intoxications - *hydrargyrismis*, or mercurialism, in slaves who mined and smelted Hg ore for several centuries in the Sisapo-Almaden mine. Occupational exposure to Hg° did not receive any noticeable attention until the 15th century, when Ulrich Ellenenborg described occupational exposure for the first time in his book, which was published posthumously in 1524. In a very extensive work entitled »The morbis artificum diatribe« (1700), Bernardo Ramazzini presented several occupational illnesses, among which he also described occupational intoxications with Hg° vapours (Goldwater, 1972). In the 16th century, several physicians described the symptoms and signs of Hg° intoxication in miners of the Idrija Mercury Mine, the most famous among them being Theophrastus von Hohenheim, otherwise known as Paracelsus, and Pierandreia Mattioli, a reputed botanist and physician who worked in the town of Gorica at the time (1544).

In his book *Von der Bergsucht und anderen Krankheiten*, published in 1527, Paracelsus described the serious condition of sick miners whom he had met during his visit to the Idrija Mine: "All the people who live there are deformed and paralyzed, asthmatic and benumbed, without any hope of ever getting well" (Lesky, 1956, p. 8). Hg° intoxication in mercury miners of the Idrija Mercury Mine was well-described by Joannes Antonius Scopoli, the first physician appointed to the Idrija Mercury Mine in 1754. Along with the symptoms of Hg° intoxication observed in miners, he also described their personality traits as well the characteristics of sleep disorders that usually appear in Hg° intoxication. Sleep disorders were also mentioned in the monographs on inorganic mercury published by WHO (1976, 1991) and the Agency for Toxic Substances and Disease Registry [ATSDR] (1999).

The observations of J. A. Scopoli in the 18th century, our observations of workers exposed to Hg° in the Idrija Mercury Mine, as well as certain biochemical interactions of Hg° in central nervous system (CNS) that were studied by many researchers in the late 20th and early 21st centuries, help to throw light on those biochemical effects of Hg in CNS that could hypothetically disturb the regulation of sleep and cause the sleep disorders occurring in occupational intoxications or increased Hg° absorption in exposed miners and smelters. In this chapter, we shall briefly present the subjective characteristics of sleep disorder observed in occupational Hg° intoxication and increased absorption, the interaction of Hg° in the body and its toxic effects in the CNS, the basic neurobiological and biochemical characteristics of sleep-wake cycles and, finally, its hypothetical interactions with Hg°.

2. Sleep disorder in occupational exposure to Hg° vapours

J. A. Scopoli presented his knowledge on occupational Hg° exposure of miners and smelters in the Idrija Mercury Mine in his book entitled DE HYDRARGYRO IDRIENSI *TENTAMINA Phisico - Chimico - Medica*, which was printed in Venice in 1761, and reprinted in 1771. In the third part of this book, *De Morbis Fossorum Hydrargyri*, he presents an in-depth description of the symptoms of mercury intoxication - mercurialism among pit and smeltery workers. He classifies mercurialism according to those symptoms that are the most pronounced in the disease pattern. Scopoli describes acute, sub-acute and chronic Hg intoxication appearing during work in the smelting plant and in the pit, in poorly ventilated sites with native ore where, according to our present-day knowledge (Kobal, 1994), mercury vapour concentrations were extremely high. Among the symptoms accompanying chronic intoxication, Scopoli mentions changes in some personality traits, such as bad temper, irritability and sadness, as well as sleep disorder. "...*somnus inquietus, somnia terrifica, artuum agitatio*..." are the key words which Scopoli uses (1771, p. 80). He finds that mercury intoxication is accompanied by restless sleep, terrible dreams with nightmares, sleep terrors, and strange, periodic contractile movements of the legs (Kobal & Kobal-Grum, 2010). The reputed clinical toxicologist, Adolph Kussmaul, presented in his book (1861, p. 227) an occupational clinical picture of mercurial intoxication in miners. Among the symptoms of eretism-increased irritability, he also mentions "restless sleep, terrible dreams and frighten awakenings".

Our observations are based on data collected from the program of health surveillance of workers exposed to Hg° in the Idrija Mercury Mine. In the first 20 years following the Second World War, the number of Hg° intoxicated workers was very high (ranging from 10 to 14% of workers in the mine and smelting plant). After 1975, no new cases of intoxication were observed thanks to the introduction of preventive-target medical examinations, which, after 1968, also included biological monitoring of exposure. Subjective descriptions of sleep disturbances and other potential, known, subjective troubles associated with Hg° exposure were always evaluated directly by the physician during contact with intoxicated or exposed workers in the course of preventive target examinations. No polysomnographic recording was used to define the stages of sleep in intoxicated workers, or in workers with increased Hg° absorption. Some disordered sleep, such as fragmentation of sleep accompanied with dreaming and awakening, as well as periodic leg contractile movements, were often observed as some important early symptoms that announced the critical absorption of Hg^{o} vapours in miners working in the pit where native Hg ore was mined, with substantially elevated air Hg^{o} vapour levels. During the target medical surveillance and biological monitoring of miners intermittently exposed to native Hg, the previously mentioned sleep disorder appeared in 30% of exposed miners, associated with increased urinary Hg excretion. In these miners, the urine Hg concentrations were usually within a range of 100-400 μg/L, which is, at intermittent type of exposure, associated with blood Hg levels from 60 to 260 μg/L (Kobal, 1975a, 1991), which are substantially above the blood Hg level of 35 μg/L usually accompanied with the earliest nonspecific symptoms (WHO, 1976). In cases of subacute mercurialism with classical signs of intoxication, such as stomatitis, limb tremor, and other known symptoms and signs, the sleep disorders were much more pronounced, and the urinary Hg excretions were very high, in some cases even over 700 μg/L (Kobal, 1975b, 1991). The periodic leg movement index was not evaluated in these miners (calculated by dividing the total number of periodic leg movements by sleep time in hours).

In the cases of increased Hg^{o} absorption, the sleep disorder decreased usually in one to two months after the interruption of exposure associated with decreased urine Hg level. In the cases of Hg^{o} intoxication, sleep disorders with terrible dreams and and periodic leg movements were much more obstinate and disappeared very slowly in association with other symptoms and clinical signs of mercurialism; the urine Hg level decreased after 3 to 6 months. A subclinical peripheral nerve function with lower motor conduction velocities of the median nerve and lower sensory conduction velocities of the ulnar nerve was observed in the subgroup of miners with long-term intermittent exposure and increased Hg° absorption (urine Hg excretion > 100μg/L). In contrast to sleep disorder, these subclinical pripheral nerve function changes usually persist many years after the cessation of exposure (Gabrovec-Nahlik et al., 1977; Kobal et al., 2004), which is also in agreement with some other observations (Albers et al., 1982).

As already mentioned above, sleep disorders were also mentioned in the monographs on inorganic-elemental mercury published by WHO (1976, 1991) and ATSDR (1999), which place them among the symptoms of erethism. However, no disorders of sleep structure or any possible neurobiological or biochemical mechanisms and EEG changes that could accompany sleep disorders in intoxicated subjects exposed to Hg° are described in these monographs.

3. The toxicology of elemental mercury-Hg°

3.1 Absorption, disposition in the body, and elimination

Hg° is the only metal that takes the form of liquid at room temperature, and releases monoatomic vapours (Hg° vapours) that are very stable and may remain in the atmosphere for months or even years on end. Their pressure is in equilibrium with the metal, and their concentrations attain a value of 18.3 mg/m^3 at a room temperature of 24°C, which is 360 times above the "permissible level" for occupational exposure (0.05 mg Hg°/m^3) prescribed in the Environmental Health Criteria 1, Mercury (WHO, 1976). We know today that Hg° vapours enter the body mainly through inhalation. As much as 80% of the inhaled amount of Hg° is absorbed in the lungs and then passes across the alveolar membrane very quickly into the plasma and erythrocytes, and through blood circulation into CNS, kidneys and other organs. In the tissue, Hg° oxidizes into the ionic divalent form (Hg++), which takes place by way of the hydrogen peroxide-catalase compound I enzyme system. The oxidation of Hg° in blood, although rapid, is sufficiently prolonged so that the Hg° dissolved in blood can be conveyed to the brain, where it passes the blood-brain barrier and cell membranes. Only a small amount of Hg° is oxidized during the transit time from the lungs to the brain, so that over ninety percent of dissolved Hg° arrives in the brain unoxidized. It is then oxidized in brain cells and complexed to the SH-group of the cell (Hursh et al., 1988; Magos et al., 1978). The divalent ionic Hg++ accumulates primarily in astrocytes, where it mostly binds to reduced glutathione (GSH), cystein, and metallothioneins (MTs) (Aschner, 1997; Tušek-Žnidarič et al., 2007). After Hg° vapour exposure of animals, a marked accumulation of Hg was observed in the cerebellum, nucleus olivarius inferior in the brainstem, and in the nucleus subtalamicus (Berlin et al., 1969). In autopsy samples of retired and ex-miners previously intermittently exposed to Hg°, substantially higher accumulations and retention of Hg were observed in the pituitary gland, pineal gland, hippocampus, nucleus dentatus, and in the cereballar cortex in comparison with the control group (Falnoga et al., 2000; Kosta et al., 1975) (Tab.1). Hg is eliminated in the urine, feces, expired air, sweat, saliva, and milk. In long-term occupational exposure, the kidneys are the major pathway of Hg excretion, and are not only an indicator of kidney burden, but may also be a rough indicator of total body burden. The retention of Hg in the brain observed several years after remote exposure in retired mercury miners suggests that the brain does not follow the some kinetics of elimination as the kidneys (Falnoga et al., 2000; Kosta et al., 1975; WHO, 1991). In the case of intermittent exposure to Hg°, blood Hg was very positively correlated with the spot urine

Hg mercury concentration (r=0.68, $p < 0.001$), which, in such types of exposure, allows use of urine Hg as a biological indicator of recent exposure (Kobal, 1991).

	Ex-miners	Controls
Pituitary gland (ng/g)	39100 (N-1)	36.9 ± 62 (N-13)
Piniel gland (ng/g)	1109 (N-1)	9.5 ± 9.2 (N-15)
Hyppocampus (ng/g)	251, 309, 337 (N-3)	3.9 ± 1.6 (N-6)
Nucleus dentatus (ng/g)	2090, 2363, 4428 (N-3)	137 ± 77 (N-7)
Cerebellar cortex (ng/g)	43, 108, 110, 301 (N-4)	2.1, 2.5, 2.9 (N-3)

Table 1. Total Hg concentration in autopsy samples (homogenised tissue) of pituitary gland, pineal gland, hippocampus, nucleus dentatus and cereballar cortex (ng/g fresh weight) in ex-miners of the Idrija Mercury Mine and controls (data adapted by Falnoga et al., 2000).

3.2 Toxic effects of Hg°

Various Hg species, as Hg°, methyl-Hg ore ethyl-Hg, accumulates in the central nervous system (CNS) and has extremely neurotoxic effects, including the appearance of well-known clinical symptoms and signs. In case of occupational exposure to Hg°, the most frequent symptoms and signs include "erethism", increased irritability, depression and other neurobehavioral changes, sleep disturbances, oral disturbances, gingivitis and stomatitis with excessive salivation, intentional tremor, peripheral neuropathy (lower sensor and motor conduction velocities), and renal impairment. In vitro and in vivo studies showed that Hg can stimulate free radical generation as a catalyst in Fenton-type reactions and through some other mechanisms, and can promote oxidative stress, peroxidation of lipids and DNA bases, disturbances in cell membrane permeation and calcium homeostasis in cells, impairment and even apoptosis of monocytes, T cells, glial cells and neurons, disturb the functioning of neurotransmitters, and cause immune disorders (Aschner, 2000; ATSDR, 1999; Castoldi et al., 2001; Clarkson & Magos, 2006; Kobal et al., 2004; Kobal-Grum et al., 2006; Lund et al., 1993; Magos, 1997; Pollard & Hultman, 1997; Schara et al., 2001; WHO, 1991).

3.2.1 Interaction with neurotransmitters

Various Hg species presynaptically blocks sodium and calcium channels and thus inhibits the uptake of some neurotransmitters, especially *glutamate* into astrocytes, which increases their extracellular concentration, thus increasing the sensitivity of neighbouring neurons for *stimulating excitotoxic effects* (Aschner et al., 2007; Brookes, 1996; Castoldi et al., 2001; Sirois & Atchison, 1991; Trotti et al., 1997). Many studies reviewed by Mottet et al. in 1997 showed that astrocytes, which accumulate a high level of Hg++, play a fundamental role in regulating glutamate level. In cases of methyl-Hg exposure, it seems that the Hg++ ions formed after the demethylation of methyl-Hg may also be responsible for the disruption of normal Ca++ ion channels.

Hg may affect sleep because it can: (i) increase extra-cellular glutamate concentrations associated with the activation of some cytokines, which can reduce the serotonin level by lowering the availability of its precursor, tryptophan, through the activation of its metabolizing enzyme, indoleamine 2,3-dioxigenase (McNally et al., 2008); (ii) increase the production of nitrogen oxide (NO) (Ikeda et al., 1999), which can directly, or in interaction with melatonin, decrease the active form of serotonin (Fossier et al., 1999; Kopczak et al., 2007); and (iii) Hg can also increase the consumption of serotonin and melatonin because of its potential oxidation in interaction with the increased production of free radicals observed in microglial cell cultures (Huether et al., 1997; Tan et al., 2000).

It is suggested that inorganic Hg potentiate and inhibite the neuronal nicotinic acetylcholine receptors, depending on its concentration (Mirzoian & Luetje, 2002). Another animal study shows that up-regulation of cerebral acetylcholine receptor can occur in chronic methyl-Hg exposure to compensate the early stage reduction of brain acetylcholine, as a consequence of acetylcholinesterase inhibition (Basu et al., 2006). It is evident from some studies on occupationally and environmentally Hg°-exposed subjects that Hg enhances the *dopaminergic effect* in CNS, which otherwise leads to cortical hyperexcitability and changes in the control of locomotor function, emotions, and behaviour (Burbure et al., 2006; Entezari-Taher et al., 1999; Lucchini et al., 2003; Missale et al., 1998).

3.2.2 Subcellular protective mechanism

Particularly significant in reducing the effects of Hg binding with SH groups of GSH and its biochemical precursors, cystine and cysteine, as well as its binding with MTs a cysteine rich low molecular weight proteins and with selenium (Se) an essential element and an integral part of a type of Se-proteins. The two major thiols, GSH and MTs, appear to be most important in regulating the accumulation and detoxification of Hg in CNS. The induction of GSH and MTs in astrocytes leads to greater detoxification of Hg and protection of CNS. Astrocytes represent the first line of CNS's defence against Hg (Aschner et al., 2007; Dringen et al., 2000). GSH (L-γ-glutamyl-L-cysteinyl-glycine) is synthesized from its precursors, glutamate, cysteine and glycine, in the cytosol of cells by the ATP-requiring enzymes γ-glutamilcysteine ligase and GSH synthetase (Meister & Andersen, 1983). Most of the free intracellular GSH (98%) is in thiol-reduced form (GSH) rather than in disulfide form (GSSG). From the cytosol, GSH is delivered into the mitochondria, endoplasmatic reticulum and nucleus, but much of it is delivered to extracellular spaces, where its degradation begins to occur on the surface of cells that express the enzyme γ-glutamil transpeptidase. GSH, as a nonenzymatic antioxidant, participates in a variety of detoxification, transport, and metabolic processes (Ballatri et al., 2009; Rossi et al., 2002). It is speculated that GSH may also function as a neuromodulator and neurotransmitter, since the degradation of extracellular GSH by γ-glutamil transpeptidase liberates glutamate and, subsequently, the hydrolysis of cysteinylglicine liberates cysteine and glycine, which function as a source of neuroactive amino acid (Oja et al., 2000).

Some other protective mechanisms, such as Se, antioxidative enzymes and melatonin, are also important in the detoxification of Hg and its peroxidative effect on the body, and particularly CNS. Se that binds with Hg in CNS in a molecular ratio of 1:1 into a nontoxic complex, which in lysosomes represents the last stage of detoxification of Hg (Falnoga et al., 2002; Kosta et al., 1975;).

It is evident from the study of ex-mercury miners that the Hg accumulated in the pineal gland and bound to Se did not impair its function, while the blood melatonin level was still high, probably due to the slow release of Hg from the gland and the adaptive response to free radical production induced by Hg (Kobal et al., 2004). Melatonin and free radicals form stable secondary and tertiary products, biogene amines, which also enter into reactions with free radicals. So melatonin inhibits the excessive formation of NO and its free radicals, peroxinitrites, and in this way also reduces the excitotoxic effects of glutamate (Sener et al., 2003; Tan et al., 2000).

The main enzymes that provide cellular protection against damage by reactive oxygen species mediated by Hg^{++} are Cu/Zn superoxide dismutase, catalase and the selenoenzyme glutathion peroxides, which transform the superoxide anion radical into hydrogen peroxide and then into oxygen and water (Lund et al., 1993). It is evident from some studies that repeated-intermittent occupational Hg° exposure induced an adaptive response and increase of GSH and catalase activity in erythrocytes, as well as the melatonin level in blood. The actual levels of GSH and catalase in erythrocytes depend on the actual level of blood Hg, both of these decreasing at higher blood Hg concentrations during actual exposure (Kobal, 1991; Kobal et al., 2004, 2008).

4. Some basic neurobiological characteristics of sleep-wake cycles

A study conducted by Qiu and colleagues in 2010 presented the main overall neurobiological activity of basal ganglia neurons associated with the sleep-wake state. The differences in firing patterns across the basal ganglia suggest multiple input sources, such as the cortex, thalamus, and the dopamine system, as well as some other intra basal ganglia inputs, such as the globus pallidus-subtalamic nucleus, and striatum-globus pallidus interactions. The largest nucleus striatum of the basal ganglia is mostly comprised of γ-aminobutiric acid ergic spiny neurons, whose activity is influenced by excitatory glutaminergic projection from the neocortex and thalamus, and dopaminergic projection from the midbrain ventral tegmental area and other known parts. The striatum receiving cortical inputs projects to the globus pallidus, which then projects to the cerebral cortex directly ore by the thalamus (mainly the mediodorsal thalamic nucleus). It was suggested that the lesion of globus pallidus produced a higher increase in wakefulness and frequent sleep-wake transitions, as well as a concomitant decrease in non-REM sleep duration. The results of the study also suggest that the cortico-striato-pallidal loop may be critically involved in the basal ganglia control of arousal.

There are four stages of sleep, which include the brain-active period associated with rapid eye movements called REM sleep (emergent stage 1 EEG), preceded by progressively deeper sleep stages (stages 2, 3, 4) graded on the basis of increasingly slower EEG patterns, called non-REM sleep. Stages 3 and 4 are referred to as slow-wave sleep (SWS) characterized by delta waves (high amplitude and low-frequency). REM sleep and wakefulness are characterized by increased activity in the cerebral cortex with low-amplitude and high-frequency EEG (alpha waves) and in REM by the inhibition of peripheral neurons displayed in the postural muscle atonia. Increased cerebral activity during REM sleep is associated with higher oxygen consumption, blood flow and neural firing (Madsen et al., 1991).

Acetylcholine, norepinephrine, serotonin, histamine and hypocretin levels are increased in wakefulness and low in non-REM sleep, whereas during REM sleep the noradrenergic, serotonergic and histaminergic cells become silent (Jones, 2005). A high cholinergic tone in the pontine reticular formation combined with a low GABAergic tone contributes to the generation of REM sleep (Vanini et al., 2011). Animal studies showed that the neurotransmitter glutamate enhances REM sleep by activation of the kainite receptor within the cholinergic cell compartment of the brainstem pedunculo pontine tegmentum of cat and rat (Datta, 2002). During REM sleep and waking, the release of acetylcholine activated dopamine in the ventral tegmental neurons, which were higher in the prefrontal cortex and nucleus accumbens. It was also suggested that glutamate and asparate release can reciprocally affect dopamine release (Forster and Blaha, 2000; Morari et al., 1998). The animal study of Lena and colleagues in 2005 also showed elevated levels of dopamine during waking and REM sleep in the medial prefrontal cortex and nucleus accumbens.

The impairment of the subcortical dopaminergic system may cause disinhibition of the GABAergic inhibitory circuitry at the motor cortex level (Entazry-Taher et al., 1999; Ziemann et al., 1996). It is suggested that the diencephalon-spinal dopaminergic tract could be important as a potential anatomic site of dopaminergic dysfunction in restless leg syndrome, and of periodic leg contractile movements in sleep. The diencephalon-spinal dopaminergic tract projects to the limbic system, sensory cortex and spinal cord (Ondo et al., 2000). The periodic leg contractile movements occur mainly during non-REM sleep. The results of the study of Rijsman et al. in 2005 indicate diminished inhibition at spinal level in subjects with periodic leg movements disorder, probably because of the altered function of the descending spinal tracts and peripheral changes in the inter-neural circuitry at the spinal level. Dreams and nightmares occur usually at the end of the night, when REM sleep is longer. On the other side, sleep terrors occur more often in children than in adults, while children have more delta sleep (Pinel, 2009; Lee & Douglass, 2010).

Another recent animal study (John et al., 2008) showed a rapid increase in the glutamate level during REM sleep and awakening in the histamine-containing posterior hypothalamic region and the perifornical-lateral hypothalamus, and its reduction shortly after the termination of REM sleep and awakening. In the animal study of Dash and colleagues conducted in 2009, which employed a very sensitive method (in vivo amperometry) to measure cortical extracellular glutamate, a progressive increase was observed in the cortical extracellular glutamate concentration during REM sleep and waking. It was suggested that extrasynaptic glutamate is released from astrocytes and neurons in extracellular space, where it is accumulated, and then declines during non-REM sleep due to the intracellular re-uptake mediated by glutamate/asparate transporters. The rate of glutamate decline during non-REM sleep positively correlated with the levels of slow wave activity (SWA) (Fig. 1). The authors of the study concluded that perhaps the glutamate-decreasing effect of non-REM sleep is especially relevant in a pathological condition.

It is thought that the pineal gland itself takes part in regulating the rhythm of sleep and wakefulness, entrained by the light/dark cycle. Neural impulses from the retina enter the pineal gland, which coordinates the formation and secretion of serotonin and melatonin, through the suprachiasmic nuclei (SCN) of the hypothalamus. Light induces serotonin secretion, while melatonin is produced at night directly from serotonin by acetylation. However, melatonin production can be acutely interrupted by light exposure during the night. Norepinephrine, which is released at night in response to stimulatory signals

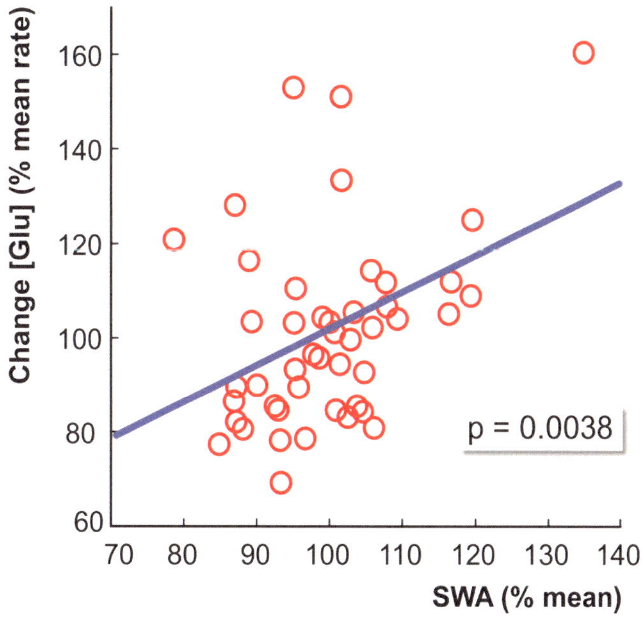

Fig. 1. The rate of glutamate decline during non-REM sleep positively correlated ($r = 0.41$, $p < 0.01$) with the amount of SWA. Each data point represents the average SWA and the change in glutamate concentration during non-REM sleep (Adapted from Dash, et al. 2009, The Journal of Neuroscience, Vol. 29, No. 3, pp. 620-629. Copyright 2009, Society for Neuroscience. Adapted with permission.)

originating in SCN, also regulates pineal gland activity. Melatonin can influence the sleep-promoting and sleep-wake rhythm regulating actions through the specific activation of melatonin receptors type 1 and 2, which are highly concentrated in SCN, and are also expressed in the peripheral organs and cells regulating other physiological functions of the so-called circadian 24-hour rhythms. The activation of type 1 occurs by inducing a receptor-suppressed neuronal firing rate in CNS, while type 2 induces a circadian phase shift. The increased secretion of melatonin is also accompanied by other circadian 24-hour rhythms of humans, and in rats studies associated with decreased production of neurotransmitter nitric oxide (NO) (Fig. 2) (Dubocovich et al., 2003; Ebadi, 1992; Geoffriau et al., 1998; Leon et al., 1998; Murphy & Delanty, 2007; Starc, 1998). Some studies do not confirm the influence of melatonin on the duration of sleep (Hughes et al., 1998), while others support the effect of melatonin on the duration and quality of REM sleep because they assume that it either directly influences cholinergic activity in REM sleep, or indirectly influences REM sleep by the elimination of serotonergic or aminergic activity (Jones, 1991; Kunz et al., 2004). It seems that melatonin modulates the release of acethylcholine in the nucleus accumbens and the motor activity of rats (Paredes et al., 1999). Some animal studies suggest that the daily changes in melatonin production may regulate the day-night variation in glutamate and GABA in the neostriatum (Marquez de Prado et al., 2000). It seems that the glutaminergic system negatively regulates norepinephrine-dependent melatonin synthesis in the rat's pineal gland (Yamada et al., 1998). In rats studies melatonin inhibits the glutamate-mediated response of the striatum to motor cortex stimulation and decrease NO content in parieto-temporal cortex, striatum and brainstem of rats due to the inhibition of neuronal nitric oxide synthase activity. On the other site the administration of high doses of melatonin have paradoxal effect and can decrease GABA and increase glutamate levels (Bikjdaouene et al., 2003; Leon et al., 1998). The synaptically released glutamate is taken up into astrocytes, where it is degraded into glutamine by the glutamate-metabolizing enzyme, glutamate synthetase. It is suggested that astrocytes are primarily responsible for controlling the extracellular level of glutamate, and melatonin seems to have a direct effect on astrocytes (Marquez de Prado et al., 2000; Segovia et al., 1999).

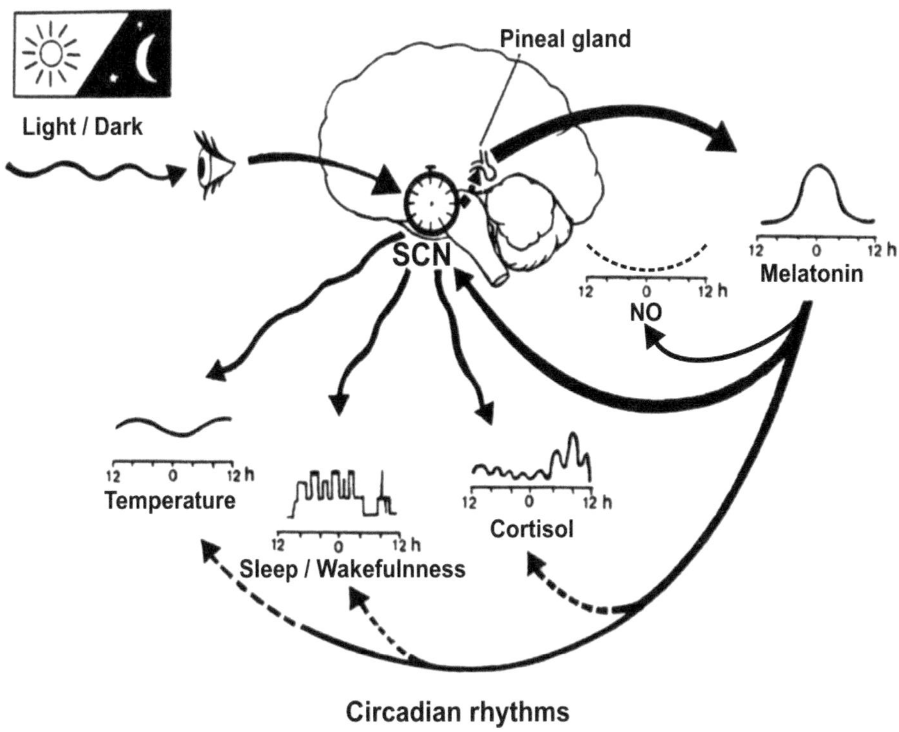

Fig. 2. Melatonin rhythm acts as an endogenous synchroniser adjusted to the 24-hour light/dark cycle, which (rats studies) regulates also the NO production (Adapted from Geoffrieau et al., 1998 ; Leon et al., 1998, *Hormone Research*, Vol. 49, pp. 136-141. Copyright 1998, S. Karger AG, Medical and Scientific Publishers. Adapted with permission.)

5. Conclusion

In the above-mentioned studies, we assumed that the increased uptake of Hg^o into CNS could affect sleep: (i) due to the further increase of extracellular concentrations of glutamate, which leads to the induction of excitotoxic effects that can have an impact on disbalance of cholinergic, glutaminergic and dopaminergic activity and other neuronal activity which otherwise regulate non-REM sleep, REM sleep and awakening , and (ii) due to the decreased night-time melatonin level, which also seems to be involved in day-night glutamate regulation and sleep-wake regulating actions by the activation of melatonin receptors in SCN and in the peripheral organ cells regulating other circadian 24-hour rhythms.

In vitro and in vivo studies have shown that due to the increased production of free radicals as well as blocked sodium and calcium channels, Hg inhibits the uptake of some neurotransmitters, especially glutamate, into astrocytes, which increases their extracellular concentration, thus increasing the sensitivity of neighbouring neurons for stimulating excitotoxic effects (Aschner et al., 2007; Castoldi et al., 2001). The increased production of the neurotransmitter nitrogen oxide (NO) mediated by Hg (Ikeda et al., 1999) is also indirectly included in the excitotoxic effects of glutamate (Dawson et al., 1991). Hg^{o} thus additionally increases the physiological level of extracellular glutamate and its glutaminergic activity during REM sleep and awakening. It is not expected that Hg++-mediated glutamate accumulation in extracellular space can decline during non-REM-SWA sleep through intracellular-astrocyte uptake by glutamate/asparate transporters and its degradation into glutamine, whose capacity is satisfactory in physiological conditions (Dash et al., 2009), but probably not in Hg++-enhanced glutaminergic activity. It seems that the decrease of melatonin mediated by interaction with Hg++ can also decrease the uptake of glutamate in astrocytes, which additionally contributes to pathological glutaminergic overactivity at increased Hg++ concentrations in CNS.

Given the results of some animal studies (Lena et al., 2005; Morari et al., 1998) and human data (Burbure et al., 2006; Entezari-Taher et al., 1999; Lucchini et al., 2003; Missale et al., 1998), it is expected that Hg++ enhances the dopaminergic effect in CNS, otherwise associated with cortical hyperexcitability and changes in the control of locomotor function. The impaired subcortical dopaminergic system, which may cause disinhibition at motor cortex level, could be associated with periodic contractile movements of the legs in the sleep (Entezari-Taher et al., 1999; Ondo et al., 2000; Rijsman et al., 2005; Ziemann et al., 1996) observed in miners during increased Hg^{o} absorption and intoxication. We can not completely exclude the potential additive effect of sub-clinical peripheral neuropathy observed in miners, which can trigger and modify the appearance of periodic leg contractile movements in sleep.

Melatonin is decreased in the night-time, either because of decreased synthesis under the influence of Hg-mediated, increased NO production, which in SCN operates similarly to a light signal (Ding et al., 1994; Ikeda et al., 1999), or by lowering its precursor tryptophan through its increased metabolizing, and because of its consumption in interaction with free radicals (McNally et al., 2008; Sener et al., 2003; Tan et al., 2000). A lower melatonin level is, at the same time, associated with the increased production of NO and its free radicals, peroxyntrites, which also increase the excitotoxic effects of glutamate (Acuna-Castroviejo et al., 1995; Leon et al., 1998). However, it has been established in many studies that melatonin plays a role in mediation between the circardian pacemaker and sleep-wake behaviour, and may have soporiphic properties and induce sedation, as well as the decreased nocturnal melatonin level labilised circadian rhythm function (Rodenbeck & Hajak, 2001; Stone et al., 2000; Turek & Gillette, 2004).

Increased extracellular glutamate and its decreased uptake in astrocytes (Dash et al., 2009) could hypothetically lead to longer REM periods and more frequent awakening associated with more frequent dreaming during increased Hg^{o} absorption or intoxication. Hypothetically, persistent glutaminergic activity can also disrupt delta wave sleep, which could be associated with the sleep terrors observed in intoxicated miners. Further animal studies would be very helpful in elucidating the potential effects of Hg on the uptake of extracellular glutamate into astrocytes during the non-REM sleep, which could be relevant for sleep disorders observed in states of increased Hg^{o} absorption or intoxication.

6. References

Acuna-Castroviejo, D., Escames, G., Macias, M., Munoz-Hoyos, A., Molina-Carballo, A., Arauzo, M., Montes, R., & Vives, F. (1995). Cell protective role of melatonin in the brain. *Journal of Pineal Research*, Vol. 19, No. 2, pp. 57-63.

Albers, J. W., Avender, G. D., Levine, S. P., & Langolf, G. D. (1982). Asymptomatic sensory motor polyneuropathy in workers exposed to elemental mercury. *Neurology*, Vol. 32, No. 10, pp. 1168-1174.

Aschner, M. (1997). Astrcyte metallothioneins (MTS) and their neuroprotective role. *Annals of the New York Academy of Sciences*, Vol. 825, No. 1, pp. 334-347.

Aschner, M. (2000). Possible mechanisms of methylmercury cytotoxicity. *Molecular Biology Today*, Vol. 1, No. 2, pp. 43-48.

Aschner, M., Syversen, T., Souza, D. O., Rocha, J. B. T., & Farina, M. (2007). Involvement of glutamate and reactive oxygen species in methylmercury neurotoxicity. *Brazilian Journal of Medical and Biological Research*, Vol. 40, No. 3, pp. 285-291.

ATSDR (1999). *Toxicological Profile for Mercury*. Agency for Toxic Substances and Disease Registry, Public Health Service, US Department of Health and Human Services, Atlanta.

Ballatori, N., Krance, S. M., Notenboom, S., Shi, S., Tieu, K., & Hammond, C. L. (2009). Glutathione dysregulation and the etiology and progression of human diseases. *Journal of Biological Chemistry*, Vol. 390, No. 3, pp. 191-214.

Basu, N., Scheuhammer, A. M., Rouvinen-Watt, K., Grochowina, N., Klenavic, K., Evans, R. D., & Chan, H. M. (2006). Methylmercury ipairs components of the cholinergic system in captive mink (Mustla vision). *Toxicological Sciences*, Vol. 91, No. 1, pp. 202-209.

Berlin, M., Fzarkerley, J., & Nordberg, G. (1969). The uptake of mercury in the brains of mammals exposed to mercury vapor and to mercuric salts. *Archives of Environmental Health*, Vol. 18, No. 5, pp. 719-729.

Bikjdaouene, L., Escames, G., Leon, J., Ferrer, M., R., Khaldy, H., Vives, F., & Acuna-Castroviejo, D. (2003). Changes in brain amino acids and nitric oxide after melatonin administration in rats with pentylenetetrazole-induced seizures. *Journal of Pineal Research*, Vol. 35, No. 1, pp. 54-60.

Brookes, N. (1996). In vitro evidence for the role of glutamate in the CNS toxicity of mercury. *Toxicology*, Vol. 76, No. 3, pp. 245-256.

Burbure, C., Buched, J. P., Leroyer, A., Nisse, C., Haguenoer, J. M., Mutti, A., Smerhovsky, Z., Cikrt, M., Trzcinka-Ochocka, M., Razniewska, G., Jakubowsky, M., & Bernard, M. (2006.) Renal and neurologic effects of cadmium, lead, mercury and arsenic in children: evidence of early effects and multiple interactions at the environmental exposure level. *Environmental Health Perspectives*, Vol. 114, No. 4, pp. 584-590.

Castoldi, A. F., Cocchini, T., Ceccatelli, S., & Manzo, L. (2001). Neurotoxicity and molecular effects of methylmercury. *Brain Research Bulletin*, Vol. 55, No. 2, pp. 197-203.

Clarkson, T. W., & Magos, L. (2006). The toxicology of mercury and its chemical compounds. *Critical Reviews in Toxicology*, Vol. 36, No. 8, pp. 609-662.

Dash, M. B., Douglas, C. L., Vyazovsky, V. V., Cirelli, C., & Tononi, G. (2009). Long-term Homeostasis of extracellular glutamate in the rat cerebral cortex across sleep and waking states. *The Journal of Neuroscience*, Vol. 29, No. 3, pp. 620-629.

Datta, S. (2002). Evidence that sleep is controlled by the activation of brain stem pedunculop. *Journal of Neurophysiology*, Vol. 87, pp. 1790-1798.

Dawson, V. L., Dawson, T. M., London, E. D., Bredt, D. S., & Snyder, S. H. (1991). Nitric oxide mediates glutamate neurotoxicity in primary cortical cultures. *Proceedings of the National Academy of Sciences USA*, Vol. 88, No. 14, pp. 6368-6371.

Ding, J. M., Chen, D., Weber, E. T., Faiman, L. E., Rea, M. A., & Gillette, M. (1994). Resetting the biological clock: mediation of nocturnal circadian shift by glutamate and No. *Science*, Vol. 266, No. 5191, pp. 1713-1717.

Dringen, R., Gutterer, J. M., & Herrlinger, J. (2000). Glutathione metabolism in brain, metabolic interaction between astrocytes and neurons in the defense against reactive oxygen species. *European Journal of Biochemistry*, Vol. 267, No. 16, pp. 4912-4916.

Dubocovich, M. L., Rivera-Bermudez, M. A., Gerdin, M. J., & Masana, M. I. (2003). Molecular pharmacology, regulation and function of mammalian melatonin receptors. *Frontiers in Bioscience*, Vol. 8, pp. 1093-1108.

Ebadi, M. (1992). Multiple pineal receptors in regulating melatonin synthesis, In: *Melatonin: Biosynthesis, Physiological Effects and Clinical Applications*, Yu, H. S., & Reiter, R. J. (Eds), pp. 39-71, CRC Press, Boca Raton, Florida.

Entezari-Taher, M., Singleton, J. R., Jones, C. R., Meekins, G., Petajan, J. H., & Smith, A. G. (1999). Changes in excitability of motor cortical circuitry in primary restless legs syndrome. *Neurology*, Vol. 53, No. 6, pp. 1201-1207.

Falnoga, I., Tušek-Žnidarič, M., Horvat, M., & Stegnar, P. (2000). Mercury, selenium and cadmium in human autopsy samples from Idrija residents and mercury mine workers. *Environmental Research*, Vol. 84, No. 3, pp. 211-218.

Falnoga, I., Kobal, A. B., Stibilj, V., Horvat, M., & Stegnar, P. (2002). Selenoprotein P in subject exposed to mercury and other stress situatuons sach as phisical load or metal chelation tretment. *Biological Trace Element Research*, Vol. 89, No. 1, pp. 25-33.

Fossier, P., Blanchard, B., Ducrocq, C., Leprince, C., Tauc, L., & Baux, G. (1999). Nitric oxide transforms serotonin into an inactive form and this affects neuromodulation. *Neuroscience*, Vol. 93, No. 2, pp. 597-603.

Forster, G. L., & Blaha, C. D. (2000). Laterodorsal tegmental stimulation elicits dopamine elux in the rat nucleus accumbens by activation of acetylcholine and glutamate receptors in the ventral tegmental area. *European Journal of Neuroscience*, Vol. 12, pp. 3596-3604.

Gabrovec-Nahlik, N., Jank, M., & Kobal, A. B. (1977). *Okvare perifernega živčevja pri delavcih, izpostavljenih živemu srebru v Rudniku Živega Srebra Irija - Peripheral neuropathy in workers exposed to mercury in Idrija mercury mine* [in Slovene], Master of Science Thesis, University of Ljubljana, Ljubljana, Slovenia.

Geoffriau, M., Brun, J., Chazot, G., & Claustrat, B. (1998). The physiology and pharmacology of melatonin in humans. *Hormone Research*, Vol. 49, pp. 136-141.

Goldwater, L. J. (1972). *Mercury: A History of Quicksilver*, York Press, Baltimore, Maryland.

Hirschhorn, N., Feldman, R. G., & Greaves, I. A. (2001). Abraham Lincoln's blue pills. Did our 16th president suffer from mercury poisoning? *Perspectives in Biology and Medicine*, Vol. 44, No. 4, pp. 631-632.

Hornyak, M., Feige, B., Rieman, D., & Voderholzer, U. (2006). Periodic leg movements in sleep and periodic limb movement disorder: Prevalence, clinical significance and treatment. *Sleep Medicine Reviews*, Vol. 10, No. 3, pp. 169-77.

Huether, G., Fettkötter, I., Keilhoff, G., & Wolf, G. (1997). Serotonin acts as a radical scavenger and is oxidised to a dimer during the respiratory burst of activated microglia. *Journal of Neurochemistry*, Vol. 69, No. 5, pp. 2096-2101.

Hughes, R. J., Sack, R. L., & Lewy, A. J. (1998). The role of melatonin and circadian phase in age-related sleep-maintenance insomnia: assessment in a clinical trial of melatonin replacement. *Sleep*, Vol. 21, No. 1, pp. 52-68.

Hursh, J. B., Sichak, S. P., & Clarkson, T. W. (1988). In vitro oxidation of mercury by the blood. *Pharmacology & Toxicology*, Vol. 63, No. 4, pp. 266-273.

Ikeda, M., Komachi, H., Sato, I., Himi, T., Yuasa, T., & Murota, S. (1999). Induction of neuronal nitric oxide synthase by methylmercury in the cerebellum. *Journal of Neuroscience Research*, Vol. 55, No. 3, pp. 352-356.

John, J., Ramanathan, L., & Siegel, J. M. (2008). Rapid changes in glutamate levels in the posteror hypothalamus across sleep-wake states in freely behaving rats. *American Journal of Physiology - Regulatory, Integrative and Comparative Physiology*, Vol. 295, No. 6, pp. 2041-2049.

Jones, B. E. (1991). Paradoxical sleep and its chemical/structural substrates in the brain. *Neuroscience*, Vol. 40, No. 3, pp. 37-56.

Jones, B. E. (2005). From waking to sleeping: neuronal and chemical substrates. *Trends in Pharmacological Sciences*, Vol. 26, No. 11, pp. 578-586.

Kobal, A. B. (1975a). Beurteilung der Wirksamkeit von persönlichen Schutzausrüstungen an Arbeisplätzen mit hohen Konzentrationen von Quecksilberdämpfen [summary in English]. *Zentralblatt für Arbeitsmedizin, Arbeitsschutz und Ergonomie*, Vol. 12, pp. 366-371.

Kobal, A. B. (1975b). *Profesionalna ekspozicija anorganskemu živemu srebru in spremembe v serumskih proteinih - Professional exposure to inorganic mercury and the alternations in serum protein* [in Slovene], Master of Science Thesis, University of Zagreb, Zagreb, Croatia.

Kobal, A. B. (1991). *Occupational exposure to elemental mercury and its influence on mercury in blood, erythrocytes, plasma, exhaled breath and urine, and catalase activity in erythrocytes* [summary in English], PhD Thesis, Faculty of medicine, University of Ljubljana, Ljubljana, Slovenia.

Kobal, A. B. (1994). Quecksilber aus Idria - Historisch und aktuell - eine arbeitmedizinische Betrachtung [summary in English]. *Zentralblatt für Arbeitsmedizin, Arbeitsschutz und Ergonomie*, Vol. 44, pp. 200-210.

Kobal, A. B., Horvat, M., Prezelj, M., Sesek-Briški, A., Krsnik, M., Dizdarevič, T., Mazej, D., Falnoga, I., Stibilj, V., Arnerič, N., Kobal, D., & Osredkar, J. (2004). The impact of long-term past exposure to elemental mercury on antioxidative capacity and lipid peroxidation in mercury miners. *Journal of Trace Elements in Medicine and Biology*, Vol. 17, No. 4, pp. 261-274.

Kobal, A. B., & Kobal-Grum, D. (2010). Scopoli's work in the field of mercurialism in light of today's knowledge: Past and present perspectives. *American Journal of Industrial Medicine*, Vol. 53, No. 5, pp. 535-547.

Kobal, A. B., Prezelj, M., Horvat, M., Krsnik, M., Gibičar, D., & Osredkar, J. (2008). Glutathione level after long-term occupational elemental mercury exposure. *Environmental Research*, Vol. 107, No. 1, pp. 115-123.

Kobal-Grum, D., Kobal, A. B., Arnerič, N., Horvat, M., Ženko, B., Džeroski, S., & Osredkar, J. (2006). Personality traits in miners with past occupational elemental mercury exposure. *Environmental Health Perspectives*, Vol. 114, No. 2, pp. 290-296.

Kopczak, A., Korth, H. G., de Grot, H., & Kirsch, M. (2007). N-nitroso-melatonin release nitricoxide in the presence of serotonin and derivates. *Journal of Pineal Research*, Vol. 43, No. 4, pp. 343-350.

Kosta, L., Byrne, A. R., & Zelenko, V. (1975). Correlation between selenium and mercury in man following exposure to inorganic mercury. *Nature*, Vol. 254, No. 5497, pp. 238-239.

Kunz, D., Mahlberg, R., Muller, C., Tilmann, A., & Bes, F. (2004). Melatonin in patients with reduced REM sleep duration: two randomized controlled trials. *The Journal of Clinical Endocrinology & Metabolism*, Vol. 89, No. 1, pp. 128-134.

Kussmaul, A. (1861). *Untersuchungen uber den Constitutionellen Mercurialismus und sein verhaltniss zur Constitutionallen Syphilis*, Wurzburg.

Lee, E., K., & Douglass, A., B. (2010). Sleep in psychiatric disorders: Where are we now? *Canadian Journal of Psychiatry*, Vol. 55, No. 7, pp. 403-412.

Leon, J., Vives, F., Gomez, I., Camacho, E., Gallo, M. A., Espinosa, A., Escames, G., & Acuna-Castroviejo, D. (1998). Modulation of rat striatal glutamatergic response in search for new neuroprotective agents: Evaluation of melatonin and some kynurenine derivates. *Brain Research Bulletin*, Vol. 45, No. 5, pp. 525-530.

Lena, I., Parrot, S., Deschaux, O., Muffat-Joly, S., Sauvinet, V., Renaud, B., et al. (2005). Variation in extracellular levels of dopamine, noradrenaline, glutamate, and asparate across the sleep-wake cycle in the medial prefrontal cortex and nucleus accumbens of freely moving rats. *Journal of Neuroscience Research*, Vol. 81, No. 6, pp. 891-899.

Lesky, E. (1956). *Arbeitsmedizin im 18. Jahrhundert: Werksarzt und Arbeiter im Quecksilberbergwerk Idria* [in German], Verlag des Notringes der wissenschaftlichen Verbände Österreichs, Wien.

Lucchini, R., Calza, S., Camerino, D., Carta, P., Decarli, A., Prrinello, G., Soleo, L., Zefferino, R., & Alessio, L. (2003). Application of a latent variable model for a multicentric study on early effects due to mercury exposure. *Neurotoxicology*, Vol. 24, No. 4-5, pp. 605-616.

Lund, B. O., Miller, D. M., & Woods, J. S. (1993). Studies on Hg (II)-induced H_2O_2 formation and oxidative stress in vivo and vitro in rat kidney mitochondria. *Biochemical Pharmacology*, Vol. 45, No. 10, pp. 2017-2024.

Madsen, P. L., Schmid, H., Wildschiedtz, G., Friberg, L., Holm, S., Vorstrup, S., & Lassen, N. (1991). Cerebral 02 metabolism in cerebral blood flow in humans during deep and rapid eye movement sleep. *Journal of Applied Physiology*, Vol. 70, No. 6, pp. 2597-2601.

Magos, L., Halbach, S., & Clarkson, T. W. (1978). Role of catalase in the oxidation of mercury vapor. *Biochemical Pharmacology*, Vol. 27, No. 9, pp. 1373-1377.

Magos, L. (1997). Physiology and toxicology of mercury. *Metal Ions in Biological Systems*, 34, pp.321-370.

Marquez de Prado, B., Castaneda, T. R., Galindo, A., del Arko, A., Segovia, G., Reiter, R. J., & Mora, F. (2000). Melatonin disrupt circardian rhythms of glutamate and GABA in the neostriatum of awake rat: A microdialysis study. *Journal of Pineal Research*, Vol. 29, No. 4, pp. 209-216.

McNally, L., Bhagwagar, Z., & Hannestad, J. (2008). Inflammatio glutamate, and glia in depression: A literature review. *CNS Spectrums*, Vol. 13, No. 6, pp. 501-510.

Meister, A., & Anderson, M. E. (1983). Glutathione. *Annual Review of Biochemistry*, Vol. 52, pp. 711-60.

Mirzoian, A., & Luetje, C. W. (2002). Modulation of neuronal nicotinic acetylcholine receptors by mercury. *Journal of Pharmacology and Experimental Therapeutics*, Vol. 302, No. 2, pp. 560-567.

Missale, C., Nash, S. R., Robinson, S. W., Jaber, M., & Caron, M. G. (1998). Dopamine receptors: from structure to function. *Physiological Reviews*, Vol. 78, No. 1, pp. 189-225.

Morari, M., Marti, M., Sbrenna, S., Fuxe, K., Bianchi, C., & Beani, L. (1998). Reciprocal dopamine-glutamate modulation of release in the basal ganglia. *Neurochemistry International*, Vol. 33, No. 5, pp. 383-397.

Mottet, N. K., Vahter, M. E., Charleston, J. S., & Friberg, L.T. (1997). Metabolism of methylmercury in the brain and its toxicological significance, In: *Metal ions in biological systems*, Sigel & Sigel, H. (Eds), pp. 371-392, Marcel Dekker, INC, New York.

Murphy, K., & Delanty, N. (2007). Sleep deprivation. A clinical perspective. *Sleep and Biological Rhythms*, Vol. 5, No. 1, pp. 2-14.

Oja, S. S., Janaki, R., Varga, V., & Saransaari, P. (2000) Modulation of glutamate receptor functions by glutatthione. *Neurochemistry International*, Vol. 37, No. 2-3, pp. 299-306.

Ondo, W. G., He, Y., Rajasekaran, S., & Le, W. D. (2000). Clinical correlates of 6-hydroxydopamine injections into A11 dopaminergic neurons in rats: A possible model for restless legs syndrome. *Movement Disorders*, Vol. 15, No. 1, pp. 154-158.

Paredes, D., Rada, P., Bonila, E., Gonzales, L. E., Parada, M., & Hernandez, L. (1999). Melatonin acts on the nucleus accumens to increase acetylcholine release and modify the motor activity pattern of rats. *Brain Research*, Vol. 850, No. 1-2, pp. 14-20.

Pinel, J.P.J. (2009). *Biopsychology* (7th edition), Pearson Education, Boston.

Pollard, K. M., & Hultman, P. (1997). Effects of mercury on immune system, In: *Metal ions in biological systems*, Sigel & Sigel, H. (Eds), pp. 421-434, Marcel Dekker, INC, New York.

Qiu, M. H., Vetrivelan, R., Fuller, P. M., & Lu, J. (2010). Basal ganglia control of sleep-wake behavior and cortical activation. *European Journal of Neuroscience*, Vol. 31, No. 3, pp. 499-507.

Rijsman, R. M., Stam, C. J., & de Weerd, A. W. (2005). Abnormal H-reflexes in periodic limb movement disorder; impact on understanding the pathphysiology of the disorder. *Clinical Neurophysiology*, Vol. 116, No. 1, pp. 204-210.

Rodenbeck, A., & Hajak, G. (2001). Neuroendocrine dysregulation in primary insomnia. *Neurology Reviews*, Vol. 157, No. 11, pp. 57-61.

Rossi, R., Milzani, A., Dalle-Donne, I., Giustarini, D., Lusini, L., Colombo, R., et al. (2002). Blood glutathione dissulfide: In vivo factor or in vitro artifact? *Clinical Chemistry*, Vol. 48, No. 5, pp. 742-753.

Scopoli, J. A. (1771). *De hydrorgyro Idriensi Tentamina Physico-Chymico-Medica, I. De Minera Hydrargyri, II. De Vitrioli Idriensi, III. De Morbis Fossorum Hydrargyri* (2nd ed), Janae et Lepsiae, Joann Guil Hartung.

Segovia, G., Del Arko, A., & Mora, F. (1999). Role of glutamate receptors and glutamate transporters in the regulatio of the glutamate-glutamate cycle in the awake rat. *Neurochemical Research*, Vol. 24, No. 6, pp. 779-783.

Sener, G., Sehirli, A. O., & Ayanog-lu-Durler, G. (2003). Melatonin protects against mercury (II)-induced oxidative tissue damage in rats. *Pharmacology & Toxicology*, Vol. 93, No. 6, pp. 290-296.

Schara, M., Nemec, M., Falnoga, I., Kobal, A. B., Kveder, M., & Svetek, J. (2001). The action of mercury on cell membranes. *Cellular & Molecular Biology Letters*, Vol. 6, No. 2A, pp. 299-304.

Sirois, J. E., & Atchinson, W. D. (1996). Effects of mercurials on ligand- an voltage-gatedion chanels: A review. *Neurotoxicology*, Vol. 17, No. 1, pp. 63-84.

Starc, V. (1998). Circadian rhythms and readiness to work II. Impact of sleep on circadian rhythms [abstract in English]. *Zdravniški vestnik*, Vol. 67, pp. 733-743.

Stone, B. M., Tumer, C., Mils, S. L., & Nicholson, A. N. (2000). Hypnotic activity of melatonin. *Sleep*, Vol. 23, pp. 663-669.

Tan, D. X., Manchester, L. C., Reiter, R. J., Qi, W.-B., Karbovnik, M., & Calvo, J. R. (2000). Significance of melatonin in antioxidative defense system: Reactions and products. *Biological Signals and Receptors*, Vol. 9, No. 3-4, pp. 137-159.

Trotti, D., Rizzini, B. L., Rossi, D., Haugeto, O., Gacagni, G., Danbold, N. C., & Volterra, A. (1997). Neuronal and glial glutamate transporters posses and SH- based redox regulatory mechanism. *European Journal of Neuroscience*, Vol. 9, pp. 1236-1243.

Turek, F. W., & Gillette, M. U. (2004). Melatonin, sleep, and circardian rhythms: rationale for development of specific melatonin agonist. *Sleep Medicine*, Vol. 5, No. 6, pp. 523-532.

Tušek-Žnidarič, M., Pucer, A., Fatur, T., Filipič, M., Ščančar, J., & Falnoga, I. (2007). Metal binding of metallothioneins in human astrocytomas (U87 MG, IPDDC-2A). *BioMetals*, Vol. 20, No. 5, pp. 781-92.

Vanini, G., Wathen, B. L., Lydic, R., & Boghdoyan, H. A. (2011). Endogeneus GABA levels in the pontine reticular formation are greater during wakefulness than during rapid eye movement sleep. *Journal of Neuroscience*, Vol. 31, No. 7, pp. 2649-2656.

Vgontzas, A. N., Pejovic, S., & Karataraki (2010). Sleep, sleep disorders, and stress, In: *Stress Consequences: Mental, Neuropsychological and Socioeconomic*, Fink, G. (Ed), pp. 257-265, Academic Press, Elsevier.

WHO (1976). *Environmental Health Criteria I Mercury*, World Health Organization, Geneva.

WHO (1980). *Recommended health-based limits in occupational exsposure to heavy metals, Reports of a WHO Study Group*, World Health Organization, Geneva.

WHO (1991). *Environmental Health Criteria 118, Inorganic mercury*, World Health Organization, Geneva.

Yamada, H., Yatsushiro, S., Ishio, S., Hayashi, M., Nishi, T., Yamamoto, A., et al. (1998). Metabotropic glutamate receptors negatively regulate melatonin sintesis in rat pinealocytes. *The Journal of Neuroscience*, Vol. 18, No. 6, pp. 2056-2062.

5

Evaluation of the Upper Airway in Patients with Snoring and OSA

Bhik Kotecha
Royal National Throat, Nose & Ear Hospital, London
UK

1. Introduction

Snoring and obstructive sleep apnoea (OSA) both exhibit multilevel upper airway obstruction. The Importance of evaluating the dynamics of the obstructing upper airway cannot be emphasised enough. Accurate assessment and evaluation of the upper airway could potentially lead to improved surgical and non-surgical treatment outcomes. Most of these patients would have undergone an ambulatory sleep study or a polysomnography prior to deciding what treatment modality is going to be offered to them. Treatment options available include nasal continuous positive airway pressure (nCPAP), mandibular advancement splints (MAS) or surgery. In terms of selecting a treatment option, in cases where the sleep study has confirmed moderate or severe OSA, nCPAP would be favoured. In the remainder and the nCPAP failed patients, further evaluation of the upper airway is useful and necessary. This chapter will not address sleep studies but will discuss various methods of assessing the upper airway and will include clinical evaluation of the upper airway during wakefulness and sleep.

2. Clinical examination

This can be quite easily conducted in out patient setting and addresses the patency of the nasal passage as well as the assessment of different segments of the pharynx. Anterior rhinoscopy using a simple nasal speculum allows visualisation of the anterior aspect of the nasal cavity and helps in identifying problems of caudal dislocation of the septum and if the nasal valve area is compromised. However, a rigid endoscope is more useful in a more comprehensive evaluation of the nasal passage and will identify problems such as deviated nasal septum, nasal polyps (fig. 1) and rhinosinusitis. The identification of these pathological features is important as they may be a cause of failed compliance and efficacy in the nCPAP patients.

Simple oropharyngeal cavity examination provides the clinician with useful information and of note would be the size and grading of palatine tonsils, the length of the soft palate and uvula and more subtle features such as redundant pharyngeal folds. Friedman tongue position[1] and Mallampati[2] grading are also utilised by many clinicians in order to select patients who may be suitable for palatal surgery. For example in patients with Friedman tongue position 3 or 4 (figs. 2 & 3) palatal surgery is unlikely to be successful. In contrast Friedman tongue position 1(fig. 4) would yield better results following palatal surgery. One must however take in to account that as this assessment is done during wakefulness it may not truly reflect what happens to the upper airway during sleep as there must undoubtedly be some variation in the muscle tone in the state of wakefulness and different stages of sleep.

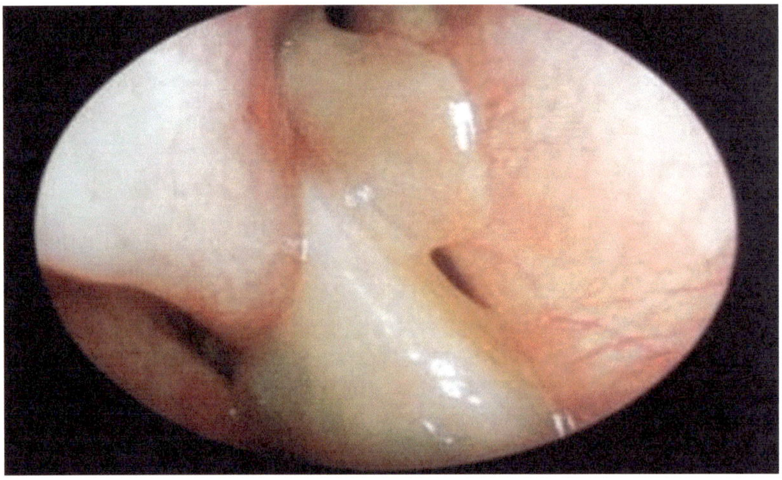

Fig. 1. Nasal Polyps

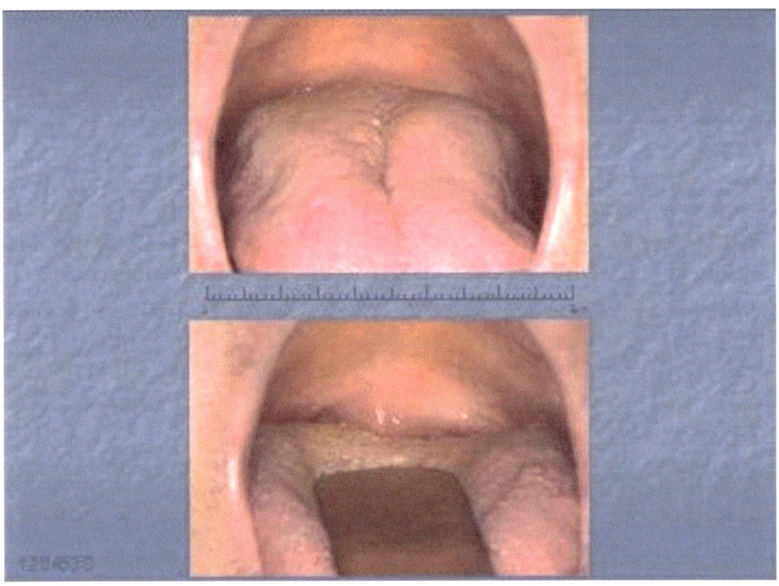

Fig. 2. Friedman tongue position 3

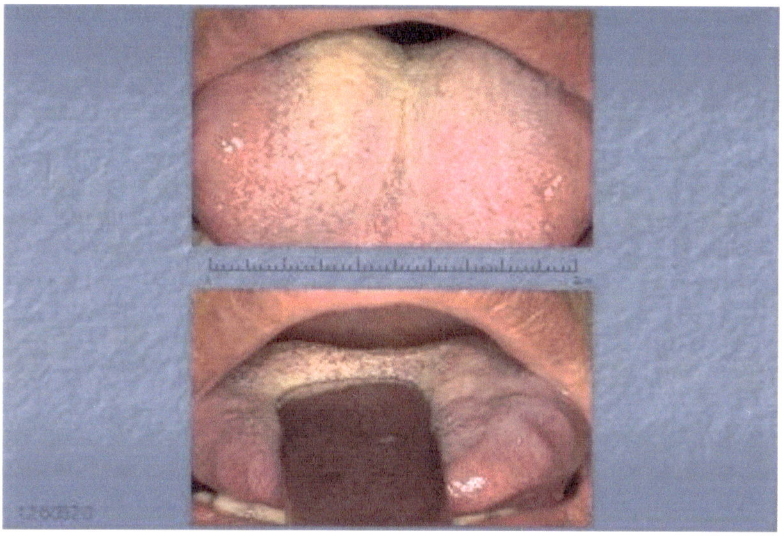

Fig. 3. Friedman tongue position 4

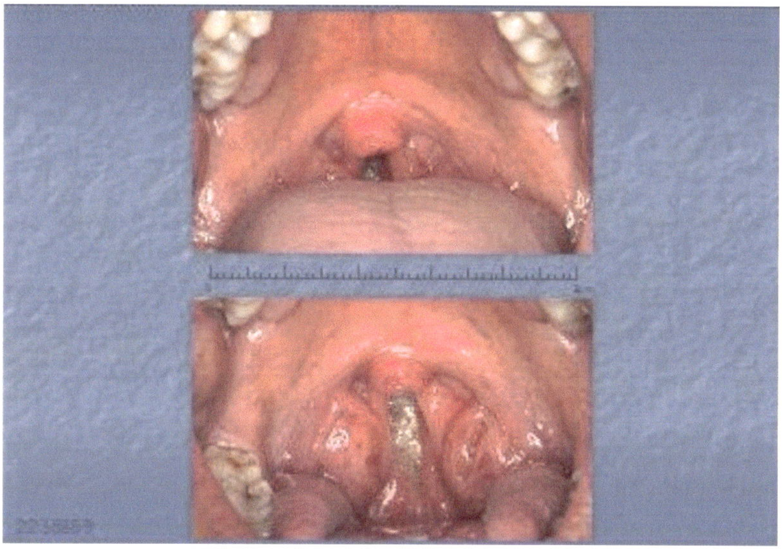

Fig. 4. Friedman tongue position 1

Probably the most useful equipment in assessing the upper airway is the flexible fibreoptic nasopharyngoscope which is widely available and allows brilliant visualisation of all aspects of the naso, oro and hypopharynx. Local anaesthesia in the form of a nasal spray can be used in allowing an easier and tolerable insertion of the scope and the different segments of the pharynx are carefully assessed. The patient could be asked to simulate a snoring sound to try and ascertain the level responsible for causing the turbulent airflow resulting in the snoring sound. Herzog[3] has reported a study based on simulating snoring sound in order to establish a model of grading upper airway obstruction. However, not all patients can simulate snoring and some may do this with mouth open or closed and these patients are usually sitting up whilst during sleep patients may be supine, prone or in lateral positions. In any case the fact that the muscle tone variation in sleep and wakefulness must also be borne in mind. Another commonly used technique during the flexible endoscopic assessment is the Mullers[4] manoeuvre. This essentially is a reversed Valsalva procedure which some patients do find difficult to perform. Furthermore, there is subjective variation in the assessment of the degree of collapse noted in different segments of the pharynx and thus the reliability of this technique may be questioned.

3. Imaging

Xrays of the maxilla and mandible in the form of cephalometry[5] may provide useful data of various parameters and dimensions controlling the upper airway. This can be particularly useful when the patient is being considered for invasive surgery such as maxillo-mandibular advancement or indeed when considering patients for MAS, though for the latter it is presently used for research purposes only. The limitation of this evaluation technique is that it provides a two dimensional image and that so during wakefulness. It also exposes the patient to considerable amount of radiation.

In contrast, computed tomography (CT) scanning and magnetic resonance imaging (MRI) provide more sophisticated imaging and allows objective cross sectional area and volumetric analysis. [6, 7] They are both more expensive than the cephalometry and the CT scans would also involve radiation. The MRI is quite noisy but is excellent at delineating soft tissue margins as well as fat deposition in the parapharyngeal space. For research reasons cine CT and dynamic MRI studies have been conducted to evaluate the upper airway but it is not considered to be practical or cost effective for routine use.

4. Acoustic analysis

This form of evaluation is safe in that there is no radiation involved and it is relatively cheap. It can be performed easily during sleep and at patient's home and simultaneously with polysomnography. Multiple night recordings can be carried out and based on sound frequency spectrum, acoustic analysis can potentially discern simple snoring from OSA.[8] Attempts have been made to correlate snoring sound frequency with different levels of obstruction and comparisons of this technique have been made to others such as drug induced sedation endoscopy.[9]

The sensitivity and specificity of this technique has often been questioned and although it can provide useful screening process, its role in helping with selecting treatment modalities is somewhat limited.[10] The other problems in studies with acoustic analysis are that of variation of software and the choice of central or fundamental frequency in determining the site of obstruction.

5. Pressure transducers

Numerous devices have been described which can measure pressure changes in different segments of the upper airway during an obstructive episode. Different numbers of transducers can be used to measure pressures at different levels of upper aerodigestive tract ranging from the nasopharynx to the oesophagus. The transducers are attached to a catheter which is introduced though the nose in a similar fashion to a nasogastric tube. This device can be left *in-situ* during sleep thus allowing an overnight recording.

One of the more recent devices illustrated in figures 5 and 6 and known as Apnea-Graph AG200 (MRA, Medical UK) seems quite promising in that it is capable of combining polysomnography data with pressure recording thus providing the clinician with information regarding the severity of OSA as well as giving some idea regarding the anatomical obstructive segment in the individual patient. Essentially, it relies on measuring pressure and airflow simultaneously at different levels in the pharynx. It stores and analyses the cardio-respiratory data of a patient with simultaneous recording of two different sites in the upper airway using a micro-pressure and temperature transducer catheter. Tvinnereim[11] *et* al published an encouraging study illustrating the importance of using this pressure catheter evaluation before embarking on surgical treatment. Singh[12] *et* al also demonstrated some usefulness of this technique, though they had some reservations about the ability of this device to accurately detect hypopharyngeal obstruction. They compared the Apnea-Graph to polysomnography. In addition they assessed correlation in some of these patients pharyngeal obstruction data to that seen whilst performing drug induced sleep endoscopy (DISE) and concluded the latter to be superior as it allowed visualisation of the upper airway and was also more useful in indentifying lateral wall collapse. They also commented that in their group of patients, some found it difficult to tolerate the catheter for the whole night and stressed that as the catheter moves during respiration the transducers would also move thus the accuracy of the levels identified could be questioned. Another point to note is that this device has fixed transducers on a catheter and has a fixed reference transducer and does not take in to account that all patients are morphologically different and therefore the positioning will not be identical in all patients.

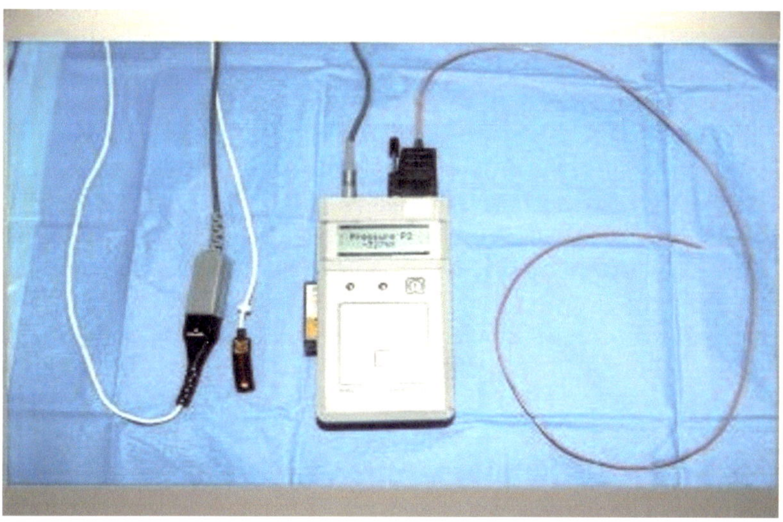

Fig. 5. The Apnea-Graph device with its components: a pulsoximeter and the fine bore nasal catheter with four transducers

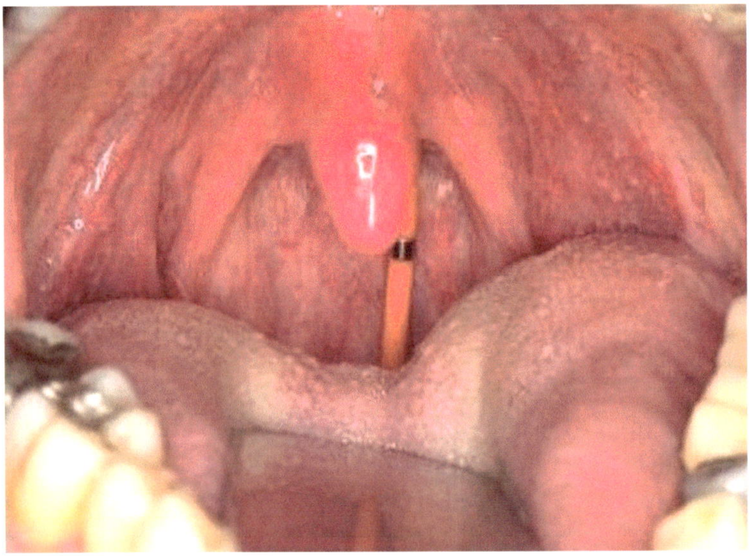

Fig. 6. Silver 'reference' marker indicating the correct position of the Apnea-Graph catheter

6. Sleep nasendoscopy

Sleep nasendoscopy (SNE) which is also known as drug induced sedation endoscopy (DISE) was pioneered at our institute.[13] The beauty of this technique lies in the fact that it allows a three dimensional visualisation of the upper airway during sleep albeit drug induced. This assessment is carried out in an operating theatre setting with the help of an anaesthetist who provides sedation to the patient and closely monitors the patients cardiovascular and respiratory parameters. The sedative agents commonly used are midazolam or propofol, however in some units both the drugs are used.

Drug induced sleep is different from natural physiological sleep but one could argue that the drug used for sedation has the same effect on the different segments of the pharynx thus it would allow us to compare the proportionate obstruction caused at each anatomical level in a similar manner that may exist in natural sleep.

An audit of 2,485 procedures performed over a period of 10 years at our institute has demonstrated that SNE correlates well with apnoea-hypopnoea index and mean oxygen desaturation.[14] We have also demonstrated the usefulness of SNE in predicting treatment success in snorers using MAS.[15,16] Similarly, SNE has allowed site specific target selection in surgical patients and improved surgical outcomes in our group of patients undergoing laser assisted palatoplasty with or without tonsillectomy has been reported.[17-19]

Sleep nasendoscopy assessment of snoring is useful as it provides evaluation of the upper airway in the dynamic mode during sleep. However, numerous controversies and debates have arisen and attempts have been made to address some of these by various authors.

For instance, criticisms made by Marais[20], whilst comparing snorers and non-snorers, it was claimed that snoring was produced during SNE in a large number of the non-snorers and was not produced in many of the snorers. This was challenged by Berry *et* al[21], demonstrating in their study using target controlled infusion of propofol during SNE that all their snorers and non-snorers responded as expected.

Similarly, questions and concerns that arose about test-retest reliability and of inter-rater reliability of SNE have been elegantly addressed by studies conducted by Rodriguez-Bruno *et* al[22] and Kezirian *et* al[23] respectively.

Bispectral index monitoring (BIS) has provided an adjunct to the assessment of sleep nasendoscopy in determining the level of sedation required for snoring assessment.[24] BIS (figs. 7 & 8) monitor is a neurophysiological monitoring device which continually analyses a patient's electroencephalogram during sedation and general anaesthesia to assess the level of consciousness and depth of anaesthesia.

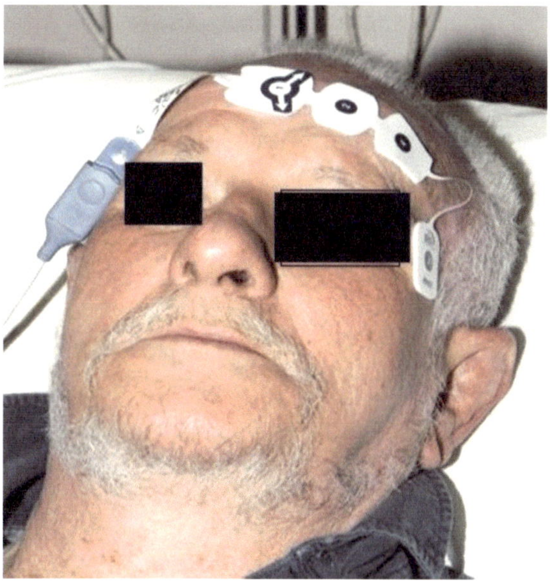

Fig. 7. Four sensor BIS electrode attached on patient's forehead

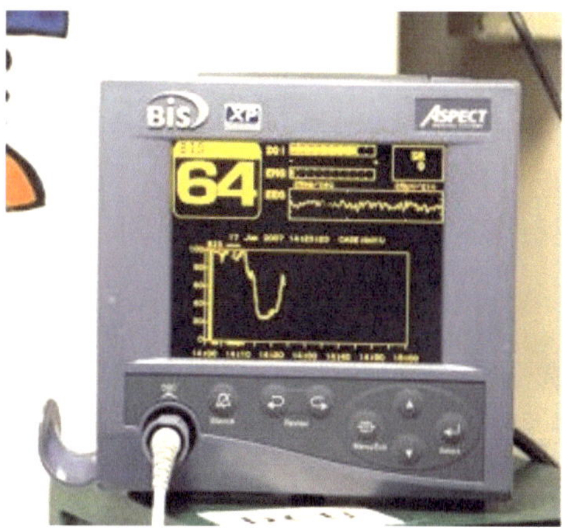

Fig. 8. BIS Monitor reading during Sleep Nasendoscopy

The issue of assessing the patient at the correct moment has not previously been addressed and this indeed is an important point as one has to bear in mind the pharmacology and the pharmacokinetics of the different drugs used during sedation. If the patient is assessed too early, the muscle relaxation effect of the drug may be over emphasised and if the patient is assessed too late then important anatomical aspect of the obstructive episodes may be missed. Thus the depth of sedation during which the assessment is conducted should be as close to the levels of depth of natural sleep. Evaluation only occurs as a snap shot of a patients whole sleep cycle. However, combining it with BIS values of patients undergoing natural sleep allows a more accurate assessment of sleep disordered breathing.

Finally, a couple of studies have compared awake assessment with SNE in the same group of patients and advocate that SNE is superior; further highlighting the point that there is muscle tone variation in control of upper airway during wakefulness and that during obstructive episodes in sleep. It appeared that hypopharyngeal or laryngeal obstruction could be missed in up to a third of the patients if the assessment was carried out in the awake state only.[25, 26]

7. Summary

In order to attain a successful outcome in treating patients with obstructive upper airway in snorers and OSA it is crucial to evaluate the upper airway dynamics very carefully. Apart from its usefulness in research, imaging has a relatively minor role to play in evaluation except in maxillo-mandibular advancement surgery.

Site specific treatment in these patients is required and therefore techniques that offer localisation of these anatomical obstructive segments would prove useful. In the author's opinion the two techniques that appear to do so are sleep nasendoscopy and the Apnea-Graph. This view has also been supported by a recent evidence based review article on assessment of obstruction level and selection of patients for obstructive sleep apnoea surgery.[27]

Sleep nasendoscopy appears somewhat superior as it allows visualisation of the upper airway whereas the Apnea-Graph merely looks at the pressure values and relies on correct positioning of the transducers. Out-patient clinical examination of the nose and the oropharynx is of paramount importance as it will help identifying potential nCPAP patients who may fail this form of therapy if there is an obvious anatomical problem.

8. References

[1] Friedman M, Ibrahim H, Bass L. Clinical staging for sleep-disordered breathing. Otolaryngol Head Neck Surg 2002; 127:13-21.

[2] Mallampati SR, Gatt SP, Gugino LD, Desai SP, Waraksa B, Freiberger D et al. A clinical sign to predict difficult tracheal intubation: A prospective study. Can Anaesth Soc J 1985; 32(4):429-434.

[3] Herzog M, Metz T, Schmidt A, et al. The prognostic value of simulated snoring in awake patients with sleep-disordered breathing: introduction of a new technique examination. Sleep 2006;29:1456-62.

[4] Ritter CT, Trudo FJ, Goldberg AN et al. Quantitative evaluation of the upper airway during nasopharyngoscopy with the Muller manoeuvre. Laryngoscope 1999;109:954-63.

[5] Mayer G, Meier-Ewert K. Cepahlometric predictors for orthopaedic mandibular advancement in obstructive sleep apnoea. Eur J Orthod1995;17:35-43

[6] Sheperd JW Jr, Stanson AW, Sheedy PF, et al. Fast-CT evaluation of the upper airway during wakefulness in patients with obstructive sleep apnoea. Prog Clin Biol Res 1990;345:273-9.

[7] Schwab RJ, Gefter WB, Hoffman EA, et al. Dynamic upper airway imaging during awake respiration in normal subjects and patients with sleep disordered breathing. Am Rev Respir Dis 1993;148:1385-400.

[8] Hara H, Murakami N, Miyauchi Y, Yamashita H. Acoustic analysis of snoring sounds by a multidimensional voice program. Laryngoscope 2006;116:379-81

[9] Saunders NC, Tassone P, Wood G, Norris A, Harries M, Kotecha B. Is acoustic analysis of snoring an alternative to sleep nasendoscopy? Clinical Otolaryngology Allied Sci 2004;29:242-6.

[10] Brietzke SE, Mair EA. Acoustic analysis of snoring: can the probability of success be predicted? Otolaryngol Head Neck Surg 2006;135:417-20.

[11] Tvinnereim M, Mitic S, Hansen RK. Plasmaradiofrequency preceded by pressure recording enhances success for treating sleep-related breathing disorders. Laryngoscope 2007;117:731-6.

[12] Singh A, Al-Reefy H, Hewitt R, Kotecha B. Evaluation of Apnea-Graph in the diagnosis of sleep-related breathing disorders. Eur Arch Otorhinolaryngol 2008;265:1489-94.

[13] Croft CB, Pringle M. Sleep nasendoscopy: a technique of assessment in snoring and obstructive sleep apnoea. Clin Otolaryngol 1991;16:504-509.

[14] Kotecha BT, Hannan AS, Khalil HMB, Georgalas C, Bailey P. Sleep nasendoscopy: a 10-year retrospective audit study. Eur Arch Otorhinoloaryngol 2007;264:1361-1367.

[15] Battagel J, Johal A, Kotecha BT. Sleep nasendoscopy as a predictor of treatment success in snorers using mandibular advancement splints. J Laryngol Otol 2005;119:106-112.

[16] Johal A, Hector MP, Battagel J, Kotecha B. Impact of sleep nasendoscopy on the outcome of mandibular advancement splint therapy in subjects with sleep-related breathing disorders. J Laryngol Otol 2007;121:668-75

[17] Kotecha B, Paun S, Leong P, Croft C. Laser assisted uvulopalatoplasty: an objective evaluation of the technique and results. Clin Otolaryngol 1998; 23: 354-359.

[18] Iyangkaran T, Kanaglingam J, Rajeswaran R, Georgalas C, Kotecha B. Long-term outcomes of laser-assisted uvulopalatoplasty in 168 patients with snoring. J Laryngol Otol 2006;120:932-8.

[19] Chisholm E, Kotecha B. Oropharyngeal surgery for obstructive sleep apnoea in cPAP failures. Eur Arch Otorhinolaryngol 2007;264:1361-1367.

[20] Marais J. The value of sedation nasendoscopy: a comparison between snoring and non-snoring patients. Clin Otolaryngol Allied Sci 1998;23:74-76.

[21] Berry S, Robin G, Williams A, Watkins A, Whittet HB. Validity of sleep nasendoscopy in the investigation of sleep related breathing disorders. Laryngoscope 2005;115:538-540.

[22] Rodriguez-Bruno K, Goldberg AN, McCulloch CE, Kezirian EJ. Test-retest reliability of drug-induced sleep endoscopy. Otolaryngology-Head and Neck Surgery 2009;140: 646-651.

[23] Kezirian EJ, White DP, Malhotra A, Ma W, McCulloch CE, Goldberg A (2010) Interrater reliability of drug-induced sleep endoscopy. Arch Otolaryngol Head and Neck Surgery 2010;Vol 136(No. 4): 393-397.

[24] Babar-Craig H, Rajani N, Bailey P, Kotecha B. Validation of sleep nasendoscopy for assessment of snoring with BIS monitoring, Clin Otolaryngol Allied Sci 2009;34: (Supp) 89-90.
[25] Hewitt RJD, Dasgupta A, Singh A, Dutta C, Kotecha B. Is sleep nasendoscopy a valuable adjunct to clinical examination in the evaluation of upper airway obstruction? Eur Arch Otorhinolaryngol 2009;266:691-697.
[26] Campanini A, Canzi P, De Vito A, Dallan I, Montevecchi F. Vicini C. Awake versus sleep endoscopy: personal experience in 250 OSAHS patients. Acta Otorhinolaryngologica Italica 2010;30:73-77.
[27] Georgalas C, Garas G, Hadjihannas E, Oostra A (2010) Assessment of obstruction level and selection of patients for obstructive sleep apnoea surgery: an evidence based approach. J Laryngol Otol 2010;124: 1-9.

6

Upper Airway Resistance Syndrome – A Twenty-Five Years Experience

Felix del Campo Matías[1], Tomas Ruiz Albi[2] and Carlos Zamarrón Sanz[3]

[1]*Division of Respiratory Medicine, Hospital Universitario Rio Hortega, Departament of Medicine, Universidad de Valladolid, Valladolid*

[2]*Division of Respiratory Medicine, Hospital Universitario Rio Hortega, Valladolid,*

[3]*Division of Respiratory Medicine Hospital Clínico Universitario de Santiago de Compostela, Santiago de Compostela, Spain*

1. Introduction

This paper will review the prevalence, pathophysiology, clinical picture, diagnostic advances, natural history, morbidity and management of upper airway resistance syndrome (UARS). The aim is to improve our knowledge about this disease and help to identify patients with UARS.

2. Background

UARS was initially used to describe a group of patients who were sleepy but did not meet the polysomnography diagnostic criteria of obstructive sleep apnoea syndrome (OSAS) (Guilleminault 1993). The first mention of the term was used about children by Guilleminault (Guilleminault 1982) in 1982 and years later also in women (Guilleminault 1995). Is UARS really a disease?. Twenty-five years after first being described, there is still significant controversy among experts as to whether UARS is a specific syndrome.

Some authors consider it to be part of the spectrum of obstructive disorders affecting the upper airway (Douglas 2000; Jhonson 2008; Cracowski 2001), while others believe that OSAS and UARS are separate entities (Gold 2008; Bao & Guilleminault 2004;Lindberg & Gislason 2000).

Normally, it is up to the clinician practitioner to screen for this syndrome. Due to its diagnostic difficulty, currently UARS is significantly under diagnosed and no standard management strategy in place in sleep labs. However, great interest exists in the literature for this entity, and many revisions have been carried out (Exar & Collop 1999; Monserrat & Badia 1999; Bao & Guilleminault 2004; Velamuri 2006; Ramar & Guilleminault 2008; Giblin 2009; Guilleminault & de los Reyes 2011).

3. Epidemiology

Epidemiologic studies estimate that SAHS affects 1-5% of adult men in western countries (Young 2002). Sleep apnoea hypopnoea syndrome is the most common form of sleep disordered-breathing. Limited data is available on the prevalence of UARS in the general population in both children and adults. Some authors consider it an uncommon disease in clinical practice. In earlier descriptions, the estimated prevalence was 6% in men and 11% in women (Votteri 1994; Guilleminault 1995). Kristo found a prevalence of 8.4% in a one year polysomnography review (Kristo 2005). In an epidemiological study conducted in Brazil, the prevalence of UARS was 18.7%, being more common in women and young people (Tufik 2009).

4. Pathophysiology

The upper airway is a very complex structure. In SAHS patients, apneas during sleep are caused by upper airway obstruction, wich leads to progressive asphyxia and awakening. The inspiratory efforts to overcome occlusion lead to arousal, sleep fragmentation, and oxyhemoglobin desaturation. From a physiological standpoint, both UARS and OSAS present intermittent upper airway collapse. This increase in upper airway resistance occasionally accompanies airflow limitation and arousals, with little desaturation. Johnson, found that even minimal airflow limitation could produce arousals that occur before alterations in gas exchange (Johnson 2005). These episodes are of short duration, about four breaths, and present negative intrathoracic pressure increases.

Another interesting difference from OSAS is that UARS patients do not present neuropathological lesions in the upper airway (Friberg 1998; Guilleminault 2002a; Boyd 2004), which could explain why these patients tend to respond more rapidly to treatment and do not develop OSAS over the long-term. Early studies did not seem to reveal differences in sleep architecture between UARS and OSAS (Loube & Andrada 1999). However, today UARS patients are considered to have unstable sleep, characterized by a cyclic alternating pattern in nonREM sleep (Guilleminault 2005a), which predisposes to the occurrence of arousals. These findings correlate with symptoms such as tiredness and fatigue, for which these patients are often referred to sleep labs. The cyclic alternating pattern has been described in many other situations (Ferré 2006), such as fibromyalgia, chronic fatigue syndrome, and OSAS (Terzano 1996). Current research suggests that nearly 50% of fibromialgia syndrome patients experience intrusive alpha wave periods. Patients with UARS present an increase in the number of cyclic alternating patterns, with a decreased phase 1 and an increased phase A2 and A3 (Guilleminault 2005c) In recent years, polysomnography has revealed that UARS patients present nonREM-sleep instability. Alpha-delta sleep is characterized by an intrusion of alpha EEG waves into slow delta waves during deep sleep, which also occurs in insomnia and non-refreshing sleep (Guilleminault 2001a).

5. Symptoms

Although OSAS and UARS share common symptoms, in most cases the clinical manifestations are different (Stoohs 2008). The most common symptoms of SAHS patients include chronic loud snoring, excessive daytime sleepiness, personality changes, depression and deterioration of quality of life (Pichel 2004). Hypersomnolence is the principal daytime manifestation of sleep disordered breathing. Excessive sleepiness resulting from increased breathing effort and sleep disruption is the guide symptom of UARS patients (Guilleminault 1993, 2001a). Drowsiness related to general exhaustion has a negative impact on quality of life. As in OSAS, snoring is a common symptom, predominantly in males, although the absence of snoring has also been described in this syndrome, the so-called silent UARS (Kristo 2005). In recent years, several studies have demonstrated strong associations between UARS and functional somatic syndromes, such as chronic fatigue syndrome, chronic insomnia, chronic pain, irritable bowel syndrome, fibromyalgia, depression, parasomnias and posttraumatic stress disorders (Gold 2003, 2011). Due to its association with chronic somatic diseases, UARS has been postulated to activate the hypothalamic-pituitary-adrenal axis (HPA) (Gold 2010), although not all studies support the association of sleep disordered breathing with these somatic functional disorders. (Vgontzas & Fernandez-Mendoza 2011, Trakada 2007).

A number of studies compare the clinical characteristics of UARS patients to those of SAHS subjects. Patients with UARS are usually younger than those with SAHS and have a lower level of obesity. There is no major difference in terms of gender prevalence, although UARS appears to be more frequent in postmenopausal women. An overall ratio of prevalence for men to women of 3.3 has been reported in SAHS patients (Bixler 2001).

UARS patients report both onset and maintenance insomnia (Guilleminault 2002b). A state of physiologic hyperarousal in UARS patients with chronic insomnia is accepted (Gold 2008). Some authors have reported complex insomnia, which paradoxically involves nighttime insomnia and daytime sleepiness (Krakov 2001; Gold 2008). This type of insomnia has been associated with parasomnias (Guilleminault 2006a), which mainly occur in young patients together with sleepwalking and night terrors. Insomnia is more common in UARS than in OSAS.

Powers (Powers 2009) found a tendency to hypersomnia in UARS patients. These patients showed altered results on the maintenance of wakefulness test that were not correlated with the Epworth scale. This author considered non-obese premenopausal women, who often consult for chronic insomnia and parasomnias, to represent a specific attention group.

Approximately half of UARS patients present symptoms of increased vagal tone such as orthostatic hypotension and coldness of the extremities (Guilleminault 2001b). Disturbances in heart rate variability have also been reported along with a decrease in the HF component (associated with increased vagal tone). In contrast, OSAS patients have an increase in the LF/HF ratio, associated with increased activity sympathetic. (Guilleminault 2005).

SAHS is widely associated with cardiovascular risk. Long-term effects can lead to severe cardiovascular and cerebrovascular diseases. However, there is little data regarding the association of cardiovascular disease and UARS. Some studies have found an association between hypertension and UARS, with a good response to CPAP treatment (Guilleminault 1996), but this association has been put into question. Notably, this controversy sheds light on the importance of hypoxia and sympathetic activation (which are not present in UARS) in OSAS as intermediary mechanisms associated with cardiovascular events.

The diagnosis of UARS is often delayed becasue of the absence of respiratory events in polysomnography. Sometimes the symptoms of UARS have been confused with other medical conditions, such as asymptomatic habitual snoring, sleep deprivation, chronic fatigue syndrome, idiopathic hypersomnia, psychiatric disorders (Lewin & Pinto 2004) and asthma (Guerrero 2001).

Some authors report a greater likelihood of traffic accidents in UARS patients (Stoohs 1994). Among drowsy drivers, UARS is associated to a higher frequency of accidents. Thus, identification of this syndrome is of great practical importance.

6. Physical examination

UARS patients differ anthropometrically from patients with SAHS. They are generally thin, young, and predominantly female. The recommended physical examination is similar to that for OSAS patients. As in OSAS, craniofacial abnormalities such as elongated face and reduced mouth opening are frequent. Guilleminault described an increase in nasal resistance, excessive pharyngeal tissue, mild retrognathia, narrowing of the oropharynx and ogival hard palate (Guillemianult 1995), with high scores on the Mallampati scale.

7. Diagnosis

UARS is defined as daytime sleepiness associated to a sleep disordered breathing and arousals related to respiratory effort (RERA) but without sufficient apneas/hypopneas for OSAS. The diagnosis is based on the association of clinical symptoms and polysomnographic findings.

Nocturnal polysomnography, which is the gold standard for diagnosing SAHS, sometimes demonstrates the presence of apneic events and non apneic breathing (hypopneas), but does not definitively diagnose UARS. Nevertheless, an increased number of RERA may lead to suspicion of UARS. Simplified polygraphic studies are not useful in this disease because they do not provide arousal information. Some laboratories have used the split-night technique followed by CPAP titration successfully. These situations require an index of over 20 RERA during the first three hours of sleep (Kristo 2009).

The continuous recording of esophageal pressure throughout the night is the gold standard for the diagnosis of UARS (Kushida 2002; Iber 2007). Esophageal manometry is a complex technique which may be affected by the placement of the probe and the position of the catheter. Moreover, it is time-comsuming, may affect patient's sleep, and is not widely available (Johnson 2008). The correct positioning of the esophageal catheter requires a lot of experience and clinical practice. The use of a small catheter has improved tolerance of the procedure. The analysis of esophageal pressure can be quantitative or qualitative, though the latter approach is more common in clinical practice (Watanabae 2000). Gold et als used the critical pressure criteria to differentiate between SAHS and UARS patients [Gold 2002].

The esophageal pressure reading may present three different patterns: a crescendo pattern that ends in arousal without achieving 3% desaturation, continuous sustained effort for at least four breaths, and finally an abrupt drop in respiratory effort indicated by a less negative peak inspiratory pressure after a sequence of increased respiratory efforts independent of the EEG patterns (Pes reversal).

Although esophageal manometry is indicated mainly for the diagnosis of UARS has also demonstrated its usefulness in studying the Cheyne-Stokes syndrome as it allows to differentiate obstructive from central apneas. However, it is a laborious technique, disruptive for patients and normal values remain to be established. The utility in the clinic is unclear and have been confined its use to research.

Indeed, the presence of RERA in the absence of apneas and hypopneas is the key polysomnography finding for diagnosing UARS (Bonnet 2007). However, the difficulty of registering respiratory effort has prompted the search for other non-invasive methods that can provide similar information (Hosselet 1998; Loube 1999; Badia 2001; Mosler 2002; Kenach 2005; Popovic 2009)(Table 1). Most systems try to develop a reliable non-invasive tecnique for respiratory effort and upper airway resistance that could represent a non-invasive alternative to esophageal pressure measurement. Of these, the most widely used and accepted by the American Academy of Sleep Medicine are nasal pressure cannulas, inductance plethysmography or diaphragmatic/intercostal EMG. The nasal cannula is the tool of choice for monitoring respiratory airflow during sleep in both clinical and research sleep studies. Nasal cannula is more sensitive than thermistor for detecting RERA The use of new technologies such as pressure probes have made it possible to identify signs of UARS in patients with high levels of arousal and airflow limitation (Krakow 2001).

The diagnostic criteria for UARS have not been established. At present, the diagnostic polysomnography of UARS is based on careful analysis of the esophageal pressure reading and nasal cannula (Guilleminault 1995, 2001; Black 2000), together with an AHI under 5 and the presence of desaturation of no more than 92%. Visual identification of intermitent flow limitation is cumbersome, subjective and trought with variability and potential error. Some authors recommend determining the length of airflow limitation episodes as well as the total percentage of airflow limitation with respect to total sleep time. Termination of flow limitation was indicated either by respiratory events related to arousal or with essofageal pressure reversal (Guilleminault 1995; 2001) without alpha EEG arousal (Guilleminault 2005b). In UARS patients these episodes of airflow limitation that is not accompanied by desaturation, are of varying lengths, and are not always associated with an increase in esophageal pressure. The coincidence of EEG arousals and Pes events is well documented. A percentage of Pes events terminate without coincident EEG activity. However, Guilleminault describes that, in patients with UARS, apnoeas accompanied by arousals have a greater tachycardic effect, even if there is only a small reduction in blood oxygen saturation (Guilleminault 2005). The shape of the inspiratory flow contour has been proposed as a noninvasive predictor of increased upper airway obstruction, increasing the potential for erroneous classification of respiratorye events (Hosselet 1998; Rees 2000; Ayyapa & Rapoport 2003). Various definitions of airflow limitation exist (Norman 2007; Mansour 2004; Kaplan 2000;Aittokallio 2001)(Table 2).

RERA is the most important event in UARS patients. In early studies, the definition of UARS included the presence of frequent arousals, indicating an RERA index >10/h as a diagnostic criteria. Owing to their relation, treating RERA tends to improve excessive daytime sleepiness. This index was established as a treatment criterion. UARS has not found its way into the International Classification of Sleep Disorders Diagnostic and Coding Manual, which is one of the main problems for the acceptance of UARS as a specific entity (AASM 1999; Iber 2007). RERA has been accepted by the American Academy of Sleep Medicine Task Force (AASM, 1999) but it has yet to be standardized. According to the AASM and a number of authors (Cracowski 2001), RERA episodes are rare and their encoding need not be mandatory. However, others consider it to be a key element, with an identifiable pathophysiology. RERAs have been incorporated into normal clinical practice, and the respiratory disturbance index used to quantify OSAS severity takes them into account together with apneas, and hypopneas.

- Pneumotachygraphy
- Nasal cannula pressure
- EMG signals
- Resistive Inductance Plethismography
- Pulse Transit Time
- Neural network
- Forced oscillation technique
- Suprasternal pressure transducer
- Presence ofalteringcyclicpattern(EEG)
- Forehead venous pressure signal
- Snore signals

Table 1. Techniques to assess respiratory effort.

Periods of high esophageal pressure swings with associated inspiratory flow limitation
Lack of increase in airflow despite increasing respiratory effort.
Flattening of the normal bell-shaped curve of normal breath with a drop in the amplitude of the curve by 2–29% compared to the normal breaths immediately preceding
Abnormal inspiratory air flow shape during partialupper airway obstruction
Abnormal contour in the nasal/presure transducer signal waveform
Presence of an inspiratory plateau or reduction in inspiratory flow independent of any increase in inspiratory efforts.
Pressure waveflattening<30% is associated with a physiological event (arousal, CAP complex, variabilidad RR, etc)
Two or more breaths (10 sec) without sinusoidal appearance and without hypopnea criteria, end abruptly, taking on the sinuidal flow aspect
At least four successive breaths reduction in amplitude simultaneously with the development of an inspiratory plateau (loss of a sinusoidal inspiratory waveform)

Table 2. Inspiratory flow limitation: Definitions.

From the standpoint of polysomnography in recent years has gained great interest to consider these patients have instability in their sleep nonREM. OSAS and UARS patients have different brain activity during sleep. Thus, in patients with UARS have described alterations in sleep architecture, such as sleep fragmentation, consequent to the presence of respiratory arousals, the presence of an alpha-delta pattern, characteristic modifications in the EEG spectral analysis and the existence of an increase of cyclic alternating pattern. Alpha-delta sleep is characterized by an intrusion of alpha EEG waves into slow delta waves during deep sleep, which also occurs in insomnia and non-refreshing sleep. It appears that cyclic alternating pattern could be a valid indicator for the persistence of some degree of sleep disturbance and instability of NREM sleep. With respect to the EEG spectral analysis in patients with UARS have less activity in slow wave sleep (delta) and a higher prevalence in the range of 7-9 Hz consequent to a different cortical activity. The development of slow wave sleep is also abnormal, with persistence of a large number of "power delta" at the end of sleep cycles. Both abnormalities may explain the symptoms of daytime sleepiness, insomnia and fatigue in patients with UARS (Guilleminault 2001a).Black et als found that visually undetectable EEG alterations may occur during breathing disturbances in the absence of arousal (Black 2000).

8. Follow up

Te long time evolution of UARS patients, within the overall spectrum of sleep disordered breathing disorders, is an area of interest. RERA may be intermediate event between snoring and hypopnea. RERA predominate in younger and thinner people than apnea and hypopnea episodes. Hypopneas becoming true apneas with increasing age and weight. Few existing studies on the matter. In a five years follow-up study of untreated UARS patients, Guilleminault report that only 10% developed a OSAS and always in the context of weight gain (Guilleminault 2006b). Jonzak, in a retrospective study,also report that obesity as an aggravating factor of severity in follow up six years (Jonzak 2009).

9. Treatment

Treatment options for UARS include lifestyle changes, Continous Positive Airway Pressure (CPAP), oral appliance therapy and surgery. All patients with UARS should be counseled about the potential benefits of therapy and the risks of going without therapy.
Obesity is a modifiable risk factor associated with OSAS so weight loss should be recommended to all overweight or obese. However, patients with UARS are often not obese, so this recommendation has less value in them. As in the treatment of OSAS, within conservative measures are recommended sleep hygiene and avoiding the supine position. Just like in OSA is advisable to multidisciplinary treatment.
Continous positive airway pressure (CPAP) is the treatment of choice for SAHS patients. CPAP was the gold standard for UARS. Initial studies described a good response to CPAP treatment which was considered to be a diagnostic criteria for the syndrome (Messner & Pelayo 2000; Guerrero 2001; Guilleminault 2006). As in mild to moderate OSAS, CPAP compliance and adherence are low. Regarding CPAP titration, it is recommend a similar protocol that for OSAS.After reaching the optimal CPAP, the esophageal peak pressure at the end of inspiration must be higher than-7 cm H_2O or the RERA index <10. If this is not achievable, CPAP may be applied at an empirical pressure level of between 8 and 10 cm of

H2O (Kristo 2009). CPAP ususally improves symptomatology and parasomnias. Some reports exist of worsening after CPAP treatment.

No studies exist about the usefulness of positional treatment or electrical stimulation of the muscles of the upper airway in patients with UARS. With respect to drug treatment, as with OSAS, the evidence on the usefulness of pharmacological treatment in UARS is scarce.

Given the poor adherence to CPAP treatment, oral devices may be a good alternative for UARS, although little research has been published (Loube 1998; Guerrero 2001; Yoshida 2002; Rose 2000). Predictable efficacy of oral appliances treatments has yet to be demonstrated.

Surgical option include laser-assisted uvulopalatoplasty,uvulectomy, snoreplasty injection, radiofrequency submucosal needle therapy and somnoplasty (Newman1996; Powell 1998; Newman 2002; Pirelli 2004). Existing data on treatment of UARS are scarce, which together with the difficulty of diagnosis makes it a priority disease research in the future.

10. Conclusions

Despite the time elapsed since its initial description, UARS remains controversial as it has yet to be accepted as its own entity. However, the literature continues to reflect interest in this disorder. Perhaps SAHS and UARS share the same pathophysiological mechanism, although their clinical expression and pathophysiologic consequences are different. We could say that UARS and OSAS are distinct entities in the spectrum of sleep-disordered breathing.

SAHS is one of the most common sleep disorders in clinical practice. It is associated to cardiovascular morbidity, and has become regarded as a public health problem. UARS is an underdiagnosed disorder with low prevalence of sleep units. It has special implications on sleep structure, especially sleepiness and tiredness, and is associated to chronic somatic diseases such as chronic fatigue syndrome, fibromialgia, irritable bowel syndrome, and tension headache. The correct diagnosis of this syndrome is essential to allow the best choice of therapy.

The identification of UARS, although not recognized by the AAMS as an entity, has improved our understanding of respiratory events and arousals, as well as increasing the search for non-invasively ways of assessing respiratory effort. Today, terms such as airflow limitation or RERAs are widely used in the polysomnographic reports.

11. References

Aittokallio T, Saaresranta T, Polo-Kantola P, Nevalainen O, Polo O. (2001).Analysis of inspiratory flow shapes inpatients with partial upper-airway obstruction during sleep. *Chest* 119:37-44

American Academy of Sleep Medicine Task Force Report. Sleep related breathing disorders in adults. Recommendations for síndrome definition and measurement techniques in clinical research. (1999). Sleep 22:667-689.

Argod J, Pepin JL, Smith RP, Levy P.(2000) Comparison of esophageal pressure with Pulse Transit Time as a measure of respiratory effort for scoring obstructive non apneic respiratory events. *Am J Respir Crit Care Med* 162: 87–93,

Ayappa I., Norman RG, Krieger AC, Rosen A, O'Malley RL. Rapoport DM. (2000) Non-invasive detection of Respiratory Effort-Related Arousals (RERAs) by a nasal cannula/pressure transducer system. *Sleep*, 23: 763-771

Ayyapa I, Rapoport DM (2003).The upper airway in sleep: physiology of the pharynx. Sleep Med Rev, 7, 9-33,

Bao G, Guilleminault C (2004) Upper airway resistance syndrome—one decade later. Curr Opin Pulm Med 10:461–467,

Badia JR, Farre R, Rigau J, Uribe ME, Navajas D, Montserrat JM. (2001) Forced oscillation measurements do not affect upper airway muscle tone or sleep in clinical studies. *Eur Respir J* 18:335–9.

Bixler EO, Vgontzas AN, Lin HM, Have TT, Rein J, Vela-Bueno A, Kales A. (2001) Prevalence of sleep disordered breathing in women. Effects of gender. *Am J Respir Crit Care Med* 163:608–613.

Black JD, Guilleminault CH, Colrain IM, Carrillo O (2000).Upper airway resistance syndrome. Central electroencephalographic power and changes in breathing effort. *Am J Respir Crit Care Med* 162:406-411.

Bonnet MH; Doghramji K; Roehrs T et al. (2007) The scoring of arousal in sleep: reliability, validity, and alternatives. *J Clin Sleep Med* 3:133-145

Boyd JH, Petrof BJ, Hamid Q et al.(2004) Upper airway muscle inflammation and denervation changes in obstructive sleep apnea. *Am J Respir Crit Care Med* 170:541–546

Cracowski C, Pepin JL, Wuyam B, Levy P. (2001) Characterization of obstructive nonapneic respiratory events in moderate sleep apnea syndrome. Am J Respir Crit Care Med 164: 944-948.

Douglas NJ. (2000). Upper airway resistance syndrome is not a distinct syndrome. Am J Respir Crit Care Med 161:1413–1416.

Exar EN, Collop N. (1999) The upper airway resistance síndrome *Chest* 115:1127-1139.

Ferré A, Guilleminault C, Lopes MC (2006) Cyclic alternating pattern as a sign of brain instability during sleep. *Neurologia.* 21:304-11

Friberg D, Gazelius B, Linblad LE et al. (1998). Habitual snorers and sleep apneics have abnormal vascular reaction of the soft palatal mucosa or afferent nerve stimulation.*Laryngoscope* 108: 431–436

Giblin, T. B (2009) Review of upper airway resistance syndrome: nursing and clinical management.*Journal of clinical nursing*, 18: 2486–2493

Gold AR, Marcus CL, Dipalo F, and Gold MS (2002). Upper Airway collapsibility during sleep in upper airway resistance syndrome. *Chest* 121;1531-1540

Gold AR, Dipalo F, Gold MS, O'Hearn D (2003) The symptoms and signs of Upper Airway Resistance Syndrome : A link to the Functional Somatic Syndromes. *Chest* 123:87-95

Gold AR, Gold MS, Harris KW et als. (2008) Hypersomnolence, insomnia and the pathophysiology of upper airway resistance síndrome *Sleep Med* 9:775-683.

Gold A. (2011) Functional somatic syndromes, anxiety disorders and the upper airway: a matter of paradigms. *Sleep Med Rev*, in press. Doi: 10.1016/j.smrv. 2010.11.004

Guerrero M, Lepler L & Kristo D (2001) The upper airway resistance syndrome masquerading as nocturnal asthma and successfully treated with an oral appliance. *Sleep breath* 5, 93–95.

Guilleminault C, Winkle R, Korobkin R, Simmons B (1982) Children and nocturnal snoring: evaluation of the effects of sleep related respiratory resistive load and daytime functioning. Eur J Pediatr.139(3):165-171.

Guilleminault C, Stoohs R, Clerk A et al. (1993). A cause of daytime sleepiness: the upper airway resistance syndrome. Chest 104: 781–787.

Guilleminault C, Stoohs R, Kim YD et al (1995). Upper airway sleep disordered breathing in women. Ann Intern Med 122: 493–501.

Guilleminault Ch, Stoohs R, Shiomi T, Kushida C, Schnittger I (1996). Upper airway resistance syndrome, nocturnal blood pressure monitoring, and borderline hypertension *Chest* 109:901-908

Guilleminault C, Kim YD, Chowdhuri S, Horita M, Ohayon M, Kushida C. (2001a) Sleep and daytime sleepiness in upper airway resistance síndrome compared to obstructive sleep apnea syndrome. *Eur Respir J* 17: 838-847

Guilleminault C, Faul JL, Stoohs R.(2001b) Sleep disordered breathing and hypotension. *Am J Respir Crit Care Med* 164: 1242-1247.

Guilleminault C, Li K, Chen NH et al. (2002a). Two-point palatal discrimination in patients with upper airway resistance syndrome, obstructive sleep apnea syndrome, andnormal control subjects. *Chest* 122: 866–870

Guilleminault C, Palombini L, Poyares D et al (2002b) Chronic insomnia, post-menopausal women, and SDB. Comparison of non-drug treatment trials in normal breathing and UARS post-menopausal women complaining of insomnia. *J Psychosomat Res* 53: 617–623

Guillemiault C, Poyares D, Rosa A, Huang YS. (2005) Heart rate variability, sympathetic and vagal balance and EEG arousals in upper airway resistance and mild obstructive sleep apnea syndromes. *Sleep Med.* 6:451-7

Guilleminault, C., Kirisoglu, C., Bao, G., Arias, V., Chan, A., & Li, K. (2005b). Adult chronic sleepwalking and its treatment based on polysomnography. *Brain,* 128: 1062-1069

Guilleminault C, Lee JH, Chan A (2005c). Pediatric obstructive sleep apnea syndrome. *Arch Pediatr Adolesc Med* 159: 775–785

Guilleminault C, Kirisoglu C, da Rosa AC, Lopes C, Chan A. (2006a) Sleepwalking, a disorder of NREM sleep instability. *Sleep Med.* 7:163-170.

Guilleminault C, Kirisoglu C, Poyares D et al.: (2006b). Upper airway resistance syndrome: a long-term outcome study. J Psychiatr Res; 40: 273–9.

Guilleminault C, Lopes MC, Hagen CC, da Rosa A (2007) The cyclic alternating pattern demonstrates increased sleep instability and correlates with fatigue and sleepiness in adults with upper airway resistance syndrome. *Sleep.* 30:641-7.

Guilleminault Ch, de los Reyes V (2011) Upper airway resistance syndrome. *Handb Clin Neurol* 98 :401-409

Hosselet J., Norman R., Ayappa A.,Rapoport D (1998). Detection of flow limitation with a nasal cannula/ pressure transducer system, *Am J Respir Crit Care Med* 157:1461-1467

Iber C., Anconi-Israel S., Chesson A. L., Qua S.F. (2007). The AASM Manual for the Scoring of Sleep and Associated Events, American Academy of Sleep Medicine, Westchester, IL.

Johnson PL, Edwards N, Burgess KR, Sullivan CE (2005) Detection of increased upper airway resistance during overnight polysomnography. Sleep 28:85-90

Jonczak, L., Pływaczewski, R., Sliwiński, P., Bednarek, M., Górecka, D., & Zieliński, J. (2009). Evolution of upper airway resistance syndrome *Journal of Sleep Research,* 18(3), 337–341

Jhonson NT. (2008). Whither the upper airway resistance syndrome? Sleep 31:14-15

Kaplan V, Zhang JN, Russi EW, Bloch KE. (2000);Detection of inspiratory flow limitation during sleep by computer assisted respiratoryinductive plethysmography. *Eur Respir J* 15:570-8.

Knaack L, Blum H, Hohenhorst W, Ryba J, Guilleminault Ch, Stoohs RA (2001), Comparison of diaphragmatic EMG and oesophageal pressure in obstructed and unobstructed reathing during sleep. *Somnologie* 9: 159–165

Krakow, B., Melendrez, D., Pedersen, B., Johnston, L., Hollifield, M., Germain, A., Koss, M., et al. (2001) Complex insomnia: insomnia and sleep-disordered breathing in a consecutive series of crime victims with nightmares and PTSD *Biological psychiatry*, 49: 948–953.

Kristo, D. A., Lettieri, C. J., Andrada, T., Taylor, Y., Eliasson, A. H (2005) Silent upper airway resistance syndrome: prevalence in a mixed military population *Chest*, 127:1654–1657.

Kristo, D. A., Shah, A. A., Lettieri, C. J., MacDermott, S. M., Andrada, T., Taylor, Y, Eliasson, A. H. (2009). Utility of split-night polysomnography in the diagnosis of upper airway resistance syndrome.*Sleep Breath.* 13: 271–275

Kushida CA, Giacomini A, Lee MK, Guilleminault Ch, Dement WC (2002) Technical protocol for the use of esophageal manometry in the diagnosis of sleep-related breathing disorders. *Sleep Medicine* 3:163–173

Lewin DS, Pinto MD (2004). Sleep disorders and ADHD: shared and common phenotypes. *Sleep* 27: 188–189

Lindberg E, Gislason T (2000). Epidemiology of related obstructive breathing. *Sleep Med Rev* 4:411-433

Loube DI, Andrada T, Howard RS (1999) Accuracy of respiratory inductive plethysmography for the diagnosis of upper airway resistance syndrome. *Chest* 115;1333-1337.

Loube DI, Andrada TF. (1999) Comparison of respiratory polysomnographic parameters in matched cohorts of upper airway resistance and obstructive sleep apnea syndrome patients *Chest* 115:1519-1524

Loube DI, Andrada T, Shanmagum N et al. (1998): Successful treatment of upper airway resistance syndrome with an oral appliance. *Sleep Breath.*; 2: 98–101.

Mansour KF, Rowley JA, Badr MS. (2004) Noninvasive determination of upperairway resistance and flow limitation, *J Appl Physiol*, 97: 1840-1848,

Meslier N, Simon I, Kouatchet A, Ouksel H ,Person C, Racineux JL (2002) Validation of a suprasternal pressure transducer for apnea classification during sleep. *Sleep* 25:753-7.

Messner AH, Pelayo R (2000) Pediatric sleep-related breathing disorders. *American Journal of Otolaryngology* 21, 98–107

Montserrat JM, Badia JR (1999) Upper airway resistance syndrome. Sleep Med Rev 3:5–21

Newman J, Moore M, Utley D et als (1996). Recognition and surgical management of the upper airway resistance síndrome. *Laryngoscope* 106; 1089-93.

Newman J (2002). Snare uvulectomy for upper airway resistance syndrome, *Operative Techniques in Otolaryngology-Head and Neck Surgery*, 13: 178-181

Norman RG, Rapoport DM, Ayappa I. (2007) Detection of flow limitation in obstructive sleep apnea with an artificial neural network. *Physiological measurement* 28(9):1089-100

Pichel F, Zamarron C, Magan F, del Campo F (2004). Health-related quality of lifein patients with obstructive sleep apnea: effects of long-term positiveairway pressure treatment. *Respir Med*, 98:968–76.

Pepin JL, Veale D, Mayer P, et al. 1996. Critical analysis of the results of surgery in the treatment of snoring, upper airway resistance síndrome (UARS), and obstructive sleep apnea (OSA). *Sleep*, 19:S90-100.

Pirelli P, Saponara M, Guilleminault C (2004). Rapid maxillary expansion in children with obstructive sleep apnea syndrome. *Sleep* 27: 761–766.

Popovic D, King Ch, Guerrero M, Levendowski DJ, Henninger D, Westbrook PR (2009). Validation of forehead venous pressure as a measure of respiratory effort for the diagnosis of sleep apnea. *J Clin Monit Comput* 23:1-10

Powell NB, Riley RW, Troell RJ, Li K, Blumen MB, Guilleminault C. (1998) Radiofrequency volumetric tissue reduction of the palate in subjects with sleep-disordered breathing. *Chest* 113:1163-1174

Powers, C. R., Frey, W. C (2009). Maintenance of wakefulness test in military personnel with upper airway resistance syndrome and mild to moderate obstructive sleep apnea *Sleep Breath* 13:253-258

Ramar K, Guilleminault Ch (2008) Upper airway resistance syndrome *Current Respiratory Medicine Reviews*, 4, 23-28

Rees K, Kingshott RN, Wraith PK, Douglas NJ. (2000). Frequency and significance of increased upper airway resistance during sleep *Am J Respir Crit Care Med* 162:1210-14.

Rose E, Frucht S, Sobanski T, Barthlen G, Schmidt R (2000). Improvement in daytime sleepiness by the use of an oral appliance in a patient with upper airway resistance syndrome. *Sleep Breath* 4:85-88.

Stoohs RA, Guilleminault C, Itoi A, Dement WC (1994). Traffic accidents in commercial long-haul truck drivers: the influence of sleep- disordered breathing and obesity. *Sleep* 17:619-23.

Stoohs RA, Knaack L, Blum HC, Janicki J, Hohenhorst W.(2008) Differences in clinical features of upper airway resistance syndrome, primary snoring, and obstructive sleep apnea/hypopnea syndrome.. *Sleep Med.* 9:121-8

Terzano MG, Parrino L, Boselli M, Spaggiari MC, Di Giovanni G (1996) Polysomnographic analysis of arousal responses in obstructive sleep apnea syndrome by means of the cyclic alternating pattern (CAP). *J Clin Neurophysiol* 13:145-55

Trakada G, Chrousos G, Pejovic S, Vgontzas A. (2007) Sleep apnea and its association with the stress system, inflammation, insulin resistance and visceral obesity. *Sleep Med Clin* 2:251-61

Tufik S, Guilleminault Ch, SilvaRS, Bittencourt LR (2009) Prevalence of upper airway resistance síndrome (UARS): a population based survey. *Sleep Med* 10, Suppl. 2 S80.

Velamuri K (2006) Upper Airway Resistance Syndrome. *Sleep Med Clin* 1:475–482.

Vgontzas, A. N., Fernandez-Mendoza, J. (2011). Is there a link between mild sleep disordered breathing and psychiatric and psychosomatic disorders. Sleep Med Rev in press doi:10.1016/j.smrv.2011.03.003

Votteri BA, Cundiff EF, Yates WA, Shabatura BB, Reichert JA (1994). The incidence of upper airway resistance syndrome (UARS) in a community-based hospital sleep disorders center. *Sleep Research* 23:339.

Watanabe T, Kumano-Go T, Suganuma N, Shigedo Y, Motonishi M, Honda H, Kyotani K, Uruha S, Terashima K, Teshima Y, Takeda M, Sugita Y (2000). The relationship between esophageal pressure and apnea hypopnea index in obstructive sleep apnea-hypopnea síndrome. *Sleep Reserach online* 3(4):169-72.

Young T, Peppard PE, Gottlieb D (2002). Epidemiology of obstructive sleep apnea: a population health perspective. *Am J Respir Crit Care Med* 165: 1217–1239.

Yoshida K. (2002) Oral device therapy for the upper airway resistance syndrome patient. *J Prosthet Dent* 87(4):427–430

7

Breathing Sleep Disturbances and Migraine: A Dangerous Synergy or a Favorable Antagonism?

C. Lovati et al*
[1]*Department of Neurology and Headache Unit, L. Sacco Hospital, Milan, Italy*

1. Introduction

Sleep and headache are two realities known to be linked in a bidirectional way [01]. Clinical research correlates specific headache diagnoses and sleep disorders with chronobiologic patterns and sleep processes, implicating that common anatomic structures and neurochemical processes are involved in the regulation of both sleep and headache. Sleep and pain perception share several structures, such as the thalamus, the hypothalamus, and a number of mesencephalic, pontine and bulbar nuclei, some of which are also involved in breathing regulation.

The respiratory parameters during sleep at night may play a important role in modifying susceptibility to various pathological conditions, including headache. Morning headache was found to be more frequent among Obstructive Sleep Apnea Syndrome (OSAS) patients with a direct relationship with the severity of the sleep breathing disorder: apnoea hypopnoea index (AHI) has been found higher in OSAS patients with morning headache compared with those without morning headaches and also mean oxygen saturation value (SpO2) during total sleep time has been found significantly lower in OSAS patients with morning headache [02]. Furthermore, it has been observed that morning headache may be largely resolved with nasal continuous positive airway pressure.

The relevance of respiratory disturbances during sleep in subjects with primary headaches has not been clearly evaluated.

Additionally, in a previous study we found that subjects with headache, and particularly those with headache-related cutaneous allodynia, had alterations in sleep behaviour [03]. Consequently, a possible link between sleep behavior disturbances, respiratory disorders during sleep and primary headaches may be hypothesized.

---

* M. Zardoni[1], D. D'Amico[3], M. Pecis[2], L. Giani[1], E. Raimondi[1], P. Bertora[1], D. Legnani[2], G. Bussone[3], C. Mariani[1]

[1]*Department of Neurology and Headache Unit, L. Sacco Hospital, Milan, Italy*

[2]*Department of Pneumology , L. Sacco Hospital, Milan, Italy*

[3]*Headache Centre, Departement of Clinical Neurosciences and Headache Unit, C. Besta Neurological Institute Foundation, Milan, Italy*

2. Objective

Based on the above reported background, we designed a study to investigate the possible relationships between nocturnal breathing disturbances and headache, particularly migraine, with and without allodynia.
The aims of the study were:

- to evaluate the prevalence of different kinds of headache in a population of subjects who underwent cardiopulmonary monitoring during sleep for presumed respiratory problems;
- to assess the frequency of allodynia among patients with headache in this population;
- to evaluate the possible relationships between the presence of headache - and of allodynia - and the respiratory parameters that reflect oxygen saturation during sleep (AHI, SpO2, T<90%).
- to compare sleep behavior parameters (sleep latency, frequency of awakenings and subjective perception of sleep quality) in subjects without headache and in headache patients, grouped by different diagnostic types.
- to compare the respiratory parameters that reflect oxygen saturation during sleep in these groups and
- to examine any relationship between headache, subjective sleep behavior and breathing quality during sleep.

3. Materials & methods

Population

We enrolled a sample of 302 subjects (225 men and 77 women) presenting consecutively at the Unit of Pneumology of the Luigi Sacco Hospital of Milan, for a full cardiopulmonary monitoring during sleep.

Methods

- History of headache was evaluated in each subject, and headache diagnosis was clinically made according to the ICHD-II criteria.
- The presence of allodynia was assessed by a set of semistructured questions, that had been used by our group in previous studies [04, 05]. This tool investigates if the patient experiences abnormal scalp sensitiveness and/or discomfort during headache episodes and which activities are able to enhance this symptom, such as touching head skin, combing hair, brushing hair, wearing glasses, and so on.
  Patients were asked to give written yes/no responses to written questions as follows: (1) Has the patient experienced abnormal scalp sensitivity or discomfort during headache attacks? If yes, does this abnormal sensitivity or discomfort arise from (a) touching head skin; (b) touching hair; (c) combing hair; (d) brushing hair; (e) wearing glasses; (f) using a hair-band, curlers or elastic for forming a ponytail; (g) lying with head resting on the pain side? Patients replying yes to the first question and at least to one of questions (a-f) were considered to have headache-associated allodynia
- Sleep behavior was evaluated through semi-structured ad hoc questionnaire exploring the mean latency of sleep onset (more or less of 30 min), the frequency of nights with nocturnal wake-up (<2 or >3 nights/month) and the subjective perception of sleep quality (satisfied/not-satisfied).

- Full cardiopulmonary monitoring with SaO2, T90 and AHI determination, was performed by SOMNO check ® effort (WEINMANN) that includes: a nasal respiratory device to reveal air flow and snoring, a pulse oxymeter to measure SaO2 and cardiac rate, an abdominal and a thoracic belt for the inductive thoraco-abdominal pletismography, and a gyroscopic body position detection device.

Statistics

Student T test with Bonferroni correction was used to compare mean ages, mean AHI, mean T<90% and mean SpO2, between groups (subjects with or without headache, with or without allodynia).
Chi square test was applied to compare the distribution of different sleep behavior aspects between different diagnostic groups.

4. Results

Among the enrolled subjects, 198 did not suffer from headache (mean age 60.3 ± 12.7 years, 159 men and 39 women) and 104 had history of headache (mean age 51.4 ± 12.3 years, 66 men and 38 women) of which 67 migraineurs (Mig - mean age 50.8 ± 14.9 years, 37 men and 30 women) and 37 with tension type headache (TTH - mean age 51.4 ± 13.3 years, 29 men and 8 women).
Out of 104 subjects with headache, 50 were allodynic. Allodynia was found in 41 out of 67 migraineurs and in 9 out of 37 patients with tension type headache.

Headache and allodynia distribution in the sample

In our population, headache was present in 34.4% of the studied subjects (104 out of 302 individuals, of which 67 with migraine and 37 with tension type headache) and allodynia during pain attacks was present in 48% of headache patients (50 out of 104 subjects). Allodynia was more frequent among migraineurs (41 out of 67) than in tension type patients (9 out of 37).
After grouping by gender, headache was present in 29,3% of men and in 49,3% of women. Migraine was found in 30 out of 39 female headache patients (30 out of 116 enrolled women, 25% of the female cohort) and in 37 out of 159 male patients with headache (37 out of 225 observed men, 16% of the male population studied). Headache distributions in the different groups are shown in Table 1.

		n°	M/F	M (%)	F (%)	Mean age (years)
Total sample		302	225/77	75	25	57,0
Without headache		198	159/39	80	20	60,3
104 with headache	migraine	67	37/30	55	45	50,8
	tension type headache	37	29/8	78	22	51,4

Table 1. Presence of headache in subjects who underwent a full cardiopulmonary monitoring for presumed respiratory problems during sleep.

Respiratory sleep parameters in different diagnostic groups

As summarized in Table 2, respiratory parameters among subjects with headache were always better than in subjects without headache.

The Apnea Hypopnea Index, that expresses the number of episodes of apnoea per hour, was 23.3 among subjects without headache and 13.8 in the headache group ($p<0.01$), without significant differences between different kinds of headache (14.2 in migraineurs and 13.1 in the tension type group).
Blood oxygenation during sleep was significantly better among headache patients (mean SpO_2 94.4% and T90 6.3%) with respect to controls (mean SpO_2 92.9% and T90 14.7%).
No differences were found between allodynic and non allodynic headache patients also with regard to specific diagnostic groups.

	n°	**AHI Apnea Hypopnea Index** (events/hour)	**SpO_2** (mean oxygen saturation) (%)	**T<90%** % of time with $SpO_2 < 90\%$ (%)
Subjects without headache,	198	23.3	92.9	14.7
Headache subjects (Mig+TTH)	104	13.8	94.4	6.3
Allodynic headache subjects	50	15.6	94.5	6.2
Non-allodynic headache subjects	54	12.1	94.3	6.4
Subjects with TTH	37	13.1	93.9	8.9
Allodynic TTH subjects	9	15.9	93.5	10.5
Non-allodynic TTH subjects	28	12.1	94.0	8.5
Subjects with Mig	67	14.2	94.7	4.8
Allodynic migraineurs	41	15.6	94.7	5.3
Non-allodynic migraineurs	26	12.0	94.7	4.0

Table 2. Distribution of respiratory parameters among the different groups

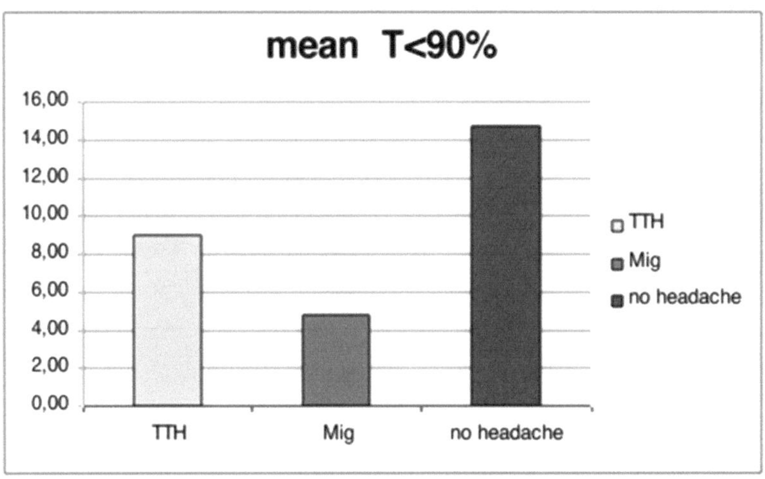

Fig. 1. Blood oxygenation was better among migraineurs. In this diagnostic group, the time period with $SpO_2 < 90\%$ was globally significantly shorter than in the other groups.

Sleep behavior in different forms of headache

As previously observed, allodynic subjects with headache, especially if migraineurs, complain of difficulties in falling asleep and of frequent awakenings that disrupt their nocturnal sleep. Tabs 3a, 3b and 3c summarize sleep characteristics in different groups of patients.

subjective satisfaction	no headache n° (%)	headache n° (%)	mig n° (%)	TTH n° (%)	allodynic subjects n° (%)	not allodynic subjects n° (%)	mig with allodynia n° (%)	mig without allodynia n° (%)	TTH with allodynia n° (%)	TTH without allodynia n° (%)
Satisfied	111 (56)	37 (36)	17 (25)	20 (54)	11 (22)	26 (48)	6 (15)	11 (42)	5 (56)	15 (54)
not satisfied	87 (44)	67 (64)	50 (75)	17 (46)	39 (78)	28 (52)	35 (85)	15 (58)	4 (44)	13 (46)
tot.	198	104	67	37	50	54	41	26	9	28

Table 3a. Sleep behavior: subjective perception of sleep quality (satisfied/not-satisfied). Migraineurs - particularly allodynic ones - have a worse perception of their sleep quality with respect to subjects without headache (chi2 test - $p < 0.01$ in both cases).

Sleep latency	no headache n° (%)	Headache n° (%)	mig n° (%)	TTH n° (%)	allodynic subjects n° (%)	not allodynic subjects n° (%)	mig with allodynia n° (%)	mig without allodynia n° (%)	TTH with allodynia n° (%)	TTH without allodynia n° (%)
<30 minutes	159 (80)	72 (69)	42 (63)	30 (81)	30 (60)	42 (78)	22 (54)	20 (77)	8 (89)	22 (79)
>30 minutes	39 (20)	32 (31)	25 (37)	7 (19)	20 (40)	12 (22)	19 (46)	6 (23)	1 (11)	6 (21)
tot.	198	104	67	37	50	54	41	26	9	28

Table 3b. Sleep behavior: sleep onset latency. Migraineurs - particularly allodynic ones - take more time to fall asleep with respect to subjects without headache (chi2 test - $p < 0.01$ in both cases).

Nocturnal awakenings	no headache n° (%)	headache n° (%)	mig n° (%)	TTH n° (%)	allodynic patients n° (%)	not allodynic patients n° (%)	mig with allodynia n° (%)	mig without allodynia n° (%)	TTH with allodynia n° (%)	TTH without allodynia n° (%)
<2 nights/month	70 (39)	26 (25)	16 (24)	10 (27)	7 (14)	19 (35)	4 (10)	12 (46)	3 (33)	7 (25)
>3 nights/month	120 (61)	78 (75)	51 (76)	27 (73)	43 (86)	35 (65)	37 (90)	14 (54)	6 (67)	21 (75)
tot.	198	104	67	37	50	54	41	26	9	28

Table 3c. Sleep behavior: nocturnal awakenings. Migraineurs - particularly allodynic ones - wake more frequently during night with respect to subjects without headache (chi2 test - $p < 0.01$ in both cases).

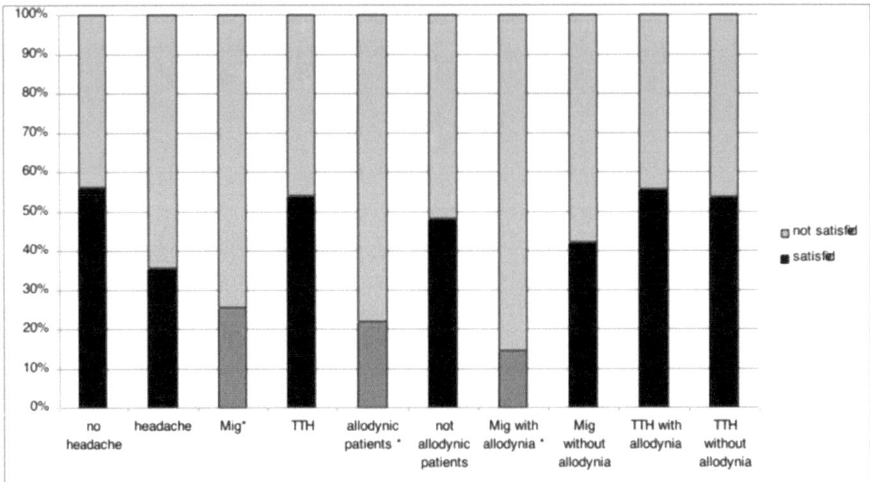

Fig. 2. Migraineurs, particularly if allodynic, are less satisfied about their subjective sleep quality.

Respiratory sleep parameters in different sleep behavior groups

As showed in tables 4a, 4b and 4c, both subjects with and without headache were grouped by sleep behaviour characteristics (satisfaction, sleep latency and presence of nocturnal awakenings). No differences in terms of respiratory parameters were found comparing, in both headache and headache-free groups, subjects satisfied vs not satisfied, subjects with short vs long sleep latency and patients with frequent vs sporadic awakenings.

	AHI	SaO2 media	T<90%
Headache subjects - satisfied by their sleep	11,4	94,6	5,4
Headache subjects - not satisfied by their sleep	15,1	94,2	6,8
Controls - satisfied by their sleep	23,3	93,1	12,8
Controls - not satisfied by their sleep	23,4	92,6	16,5

Table 4a. Sleep behavior: subjects grouped by subjective perception of sleep quality. Respiratory parameters among different groups. No significant differences between satisfied and not-satisfied in both headache and non-headache group with regard to respiratory parameters during sleep.

	AHI	SaO2 media	T<90%
Headache subjects with short sleep latency	15,6	94,3	6,8
Headache subjects with long sleep latency	9,6	94,5	4,2
Controls with short sleep latency	26,0	92,8	14,3
Controls with long sleep latency	14,8	93,7	17,7

Table 4b. Sleep behavior: subjects grouped by sleep onset latency. Apnea episodes (AHI) are meanly more frequent among subjects with rapid sleep onset in both headache and non-headache subjects (no difference after Bonferroni correction). No differences in term of blood oxygenation.

	AHI	SaO2 media	T<90%
headache subjects with sporadic nocturnal awakenings	10,6	94,8	5,1
headache subjects with frequent nocturnal awakenings	15,0	94,2	6,8
controls with sporadic nocturnal awakenings	20,6	93,0	13,2
controls with frequent nocturnal awakenings	25,3	92,8	15,1

Table 4c. Sleep behavior: subjects grouped by presence of nocturnal awakenings. Respiratory parameters do not significantly differ among groups.

5. Discussion

The study gave to somewhat unexpected results. Namely, the evidence of the significant difference observed between headache and non headache subjects in terms of mean AHI ($p < 0.01$), SpO2 ($p < 0.01$) and T <90% ($p < 0.01$) with better respiratory parameters among headache sufferers, particularly amongst the migraineurs. In fact, when we had planned the study, we were looking for possible endogenous elements able to induce and/or transform headache and we hypothesized that a sleep breathing disturbance might be one of this factors. On the contrary, it emerged that headache patients have a better respiratory condition during sleep, also in allodynic cases.

The analysis of sleep behavior in different groups showed that migraineurs took more time to fall asleep and awake more frequently during night with a reduced global sleep satisfaction. In conclusion, if compared to controls, migraineurs seem to sleep worse but to breathe better.

However, the hypothesis that there is an allostatic function of migraine and allodynia could also be made: the presence of these conditions might inhibit deep sleep, and thus avoid prolonged apneas. The observation that allodynic patients complain of a poor subjective satisfaction by sleep with frequent awakenings and difficulties in starting sleep may be the time when an allostatic load (episodic migraine) becomes an allostatic overload (allodynic migraine), or it may correspond to a further allostatic adjustment to maintain an equilibrium: migraine is "sufficient" until the metabolic unbalance is such, that allodynia is needed. Allodynia is more frequently observed among subjects with chronic/transformed migraine, but it is also present in a large portion of episodic migraineurs. Probably transformed migraine is the true manifestation of the overwhelmed allostatic capacity of migraine (allostatic overload) while the presence of allodynia is still a marker of a functional modification.

Overall, using an allostatic perspective, migraine may be considered a functional strategy to maintain equilibrium and to reverse situations potentially dangerous for the hyperexcitable and hypoenergetic migraineurs brain [08]. Transformed migraine may than represent the failure of this strategy (allostatic over-load), without the capacity to counteract the energetic unbalance.

Allodynia (the perception of pain by non-painful stimuli) is largely considered as a marker of migraine transformation, but the observation that it is frequently present also among episodic migraineurs, offers another possible way to interpret this symptom. Allodynia may be an additional manifestation of migraine in an extreme effort to correct a metabolic or energetic or homeostatic disequilibrium, nocturnal sleep related blood oxygenation included.

To explore this unexpected hypothesis, we grouped both headache and non-headache subjects by sleep subjective satisfaction, sleep latency, and presence of awakenings. Comparing groups (headache subjects with short vs long sleep latency, with frequent vs sporadic awakenings and satisfied vs non-satisfied) no significant difference emerged, at least after Bonferroni correction. Probably the relatively small cohort dimension may have influenced the analysis.

The fact that patients with chronic headaches have a high prevalence of sleep complaints is well documented [09] and a high frequency of headache among patients with pathological breathing during sleep is well defined [02], but in the transitional phase toward sleep breathing disturbances, allodynia may be a useful para-physiological modification instead of a symptom of migraine transformation/chronification.

6. Conclusions

Our convenience data found that migraineurs seem to sleep worse but to breath better than headache free patients. The possible mechanism or mechanisms underlying this observation are not clear, but an allostatic mechanism has been proposed which can be tested in future studies.

7. References

[1] Lovati C, D'Amico D, Raimondi E, Mariani C, Bertora P. Sleep and headache: a bidirectional relationship. Expert Rev Neurother. 2010;10(1):105-17.

[2] Goksan B, Gunduz A, Karadeniz D, Ağan K, Tascilar FN, Tan F, Purisa S, Kaynak H. Morning headache in sleep apnoea: clinical and polysomnographic evaluation and response to nasal continuous positive airway pressure. Cephalalgia. 2009 Jun;29(6):635-41. Epub 2009 Feb 2.

[3] Lovati C, D'Amico D, Bertora P, Raimondi E, Rosa S, Zardoni M, Bussone G, Mariani C. Correlation between presence of allodynia and sleep quality in migraineurs. Neurol Sci. 2010;31 Suppl 1:S155-8.

[4] Lovati C, D'Amico D, Bertora P, Rosa S, Suardelli M, Mailland E, Mariani C, Bussone G (2008) Acute and interictal allodynia in patients with different headache forms: an Italian pilot study. Headache 48(2):272–277

[5] Lovati C, D'Amico D, Brambilla A, Mariani C, Bussone G (2008) Personality profile and allodynic migraine. Neurol Sci 29(Suppl 1):S152–S154

[6] Stovner LJ *et al*, 2006 Stovner LJ, Zwart JA, Hagen K, Terwindt GM, Pascual J. Epidemiology of headache in Europe. Eur J Neurol. 2006 Apr;13(4):333-45. Review

[7] Lovati C, D'Amico D, Bertora P, Raimondi E, Rosa S, Zardoni M, Bussone G, Mariani C. Correlation between presence of allodynia and sleep quality in migraineurs. Neurol Sci. 2010 Jun;31 Suppl 1:S155-8.

[8] D'Andrea G, Leon A. Pathogenesis of migraine: from neurotransmitters to neuromodulators and beyond. Neurol Sci. 2010 Jun;31 Suppl 1:S1-7.

[9] Sancisi E, et al. Increased prevalence of sleep disorders in chronic headache: a case-control study. Headache. 2010 Oct;50(9):1464-72.

8

Sleep-Disordered Breathing in Neurological Diseases

Rafał Rola
Institute of Psychiatry and Neurology
Poland

1. Introduction

Episodes of hypoxia and hypercapnia occurring during apneas significantly dilate blood vessels in the brain (both hypercapnia and hypoxia are potent stimuli of cerebral blood vessels dilation - Guyton, 2005). This results, together with a concomitant increase of mean arterial pressure, in average blood flow increase in the cerebral vessels. Studies in healthy volunteers (Przybylowski, 2003) have shown that episodes of breath apneas cause an increase of cerebral blood flow compared with resting conditions (43% on average). Following an episode of apnea, hyperventilation (with normoxia and hypocapnia) significantly decreases flow in the middle cerebral artery as compared to quiet breathing by 20% (Przybylowski, 2003). In normal subjects sleep reduces the vasodilatation response to a hypoxia (Meadows, 2004). A number of different mechanisms triggered during sleep apneas can influence the blood flow in the brain. The increase in intracranial pressure, together with a negative pressure in the chest, may reduce the perfusion of the brain (Jennum, 1989). More frequent significant carotid artery stenosis (Silvestrini et al, 2002; Nachtmann et al, 2003) and flow disturbances in the intracranial arteries (Behrens et al, 2002; Nachtmann et al, 2003) were found in patients with sleep-disordered breathing as compared with a population of healthy controls. There was also found that: cerebrovascular autoregulation reserve and hypercapnia triggering cerebral blood vessels dilatation are reduced in patients with obstructive sleep apneas as compared with the control group (Balfors, 1994). Similarly, studies of cerebral blood flow autoregulation in patients with sleep disordered breathing show impaired and delayed expansion of cerebral blood vessels in response to hypoxia (Urbano, 2008). Short-term mechanisms, associated with airway obstruction and hypoxia during sleep, are of paramount importance in the pathophysiology of cerebral circulation disorders and ischemic stroke. During obstructive apnea there is a temporary increase in blood flow through the brain vessels due to hypoxia and hypercapnia, but this increase is smaller than that of healthy people. Hyperventilation which follows the apnea causes hypocapnia and normoxia with significant reduction of blood flow through the brain vessels. Obstructive sleep apnea promotes a substantial fall in cerebral blood flow (Culebras et al, 2004; Netzer et al, 1998). It seems that short-term mechanisms, associated with apnea during sleep, underlie the observed periodicity of brain ischemic stroke occurrence during the day and more frequent prevalence of ischemic stroke in the early morning hours (Mohsenin, 2003; Yaggi, 2003).

The patomechanisms described above, triggered during obstructive apneas in sleep, foster the development of several cardiovascular diseases, including stroke. One should be aware of highly complex mechanism of formation and interaction between apneas and coexisting metabolic pathological disturbances such as obesity, impaired glucose and lipid metabolism and impaired endothelial functions in cerebrovascular disorders. These patomechanisms often triggered or aggravated by apnea initiate a vicious cycle of pathological metabolic disorders, vascular and structural, that start or grow an existing cerebrovascular pathology.

2. Sleep-disordered breathing (SDB) in patients with ischemic stroke

2.1 Sleep-disordered breathing (SDB) as a risk factor for ischemic stroke

The first controlled study of sleep related breathing disorders in cerebrovascular diseases were carried out in the 80s. They concerned the snoring as a risk factor for ischemic stroke. The first studies were published by a group of Palomaki (Partinen et al, 1985). They compared the incidence of snoring in 50 men with ischemic stroke with a control group. The study was retrospective with use of a standardized questionnaire. Patients were divided into groups of regularly snoring (every night), often and seldom. Polysomnographic studies were not performed. It was shown that the relative risk of ischemic stroke is 10.8 times higher in regular snorers as compared with not snoring patients. Further results of these investigators have shown that snoring is independent of other risk factor for ischemic stroke (Palomaki 1989, 1991). Results of other studies on snoring as a risk factor of ischemic stroke, show an increased relative risk of stroke in snoring people (Koskenvuo, 1987). The largest cohort study of over 70 thousands women (Nurses Health Study), showed an increased risk of ischemic stroke in regularly snoring women (risk ratio - RR 1.88) and irregularly snoring women (RR 1.60) (Hu, 2000). It should be emphasized that the cited studies were done with the use of different questionnaires. Both the design of different survey questions, the lack of clear criteria for classification of patients as regularly, often and rarely snorers in different studies, and the self- assessment of patients (some snoring patients are not aware of it) can cause false results. The interpretation of these results should be cautious (Harbison, 2000). More recent studies (Davies, 2003) did not show an increased risk of ischemic stroke among snoring men but excessive daytime sleepiness which is associated with an increased risk of ischemic stroke with a relative RR = 3.07 (Davies, 2003).
In recent years a well-designed studies, with large number of participants, were published on the impact of snoring in other vascular diseases. It has been found, that snoring has negative effect on the incidence, clinical course and mortality of myocardial infarction (Janszky, 2008). In women with type II diabetes snoring increases the risk of hyperlipidemia and increases levels of triglycerides (Williams, 2007). Snoring also increases the risk of diabetes (Al-Delaimy, 2002). Snoring, regardless of other risk factors, increases the incidence of carotid atherosclerosis (Lee, 2008). Recent studies (Davies, 2003), however, do not prove that snoring is a direct risk factor for ischemic stroke. A series of new reports indicate the importance of snoring in the development of risk factors for cerebrovascular diseases (Williams, 2007; Lee, 2008). Snoring, especially loud and habitual, can indirectly contribute to the development of ischemic stroke.
The first studies concerning the sleep-disordered breathing in patients with ischemic stroke, with a quantitative assessment of respiratory dysfunction, were conducted in the 90s. It was shown that among 47 patients with ischemic stroke 72% have breathing problems during sleep (defined as AHI> 10), 53% of patients in this group have had AHI> 30, and 30%

of patients have had AHI > 40 (Good 1996). Mohsenin and Valor (1995) showed that, among patients with ischemic stroke SDB (AHI> 10) occur in 80% of patients. Another studies (Bassetti, 1996, 1997, 1999), conducted on 128 patients with ischemic stroke and 28 in the control group, showed the incidence of SDB (AHI> 10) in 62% of patients with ischemic stroke, compared with 12,5% in the control group. It has been also shown that the incidence of apneas is similar and significantly higher in patients with ischemic stroke and TIA than in the control group (Bassetti, 1996). These results suggest that sleep-disordered breathing is a risk factor for ischemic stroke, rather than its consequence.

Similar results for sleep-disordered breathing in patients with ischemic stroke and TIA were obtained in the group of 161 patients (Parra, 2000). The incidence of sleep-disordered breathing in the group with ischemic stroke was 74.5%, while in the TIA group, 61.5%. Another study (Wessendorf, 2001) have shown the incidence of apnea during sleep in 44% of patients with ischemic stroke, obstructive apneas were the most prominent type of SDB - 94%, central apneas occurred in 6% of patients. Turkington (2002) observed presence of SDB (AHI> 10) in 61% of patients with ischemic stroke. In other studies (Harbison, 2002), the incidence of sleep-disordered breathing in patients with acute stroke was 94% and decreased during hospitalization to 72% within 6 weeks after stroke. Results presented by Iranzo (2002) show that SDB (AHI> 10) in the first night after the stroke occurred in 62% of patients. Another study (Kaneko, 2003) showed sleep-disordered breathing in 72% of patients with ischemic stroke. A prospective study of 120 patients with excessive day sleepiness have shown the relationship between the severity of obstructive apneas and hypopneas in patients in the first day of stroke and the clinical course and functional capacities, measured using the Barthel scale (Turkington, 2002). Obstructive apneas and hypopneas were also associated with increased probability of death and disability after stroke (Turkington, 2004). Another study assessed the occurrence of sleep-disordered breathing in 139 patients with ischemic stroke within the first three days of stroke, comparing characteristics of the strokes that occur at night and during the day. It was found that strokes occurring at night were associated with higher risk of SDB prevalence (RR = 2.62) compared with strokes occurring during the day. The authors suggest pathophysiological association between apneas during sleep and nocturnal strokes (Martinez-Garcia, 2004). Another studies evaluated the relationship between arterial blood pressure values after stroke and sleep-disordered breathing and prognosis after stroke. It was found that sleep-disordered breathing is associated with elevated nocturnal arterial blood pressure and the lack of nocturnal arterial blood pressure decrease (non dippers). There was little correlation between the severity of neurological symptoms, clinical course (degree of disability assessed with Barthel scale) and the severity of apnea (Selic, 2005). A much larger relationship occurred between nocturnal blood pressure abnormalities and the severity of the clinical course of stroke (Selic, 2005). The lack of nocturnal arterial blood pressure decrease (non dippers), however, is associated with sleep-disordered breathing and increased activity of sympathetic nervous system. Prospective study of 102 patients with ischemic stroke and sleep-disordered breathing showed significantly higher risk of ischemic stroke in patients with AHI> 10 (RR = 3.5), regardless of other risk factors (Dziewas, 2005). Prospective, cohort study (follow-up of 3.4 years ; 1022 patients diagnosed with obstructive apneas and hypopneas - 68% of the total population), showed a significantly higher risk of stroke or death (RR = 1.97, p = 0.01) in patients with sleep-disordered breathing (AHI> 5) compared with the control group regardless of other risk factors (age, sex, BMI, arterial hypertension, atrial fibrillation and lipid disorders) (Yaggi, 2005). Correlation studies show a trend related to the higher risk of ischemic stroke and death in patients with more advanced sleep-disordered breathing (Yaggi, 2005). Patients with AHI <35 and AHI> 35 had a relative risk ratios respectively 1.74 and 3.3. Another prospective study of stroke risk in patients with sleep-disordered breathing based on a cohort of Wisconsin (Wisconsin Sleep Cohort Study, 1121 patients without SDB and 1475 patients with SDB (AHI> 5), showed significantly higher incidence of ischemic stroke in patients with advanced apneas (AHI> 20) compared with control group matched demographically and by other risk factors, (Arzt, 2005). The relative risk of ischemic stroke in patients with AHI> 20 in a four-year follow-up was RR = 4.33 (Arzt, 2005). Most studies conducted so far focused mainly on obstructive sleep-breathing disorders in stroke. Most of the observational studies of patients with ischemic stroke indicate a small proportion of the central type apneas (20%) (Bassetti, 1996; Parra, 2000; Yaggi, 2003; Kaneko, 2003; Selice, 2005). Respiratory disturbances of the central type (Cheyne-Stokes breathing pattern) are observed mainly in patients with ischemic stroke with concomitant heart failure (Nopmaneejumruslers, 2005). Another prospective study of elderly people (394 pts aged 70 to 100 years) during 6 year follow-up showed significantly higher incidence of ischemic stroke in patients with severe obstructive apneas and hypopneas (AHI> 30) with a relative risk ratio RR: 2.52 (Munoz, 2006). Further prospective studies assessing the mortality of patients with stroke and sleep-disordered breathing in 10-year follow-up showed a significantly higher risk of death in patients with obstructive apneas and hypopneas RR = 1.76, compared with the control group. Mortality of patients with central sleep apneas was comparable with the control group (Sahlin, 2008). Patients with ischemic heart disease and SDB (AHI> 5) were at increased risk of ischemic stroke RR = 2.69 in ten-years perspective (Valham, 2008). Accordingly, with increasing severity of sleep- disordered breathing (AHI <15 and AHI> 15), the risk of stroke was higher (RR = 2.44 and RR = 3.56).

2.2 Sleep-disordered breathing in patients in the acute phase of ischemic stroke

Sleep-disordered breathing occurs in 30 to 90% of patients in the acute phase of ischemic stroke. SDB can be divided into two types - central apneas and obstructive hypopneas and apneas. In the acute phase of ischemic stroke obstructive apneas are predominant - (Parra, 2000; Yaggi, 2003; Kaneko, 2003). Central-type apneas occurring in the acute phase of ischemic stroke are promoted by impaired consciousness, brain edema and location of ischemic lesions in the medulla. Supine position and dysphagia favor obstructive type apneas. Recently, many research groups have sought to determine the relationship between the occurrence, type and severity of apnea in the acute phase of ischemic stroke and its outcome. It was found that a quantity of central apneas since the onset of disease decreases over time (Parra, 2000; Kaneko, 2003) while obstructive apneas remain constant in patients with ischemic stroke (Parra, 2000; Kaneko, 2003; Harbison, 2002). The next stage of the research was to determine the relationship between the number of obstructive type apneas during sleep and clinical improvement in patients with ischemic stroke. It was found that the severity of SDB in the acute phase of ischemic stroke negatively correlates with the clinical improvement of neurological syndrome (Turkington, 2004; Harbison, 2002; Kaneko, 2003). The increased number of obstructive type apneas in the acute phase of ischemic stroke is highly correlated with increased mortality in patients with ischemic stroke, especially if the apneas last longer than 30 seconds (Turkington, 2004). The severity of apneas in the acute phase of ischemic stroke may be regarded as a predictor of poor neurological improvement in patients with similar severity of neurological symptoms on admission (Cherkassky, 2003) and duration of hospitalization (Kaneko, 2003). Improvement of the functional status of patients (assessed with the Barthel scale) after stroke is negatively correlated with the frequency of incidents of sleep-disordered breathing (Turkington, 2004; Kaneko, 2003).

2.3 Treatment of sleep-disordered breathing in patients with ischemic stroke

Treatment of sleep-disordered breathing in patients with ischemic stroke is strongly dependent on the patient's clinical condition (Hui, 2002). It was shown that among patients with profound neurological deficit CPAP treatment results are unsatisfactory and do not bring the improvement of respiratory parameters (Sandberg, 2001; Wessendorf, 2001). These failures are mainly due to poor tolerance of CPAP and poor compliance among patients with stroke (Sandberg, 2001; Wessendorf, 2001; Hui, 2002). Results published in 2005 regarding the introduction of CPAP treatment in patients with first episode of ischemic stroke and severe obstructive sleep apneas (AHI> 20) showed a significantly lower occurrence of subsequent vascular events (cerebral and cardiac) in patients treated with CPAP - 6 , 7% compared with 36% in patients not treated within two months of follow-up (Martinez-Garcia, 2005). Other authors did not observe statistically significant benefit from the introduction of CPAP treatment in stroke patients with severe obstructive sleep apneas (AHI> 30) (Hsu, 2006). Further prospective study on 449 patients with mild and severe OSAS and CPAP treatment, showed significantly lower risk of cardiovascular event, including stroke (Buchner, 2007). Therapy of patients with severe obstructive sleep apneas and arterial hypertension is postulated as a primary prophylaxis of ischemic stroke (Goldstein, 2006). Recent prospective study in 223 in stroke patients with concomitant obstructive sleep apneas treated with CPAP have reported that treated patients have reduced risk of death compared with not treated in 5-years follow-up (Martinez-Garcia, 2009). It should be noted that the failure of CPAP treatment is usually the result of a difficult cooperation and intolerance of treatment in patients after ischemic stroke. Although there are discrepant reports in the literature, the method of CPAP treatment appears to be effective in preventing further stroke incidents and reduces the risk of death if there is good tolerance of this type of treatment. These results should not limit the interest of researchers in the problem of obstructive sleep apnea in stroke patients. There are several recognized methods of prevention and treatment of sleep-disordered breathing, which can be used successfully in patients with a history of ischemic stroke. These methods include weight reduction, improving sleep hygiene - proper sleep position, avoiding the supine position, avoiding use of alcohol before bedtime, and very important issue - limitation of the use of sleeping pills, particularly the group of benzodiazepines, which may lead to depression of central respiratory center and worsen SDB. Surgical treatment has a prominent place in the treatment of SDB. Correction of the anatomical defects of nasopharynx results in many patients in reduction of the number and severity of obstructive sleep apneas. It is important among stroke patients to select a group with sleep-disordered breathing because of a double benefit - diagnostic and therapeutic, as it allows to modify on of the risk factor-SDB in these patients.

3. Sleep-disordered breathing disorders in neurological diseases

Respiratory disorders in patients with neurological diseases may be a result of damage to different parts of the respiratory rhythm generator and controlling structures responsible for generation of respiratory movements (neuromuscular disorders). Vascular damage to the respiratory center may lead to central respiratory disturbances. Neurodegenerative disease can damage the respiratory center (Cormican, 2004), as well as demyelinating lesions (Auer, 1996) located within the respiratory center. Damage of the axons projecting from respiratory center to spinal cord α-motoneurons (cervical spine trauma, demyelinating plaques in multiple sclerosis) can cause respiratory disorders. Damage to the α-motor neurons of the spinal cord (amyotrophic lateral sclerosis, post-polio syndrome) leads to respiratory failure (Aboussouan, 2005). Similarly, peripheral nerve conduction abnormalities (Guillian-Barre syndrome and congenital polyneuropathy) may lead to hypoventilation and respiratory failure. Disorders of the neuromuscular transmission (myasthenia gravis, botulinum toxin poisoning) and primary muscle disorders (myopathies, muscular dystrophy) can cause respiratory disorders. Physiological sleep, especially REM sleep phase, is a period vulnerable to the occurrence of respiratory disorders. Often the first sign of respiratory failure in the course of neurological diseases is sleep-disordered breathing (Katz, 2009; Landon, 2006). Due to the risk of significant respiratory complications, often fatal, in the course of certain neurological diseases (amyotrophic lateral sclerosis, glycogenosis type II), it is advisable to closely monitor the sleep-disordered breathing among such patients (Bach, 2004; Birnbaum, 2009). Early detection of sleep-disordered breathing, thanks to the possibilities of non-invasive respiratory therapy in the earlier stages of the disease, can significantly improve the quality of life of patients and their prognosis (Bourke, 2003; Farrero, 2005; Mustfa, 2006; Bourke, 2006; Katz, 2009; Ambrosino, 2009). An interesting fact is the presence and influence of breathing disorders in neurological diseases not associated in their pathophysiology with respiratory problems. Examples of such diseases include Alzheimer's disease, Parkinson's disease and epilepsy. Sleep-disordered breathing can often worsen the course of these diseases. The main group of neurological disorders often associated with respiratory disorders are neuromuscular diseases.

3.1 SDB in neuromuscular diseases

Sleep-disordered breathing and respiratory failure are a common consequence of neuromuscular diseases. Respiratory failure as a result of the underlying disease is more prominent during physiological sleep. Ventilation disorders caused by weakening of breathing muscles occur mostly in patients at REM sleep stage. Physiological relaxation of most of the body muscles (except diaphragm and oculomotory muscles, Tabachnik, 1981) and respiratory drive instability may be the cause of breathing disorders during this phase of sleep. It was confirmed in patients with neuromuscular diseases in which blood saturation was measured (Bourke, 2002; Katz, 2009). Sleep-disordered breathing in patients with neuromuscular diseases can be either of central or obstructive origin. The most common type of sleep-disordered breathing in these patients are central hypoventilation and central apneas.

3.1.1 Motor neuron disease

Motor neuron disease leads to progressive muscle weakness, including respiratory muscles. This results in decreased breathing exertion and hypoventilation (Lyall, 2001). The course and severity of respiratory distress affects the clinical course of disease. First of all, bulbar form of amyotrophic lateral sclerosis is associated with more rapid development of respiratory failure (Hadjikoutis, 2001). Respiratory failure develops in a significant majority of patients with motor neuron disease and is a major cause of mortality. Studies concerning sleep disorders and sleep-disordered breathing in motor neuron disease often differ significantly. Some studies indicate a significantly higher incidence of sleep-disordered breathing in the early stages of the disease (Santos, 2003) and fragmentation of sleep (Arnulf, 2000) with the absence or substantial reduction of the duration of REM sleep and increased number of arousals (Takekawa, 2001). Sleep-disordered breathing was mainly of central origin (Santos, 2003; Bourke, 2002). The severity of respiratory distress tended to decrease with time of disease; in patients with disease lasting less than 1 year AHI = 23, while in patients suffering from more than 2 years AHI = 16. Other studies in the early stages of the disease (Kimura, 1999; Ferguson, 1996, David, 1997) do not show significantly higher incidence of SDB. Some authors have postulated the relationship between the number of apneas during sleep and the clinical course (bulbar form) (Santos, 2003; Kimura, 1999), others did not observed similar corelations (Ferguson, 1996). The incidence of SDB in the early stages of motor neuron disease is estimated from 16 to 76.5% (Bourke, 2002). The reasons for such divergent results are due to small study groups of patients (usually not exceeding 20 persons), a different methodological approach (polysomnography vs. portable devices) and a different stage of the disease and its clinical course. Summarizing the results of these studies it is clear that sleep-disordered breathing in patients with motor neuron disease in the early stages of the disease are mostly represented in the form of shallow breaths of central origin, arising from the failure of the diaphragm muscle contraction. Obstructive disorders are rare and are associated rather with the bulbar form (Bourke, 2002). With disease progression the severity of respiratory distress during the day and during sleep increases. Most researchers (Kimura, 1999; Bourke, 2002; Bourke, 2003; Santos, 2003; Mustfa, 2006; Ozsancak, 2008; Ambrosino, 2009) suggest that early detection of major breathing problems during sleep is important and early qualification for home treatment of patients with non-invasive ventilation methods should be performed (Bourke, 2003; Santos, 2003; Mustfa, 2006; Ozsancak, 2008; Ambrosino, 2009). Along with the improvement of technical devices and their increased availability, treatment should be introduced as soon as possible (Ozsancak, 2008; Ambrosino, 2009). A number of studies in patients with motor neuron disease proved a beneficial effect of using non-invasive ventilation during sleep on the quality of life and prognosis (Bourke, 2003, 2006; Moustfa, 2006). Randomized study of 41 patients with motor neuron disease using non-invasive ventilation during sleep (Bourke, 2006) showed a significant increase in their quality of life and its prolongation, for an average 205 days compared with the control group. The greatest benefit was found in the group of patients with less severe involvement of bulbar muscles (Bourke, 2006). Due to the nature of SDB in patients with motor neuron disease (mainly central hypoventilation), the optimal screening study evaluating the severity of respiratory distress seems to be, both in terms of accessibility and sensitivity, overnight oximetry.

3.1.2 Duchenne muscular dystrophy

Sleep-disordered breathing in patients with Duchenne muscular dystrophy has a characteristic clinical course (Barbe, 1994). In children under 10 years mostly obstructive apneas occur, while in older children, with the development of disease, the apneas of central origin predominate (Smith, 1989; Suresh, 2005). The occurrence of obstructive sleep apnea and snoring at a younger age is associated with frequent enlargement of the tongue (Barbe, 1994; Suresh, 2005) and a relatively good function of the respiratory muscles. With age, symptoms of respiratory muscle failure develop and lead to sleep- apneas of central type. The study of 34 patients aged from 1 to 15 years showed the presence of daily symptoms of sleep-disordered breathing in 64%. Polysomnographic studies have shown obstructive SDB incidence in 31% (median age 8 years) and central type SDB in 32% (median age 13 years) (Suresh, 2005). The non-invasive ventilation therapy during sleep significantly reduced the number of episodes of breathing problems, an average of 11 per hour in 5 years. The authors recommend polysomnography study in patients under 10 years of age with symptoms of sleep-disordered breathing. In children above 10 years of age, with early signs of respiratory distress, polysomnographic studies must be performed. Treatment with non-invasive home night ventilation should begin as early as possible (Suresh, 2005; Katz, 2009). In children with Duchenne muscular dystrophy the best predictor of outcome is the vital capacity, respiratory parameters during sleep are of less importance. Recommendations of the American Thoracic Society (2006) include: a history of breathing problems during sleep during each visit, regardless of age, in the case of a patient immobilized in a wheelchair polysomnographic evaluation once a year. When polysomnography is not feasible it is recommended to control overnight pulse oximetry (Kirk, 2000) and evaluate arterial gasometry during follow-up visits.

There are no large systematic studies on sleep -disordered breathing in other types of muscular dystrophies. Recently published study analyses SDB in 51 patients with facioscapulohumeral muscular dystrophy (Della Marca, 2009). 22 patients had abnormal breathing during sleep, 13 of them had obstructive breathing disorders (3 of them required the CPAP treatment). In 4 patients during REM sleep hypoxia of central origin were found, 3 patients had mixed type of respiratory disorders. Other parameters such as BMI, daytime sleepiness, and neck circumference did not correlate with the occurrence of sleep-disordered breathing.

3.1.3 Myotonic dystrophy

Myotonic dystrophy (DM) is the most common neuromuscular disease in the adult population (Rowland, 2005). During sleep, individuals with DM may develop hypopneas and apneas, obstructive, central and mixed (Finnimore, 1994; Kiyan, 2009). These disorders occur in about half of patients with DM (Labanowski, 1996; Kiyan, 2009). Polysomnographic studies show a reduction in the duration and sleep efficiency, increased number of nocturnal arousals and time of light sleep (NREM1) and decrease in the time of REM sleep (Bourke, 2002). During the day, the rhythm of breathing in patients with myotonic dystrophy is irregular while awake, as well as during light sleep. The main problems are observed in the REM phase of sleep (Finnimore, 1994). Usually, symptoms of sleep-disordered breathing in patients with myotonic dystrophy are far before of signs of respiratory distress during the day (Bourke, 2002). Daytime sleepiness in patients with DM (assessed with the Epworth sleepiness scale ≥ 10) is felt by about 50% of patients (Laberge, 2009). Objective tests of daytime sleepiness (MSLT test) show excessive daytime sleepiness in 69% of the respondents (Laberge, 2009). Excessive sleepiness correlates with the degeneration of serotonergic neurons in the raphe nuclei and central superior nucleus of the reticular formation (Ono, 1998). Authors describe the decrease of orexin concentration in the cerebrospinal fluid, which indicates a similarity in the pathomechanism of sleepiness in narcolepsy and DM (Martinez-Rodriguez, 2003). Due to the progressive nature of the disease and mixed character of breathing disorders, respiratory treatment should be implemented only in specialized centers. Sometimes it is necessary to apply a positive pressure with a variable values (BiPAP, Auto-CPAP) or additional oxygen therapy. In the treatment of excessive sleepiness psychostimulants - metylfenidad and modafinil are used.

3.1.4 Myasthenia

Disorders of neuromuscular transmission in the course of myasthenia gravis may cause sleep-disordered breathing of central type, especially during REM sleep accompanied by declines in blood oxygen saturation (Quera-Salva, 1992; Manni, 1995). The nature of respiratory disorders is similar as in other neuromuscular diseases. The severity of respiratory distress is associated with disease severity. Sleep-disordered breathing in patients with myasthenia gravis is particularly pronounced before the occurrence of myasthenic crisis and precede symptoms of respiratory failure due to exhaustion of the respiratory muscles during the night. At that time hypercapnia is the most characteristic symptom. Hypoxia and hypercapnia occurring during sleep are often the case of morning headaches and progressive fatigue associated with underlying disease. Implementation of treatment reduces sleep-disordered breathing (Amino, 1998). There is no clear data to evaluate the incidence of SDB in patients with well-controlled myasthenia gravis. Some authors have shown an increased incidence of obstructive type of sleep-disordered breathing in patients with myasthenia gravis (36% compared to 15-20% expected in the population (Nicolle, 2006). Other authors (Prudlo, 2007) found no correlation between the occurrence of myasthenia gravis and the occurrence of obstructive breathing disorder during sleep. Most studies on the prevalence of SDB in myasthenia gravis was conducted on small groups (up to 30 patients). These results should therefore be carefully analyzed. Currently it seems that the periods of worsening of the disease are associated with increased risk of respiratory distress, while the periods of remission during medical treatment are not associated with an increased risk of respiratory disorders during sleep (Prudlo, 2007).

3.1.5 Glycogenosis type II-Pompe disease

Pompe disease is a chronic, progressive metabolic myopathy associated with deficiency or reduced activity of the acid alpha-glucosidase enzyme. As a result, glycogen storage occurs in tissues and impairs their functioning. Depending on the degree of enzyme defficiency clinical course of disease may be different. The infantile form is associated with a complete lack of the enzyme. Symptoms begin within the first few months of life. The usual presenting features are cardiomyopathy and hepatomegaly leading to progressive heart failure and respiratory distress. Juvenile and adult forms are due to partial enzyme deficiency. Symptoms appear later and the disease has a chronic progressive course (Lewandowska, 2008). Adult -onset type of Pompe disease is associated with progressive respiratory failure resulting from progressive respiratory muscle weakness (Wierzba-Bobrowicz, 2007). Patients with adult-onset type of Pompe disease often have sleep-disordered breathing (Bembi, 2008; Mellies, 2001). These problems usually occur before the total respiratory failure. Sleep-disordered breathing is usually present in the REM sleep phase in forms of central apneas or hypopneas (Mellies, 2001). Since Pompe is a rare disease, few studies have been published regarding the prevalence of SDB in this disease. In one study performed in 27 patients with juvenile and adult form, sleep-disordered breathing was found in 13 patients, 12 of which had diaphragm weakness (Mellies, 2001). Respiratory disorders: hypopneas and apneas, occurred primarily during REM sleep and correlated with decreased tidal volumes, as measured by spirometry during the day. In some patient overnight non-invasive mechanical ventilation were initiated (Mellies, 2001). Recommendations of treatment and diagnosis of Pompe disease suggest control polysomnography study and initiation of respiratory treatment as early as possible in patients with significant SDB (Bembi, 2008).

4. Neurodegenerative diseases of the central nervous system and SDB

4.1 Alzheimer disease

Searching for links between Alzheimer's disease and sleep-disordered breathing has already started in the eighties. Cognitive deficits observed in individuals with SDB was seen as a preliminary stage in the development of dementia. Cognitive deficits in individuals with impaired respiratory function were found on both verbal, spatial and executive functions as well as short-term memory (Naegele, 1995; Alchanatis, 2005). A number of pathomechanisms may contribute to cognitive impairment in patients with respiratory disorders. The important part play episodes of hypoxia and subsequent oxidative stress resulting in impaired cholinergic transmission in the central nervous system (Gibson, 1981; Shimada, 1981). Another pathomechanism may be associated with changes in cerebral blood flow, observed during sleep -significant hypoperfusion after an episode of apnea. Studies using magnetic resonance spectroscopy showed a decrease in metabolism in the frontal lobes in people with severe respiratory problems during sleep (Alchanatis, 2004) and a decrease in metabolism in the white matter (Kamba, 1997). However, biochemical studies, concerning the biochemical markers of neuronal damage (S-100β protein), showed no significant differences between patients with impaired breathing during sleep and the control group (Jordan, 2002). Homocysteine levels did not differ in patients with apneas compared with the control group (Svatikova, 2004). The study of magnetic resonance and computed tomography show damage to white matter in patients with apneas (Kamba, 2001; Macey, 2006) and reduction of the total intracranial brain volume (O'Donoghue, 2005). Another argument in favor of the relationship between dementia and apneas was the discovery of frequent occurrence of apolipoprotein genotype ApoE4 in people with sleep apneas (Kadotani, 2001; Gottlieb, 2004). There were several studies conducted on the effects of sleep apnea treatment on improvement of cognitive functions. In most studies a positive effect of introducing CPAP therapy was found on improvement of cognitive functions (Feuerstein, 1997; Bliwise, 2002; Zimmerman, 2006). It was also observed a beneficial effect of donepezil treatment on reducing the number of apneas during sleep and improvement of sleep architecture (Moraes, 2008). The degree of cognitive impairment observed in patients with sleep-disordered breathing, however, is significantly lower and more slowly progressive than in those with Alzheimer's disease (Bliwise, 2002). Daytime sleepiness, which is a symptom of respiratory distress has a significant impact on cognitive impairment (Feuerstein, 1997). More and more evidence points to a potential relationship between vascular dementia and sleep-disordered breathing. Early studies showed a significantly higher incidence of respiratory distress in patients with vascular dementia (Hoch, 1986; Bliwise, 1989). The authors also showed a correlation between the severity of respiratory disorders and dementia (Reynolds, 1985). These studies, however, were performed on small groups of patients (up to 30 our participants). Newer studies show a similar incidence of sleep-disordered breathing in patients with Alzheimer's disease as in the general population of similar age (Bliwise, 2002). However, vascular dementia associated with lacunar strokes and damage to white matter, occurs more frequent in patients with obstructive sleep apneas (Bliwise, 2002; Matthews, 2003).

4.2 Parkinson's disease

Parkinson's disease is associated with many sleep disorders which include excessive daytime sleepiness, insomnia, abnormal sleep architecture, restless legs syndrome and sleep disorders associated with REM sleep stage (Dhawan, 2006; Postuma, 2009). It was thought that excessive daytime sleepiness is associated with concomitant breathing disorders during sleep. Most studies did not confirm this hypothesis. Sleep-disordered breathing in patients with Parkinson's disease are at a level similar to the prevalence in the population of people in middle age and older (Diederich, 2005; Jahan, 2009). The degree of severity of Parkinson's disease does not affect the frequency and severity of respiratory distress (Young, 2002). One publication noted a higher incidence of mild obstructive breathing disorders during sleep in patients with Parkinson's disease compared with controls (Maria, 2003). Parkinson's disease patients who present with symptoms of disordered breathing during sleep should be performed diagnostic tests and the treatment should be implemented immediately. It is known that excessive daytime sleepiness, cognitive impairment and depressive reactions, caused by sleep-disordered breathing, may exacerbate the non-motor symptoms of the Parkinson's disease (Monaca, 2006).

4.3 Multiple system atrophy (MSA)

In the course of the multiple system atrophy a number of types of SDB may occur (Gilman, 2003). Obstructive (Munschauer, 1990; Glass, 2006) central (Glass, 2006), and mixed disorders of breathing pattern (Guilleminault, 1981) were found. Respiratory disorders and respiratory failure may be the first sign of disease. Glass and colleagues (2006) described 6 cases of MSA beginning with respiratory disturbances. Leading respiratory symptoms were excessive daytime sleepiness, laryngeal stridor during sleep, and dyspnea on exertion. Polysomnographic studies have shown co-existing obstructive disorders associated with laryngeal stridor (caused by paralysis of vocal cords) and the numerous apneas and hypopneas of central type. Patomechanisms which links MSA with respiratory problems, concern both neural control of breathing rhytmogenesis and respiratory airways. It has been shown in postmortem studies reduced excitatory projection from the thalamus (behavioral respiratory rhythm drive) to the dorsal inspiratory neurons (Gilman 2003) and a significant loss of neurons in the brainstem chemoreceptive neurons (metabolic respiratory drive) (Benarroch, 2007). Loss of serotonergic neurons that stimulate the nucleus ambiguous, observed in MSA (Weston, 2004), causes weakening of negative throat pressure reflexes and may be responsible for laryngeal stridor and obstructive sleep apneas (Bennaroch, 2007). The loss of dopaminergic neurons in the periventricular gray matter, probably responsible for the maintenance of wakefulness, can affect both the respiratory rhythmogenesis, as well as excessive daytime sleepiness (Bennaroch, 2009).

5. SDB in epilepsy

The increased incidence of seizures during the night has been known for a long time. Mechanisms associated with the generation of epileptic seizures during sleep are not fully understood. It has been suggested there are several mechanisms of pathological synchronization of brain bioelectrical activity, triggered by physiological stages of sleep (Gigli, 1992). The phases of sleep in which there is greatest risk of seizures include the phases associated with a higher probability of awakening - mainly phase I and II NREM sleep type. Phase of sleep associated with EEG desynchronization - REM is characterized by a lower risk of seizures. The probability of awakening during sleep increases the risk of seizure in the case of idiopathic generalized epilepsies (Bonakis, 2009). A similar mechanism was proposed in focal and secondarily generalized seizures (Manni, 2005). Also in these types of epilepsy light sleep phase (I and II NREM) may initiate abnormal synchronous epileptic discharges. The EEG patterns associated with arousal (K complexes) trigger pathological EEG hypersynchrony in the second phase of NREM sleep. Seizure during sleep is associated with the interruption of the continuity of sleep and disorder of its architecture. Seizure, both partial (Bateman, 2008) and generalized (Seyal, 2009), can cause apnea of central origin. It is probably due to the short-term disturbances of respiratory rhythmogenesis during sleep by hypersynchronic epileptic discharges. The effects of sleep-apnea during seizures, are prolonged hypoxia with a decrease in blood oxygen saturation to 58% and a significant hypercapnia and acidosis (Seyal, 2009). The mechanism of respiratory arrest, and neurogenic pulmonary edema associated with asystole are some of the hypothetical mechanisms of sudden unexpected death in epilepsy (SUDEP) (Nashef, 2007; So, 2008; Jehi, 2008; Pezzela, 2009). Descriptions of near SUDEP cases during polysomnographic studies indicate sleep apnea as an important part of the clinical picture (So, 2000; Trotti, 2009). The pathogenesis of SUDEP is probably associated with the diving reflex mechanisms, generated during apnea (So, 2008) followed by significant bradycardia to asystole and a significant increase in systemic blood pressure, which significantly increases the afterload and metabolic demands of myocardium. In literature there are two cases of patients in whom obstructive sleep apnea caused changes in the EEG and cerebral hypoxia, which in one case ended in death, and in the second with transient encephalopathy (Dyken, 2004). Animal model of SUDEP proves that central apnea and myocardial ischemic changes should be considered as the main patomechanisms of death in the course of a seizure (Johnston, 1997). The relationship between sleep-disordered breathing and epilepsy also revealed a higher incidence of obstructive sleep apneas in patients with epilepsy compared with the general population matched for age. In various studies, the incidence of sleep-disordered breathing is estimated between 5% and 63% in patients with epilepsy (Malow, 1997; Malow, 2000; Beran, 1999; Weatherwax, 2003; Malow, 2003, Hollinger, 2006). Higher incidence of obstructive apneas and hypopneas was found in patients with drug-resistant epilepsy (Malow, 2000). The co-existence of idiopathic epilepsy and obstructive sleep apneas was also observed in the elderly population (Chihorek, 2007). In the cited paper the authors suggest that the increase in the number of new cases of idiopathic epilepsy in the elderly is associated with an increased incidence of sleep-disordered breathing in these patients. A number of studies indicate the beneficial effect of treatment with CPAP method for reducing the number of seizures (Malow, 2000, Hollinger, 2006; Chihorek, 2007; Malow, 2008). Precise pathomechanisms linking apnea with seizure are unknown. There are several reasons that may come up for coexistence of the observed higher incidence of seizures with sleep-disordered breathing. Particularly interesting is the observation on the significantly higher prevalence of sleep apnea in patients with drug-resistant epilepsy (Malow, 2000). One of the pathomechanisms may be related to apnea hypoxia, which leads to decrease of the available pool of ATP in cortical neurons. It was shown that lack of ATP increases the excitability of neurons by the partial depolarization of the cell membrane (Somjen, 2001), which reduces the seizure threshold. Reducing the amount of ATP in neurons also causes increase in amplitude of the sodium ion current in neurons (Rola, 2004), which may accelerate neuron depolarization and action potential generation. Another possible pathomechanism, causing seizures during sleep apnea, is the increased number of awakenings and disturbed sleep architecture. Obstructive type of respiratory disorders are most common during light sleep (stage I and II NREM sleep), during the instability of the respiratory center. In these phases, there are also more awakenings. K complexes and sleep spindles which occur in II phase of NREM are associated with increased pathological hyper synchrony (Bonakis, 2009). Patients with sleep-disordered breathing have disturbed sleep architecture. There is an increased time of shallow sleep (stage I and II NREM) and the reduction or total absence of REM sleep stage. As mentioned above, the NREM sleep, I and Phase II contribute to the occurrence of seizures, while desynchronization of bioelectrical activity of the brain in REM stage prevents seizures (Seyal, 2009). A patient with severe sleep apneas and disturbed sleep architecture is staying longer in the NREM stages, exposed to the induction of seizures, and less in the REM stages of sleep associated with lower risk of seizure. Although the consequence of these pathomechanisms may be increased risk of seizures in patients with apneas, but thanks to the possible treatment a reduction in seizure frequency is observed. Case reports noted the reduction of symptoms of sleep-disordered breathing after surgical treatment of epilepsy (Földvary-Schaefer, 2008) and the reverse effect of vagal stimulation (Holmes, 2003) which indicates a mutual relationship of these two disease entities.

6. References

[1] Guyton AC, Hall EJ, Textbook of Medical Physiology, W.B. Saunders Company; 11th edition 2005

[2] Przybyłowski T, Bangash MF, Reichmuth K, Morgan BJ, Skatrud JB, Dempsey JA, Mechanisms of the cerebrovascular response to apnoea in humans, J. Physiol., 2003; 548: 323 - 332.

[3] Meadows GE, O'Driscoll DM, Simonds AK, Morrell MJ, Corfield DR, Cerebral blood flow response to isocapnic hypoxia during slow-wave sleep and wakefulness, J Appl Physiol, 2004; 97: 1343 - 1348.

[4] Jennum P, Borgesen SE, Intracranial pressure and obstructive sleep apnea, Chest, 1989; 95: 279 - 283.

[5] Silvestrini M, Rizzato B, Placidi F, Baruffaldi R, Bianconi A, Diomedi M, Carotid Artery Wall Thickness in Patients With Obstructive Sleep Apnea Syndrome, Stroke, 2002; 33: 1782 - 1785.

[6] Nachtmann A, Stang A, Wang YM, Wondzinski E, Thilmann AF, Association of obstructive sleep apnea and stenotic artery disease in ischemic stroke patients, Atherosclerosis, 2003; 169(2): 301-7.

[7] Behrens S, Spengos K, Hennerici M, Acceleration of cerebral blood flow velocity in a patient with sleep apnea and intracranial arterial stenosis, Sleep Breath, 2002; 6(3): 111-4.

[8] Balfors EM, Franklin KA, Impairment of cerebral perfusion during obstructive sleep apneas, Am. J. Respir. Crit. Care Med., 1994; 150: 1587 - 1591.

[9] Urbano F, Roux F, Schindler J, Mohsenin V, Impaired cerebral autoregulation in obstructive sleep apnea, J Appl Physiol, 2008; 105: 1852 - 1857.

[10] Culebras A, Cerebrovascular disease and sleep, Curr Neurol Neurosci Rep, 2004; 4(2): 164-9.
[11] Netzer N, Werner P, Jochums I, Lehmann M, Strohl KP, Blood Flow of the Middle Cerebral Artery With Sleep-Disordered Breathing: Correlation With Obstructive Hypopneas, Stroke, 1998; 29: 87 - 93.
[12] Mohsenin V, Sleep-disordered breathing: implications in cerebrovascular disease, Prev Cardiol, 2003; 6(3): 149-54
[13] Yaggi H, Mohsenin V, Sleep-disordered breathing and stroke, Clin Chest Med, 2003; 24(2): 223-37.
[14] Partinen M, Palomaki H, Snoring and cerebral infarction, Lancet, 1985; 2(8468): 1325-6.
[15] Palomaki H, Partinen M, Juvela S, Kaste M, Snoring as a risk factor for sleep-related brain infarction, Stroke, 1989; 20: 1311 - 1315.
[16] Palomaki H, Snoring and the risk of ischemic brain infarction, Stroke, 1991; 22: 1021 - 1025.
[17] Koskenvuo M, Kaprio J, Telakivi T, Partinen M, Heikkilä K, Sarna S, Snoring as a risk factor for ischaemic heart disease and stroke in men, Br Med J (Clin Res Ed), 1987; 294: 16 - 19.
[18] Hu FB, Willett WC, Manson JE, Colditz GA, Rimm EB, Speizer FE, Hennekens CH, Stampfer MJ, Snoring and risk of cardiovascular disease in women, J. Am. Coll. Cardiol., 2000; 35: 308 - 313.
[19] Harbison JA, Gibson GJ, Snoring, sleep apnoea and stroke: chicken or scrambled egg?, QJM, 2000; 93: 647 - 654.
[20] Davies DP, Rodgers H, Walshaw D, James OF, Gibson GJ, Snoring, daytime sleepiness and stroke: a case-control study of first-ever stroke, J Sleep Res, 2003; 12(4): 313-8.
[21] Janszky I, Ljung R, Rohani M, Hallqvist J, Heavy snoring is a risk factor for case fatality and poor short-term prognosis after a first acute myocardial infarction. Sleep, 2008; 31(6): 801-7.
[22] Williams CJ, Hu FB, Patel SR, Mantzoros CS, Sleep Duration and Snoring in Relation to Biomarkers of Cardiovascular Disease Risk Among Women With Type 2 Diabetes, Diabetes Care, 2007; 30: 1233 - 1240.
[23] Al-Delaimy WK, Manson JE, Willett WC, Stampfer MJ, Hu FB, Snoring as a Risk Factor for Type II Diabetes Mellitus: A Prospective Study, Am. J. Epidemiol., 2002; 155: 387 - 393.
[24] Lee SA, Amis TC, Byth K, Larcos G, Kairaitis K, Robinson TD, Wheatley JR, Heavy snoring as a cause of carotid artery atherosclerosis. Sleep, 2008; 31(9): 1207-13.
[25] Good DC, Henkle JQ, Gelber D, Welsh J, Verhulst S, Sleep-Disordered Breathing and Poor Functional Outcome After Stroke, Stroke, 1996; 27: 252 - 259.
[26] Mohsenin V, Valor R. Sleep apnea in patients with hemispheric stroke. Arch Phys Med Rehabil, 76: 71-76. 1995
[27] Bassetti C , Aldrich MS, Sleep apnea in acute cerebrovascular diseases: final report on 128 patients. Sleep, 1999; 22(2): 217-23.
[28] Bassetti C, Aldrich MS, Chervin RD, Quint D, Sleep apnea in patients with transient ischemic attack and stroke: A prospective study of 59 patients, Neurology, 1996; 47: 1167 - 1173.
[29] Bassetti C, Aldrich MS, Quint D, Sleep-Disordered Breathing in Patients With Acute Supra- and Infratentorial Strokes : A Prospective Study of 39 Patients, Stroke, 1997; 28: 1765 - 1772.

[30] Parra O, Arboix A, Bechich S, Garcia-Eroles L, Mentserrat JM, Lopez JA, Ballester E, Guerra JM, Sopena JJ, Time Course of Sleep-related Breathing Disorders in First-Ever Stroke or Transient Ischemic Attack, Am. J. Respir. Crit. Care Med., 2000; 161: 375 - 380.
[31] Wessendorf TE,. Wang YM, Thilmann AF, Sorgenfrei U, Konietzko N, Teschler H, Treatment of obstructive sleep apnoea with nasal continuous positive airway pressure in stroke, Eur. Respir. J., 2001; 18: 623 - 629.
[32] Turkington PM, Bamford J, Wanklyn P, Elliott MW, Prevalence and Predictors of Upper Airway Obstruction in the First 24 Hours After Acute Stroke, Stroke, 2002; 33: 2037 - 2042.
[33] Harbison J, Ford GA, James OFW, Gibson GJ, Sleep-disordered breathing following acute stroke, QJM, 2002; 95: 741 - 747.
[34] Iranzo A, Santamaría J, Berenguer J, Sánchez M, Chamorro A, Prevalence and clinical importance of sleep apnea in the first night after cerebral infarction, Neurology, 2002; 58: 911 - 916.
[35] Kaneko Y, Floras JS, Usui K, Plante J, Tkacova R, Kubo T, Ando SI, Bradley TD, Cardiovascular Effects of Continuous Positive Airway Pressure in Patients with Heart Failure and Obstructive Sleep Apnea, N. Engl. J. Med., 2003; 348: 1233 - 1241.
[36] Kaneko Y, Hajek VE, Zivanovic V, Raboud J, Bradley TD, Relationship of sleep apnea to functional capacity and length of hospitalization following stroke. Sleep, 2003; 26(3): 293-7.
[37] Turkington PM, Allgar V, Bamford J, Wanklyn P, Elliott MW, Effect of upper airway obstruction in acute stroke on functional outcome at 6 months, Thorax, 2004; 59: 367 - 371.
[38] Martinez-Garcia MA, Galiano Blancart R, Cabero Salt L, Soler Cataluna JJ, Escamilla T, Roman Sanchez P, Prevalence of sleep-disordered breathing in patients with acute ischemic stroke: influence of onset time of stroke, Arch Bronconeumol, 2004; 40(5): 196-202.
[39] Selic C, Siccoli MM, Hermann DM, Bassetti CL, Blood Pressure Evolution After Acute Ischemic Stroke in Patients With and Without Sleep Apnea, Stroke, 2005; 36: 2614 - 2618.
[40] Dziewas R, Humpert M, Hopmann B, Kloska SP, Ludemann P, Ritter M, Dittrich R, Ringelstein EB, Young P, Nabavi DG, Increased prevalence of sleep apnea in patients with recurring ischemic stroke compared with first stroke victims. J Neurol, 2005; 252(11): 1394-8.
[41] Yaggi HK, Concato J, Kernan WN, Lichtman JH, Brass LM, Mohsenin V, Obstructive Sleep Apnea as a Risk Factor for Stroke and Death, N. Engl. J. Med., 2005; 353: 2034 - 2041.
[42] Arzt M, Young T, Finn L, Skatrud JB, Douglas Bradley T, Association of Sleep-disordered Breathing and the Occurrence of Stroke, Am. J. Respir. Crit. Care Med., 2005; 172: 1447 - 1451.
[43] Nopmaneejumruslers C, Kaneko Y, Hajek V, Zivanovic V, Douglas Bradley T, Cheyne-Stokes Respiration in Stroke: Relationship to Hypocapnia and Occult Cardiac Dysfunction, Am. J. Respir. Crit. Care Med., 2005; 171: 1048 – 1052
[44] Munoz R, Duran-Cantolla J, Martínez-Vila E, Gallego J, Rubio R, Aizpuru F, De La Torre G, Severe Sleep Apnea and Risk of Ischemic Stroke in the Elderly, Stroke, 2006; 37: 2317 - 2321.

[45] Sahlin C, Sandberg O, Gustafson Z, Bucht G, Carlberg B, Stenlund H, Franklin KA, Obstructive Sleep Apnea Is a Risk Factor for Death in Patients With Stroke: A 10-Year Follow-up, Arch Intern Med, 2008; 168: 297 - 301.

[46] Valham F, Mooe T, Rabben T, Stenlund H, Wiklund U, Franklin KA, Increased Risk of Stroke in Patients With Coronary Artery Disease and Sleep Apnea: A 10-Year Follow-Up, Circulation, 2008; 118: 955 - 960.

[47] Cherkassky T. Oksenberg A. Froom P. Ring H., Sleep-related breathing disorders and rehabilitation outcome of stroke patients: a prospective study, American Journal of Physical Medicine & Rehabilitation. 2003; 82(6):452-5.

[48] Hui DSC, Choy DKL, Lawrence KS, Wong, Fanny WS Ko, Thomas ST Li, Jean Woo, Kay R, Prevalence of sleep-Disordered Breathing and Continuos Positive Airway Pressure Compliance, Chest 2002; 122 (3).

[49] Sandberg O, Franklin KA, Bucht G, Eriksson S, Gustafson Y, Nasal continuous positive airway pressure in stroke patients with sleep apnoea: a randomized treatment study, Eur. Respir. J., 2001; 18: 630 - 634.

[50] Wessendorf TE,. Wang YM, Thilmann AF, Sorgenfrei U, Konietzko N, Teschler H, Treatment of obstructive sleep apnoea with nasal continuous positive airway pressure in stroke, Eur. Respir. J., 2001; 18: 623 - 629.

[51] Martínez-García MA, Galiano-Blancart R, Román-Sánchez P, Soler-Cataluña JJ, Cabero-Salt L, Salcedo-Maiques E, Continuous Positive Airway Pressure Treatment in Sleep Apnea Prevents New Vascular Events After Ischemic Stroke, Chest, 2005; 128: 2123 - 2129.

[52] Hsu CY, Vennelle M, Li HY, Engleman HM, Dennis MS, Douglas NJ, Sleep-disordered breathing after stroke: a randomised controlled trial of continuous positive airway pressure, J. Neurol. Neurosurg. Psychiatry, 2006; 77: 1143 - 1149.

[53] Buchner NJ, Sanner BM, Borgel J, Rump LC, Continuous Positive Airway Pressure Treatment of Mild to Moderate Obstructive Sleep Apnea Reduces Cardiovascular Risk, Am. J. Respir. Crit. Care Med., 2007; 176: 1274 - 1280.

[54] Goldstein LB, Adams R, Alberts MJ, Appel LJ, Brass LM, Bushnell CD, Culebras A, DeGraba TJ, Gorelick PB, Guyton JR, Hart RG, Howard G, Kelly-Hayes M, Nixon JVI, Sacco RL, Primary Prevention of Ischemic Stroke: A Guideline From the American Heart Association/American Stroke Association Stroke Council: Cosponsored by the Atherosclerotic Peripheral Vascular Disease Interdisciplinary Working Group; Cardiovascular Nursing Council; Clinical Cardiology Council; Nutrition, Physical Activity, and Metabolism Council; and the Quality of Care and Outcomes Research Interdisciplinary Working Group: The American Academy of Neurology affirms the value of this guideline. Circulation, 2006; 113: e873 - e923.

[55] Martínez-García MA, Soler-Cataluña JJ, Ejarque-Martínez L, Soriano Y, Román-Sánchez P, Illa FB, Montserrat Canal JM, Durán-Cantolla J, Continuous Positive Airway Pressure Treatment Reduces Mortality in Patients with Ischemic Stroke and Obstructive Sleep Apnea: A 5-Year Follow-up Study, Am. J. Respir. Crit. Care Med., 2009; 180: 36 - 41.

[56] Cormican LJ, Higgins S, Davidson AC, Howard R, Williams AJ, Multiple system atrophy presenting as central sleep apnoea, Eur. Respir. J., 2004; 24: 323 - 325.

[57] Auer RN, Rowlands CG, Perry SF, Remmers JE, Multiple sclerosis with medullary plaques and fatal sleep apnea (Ondine's curse). Clin Neuropathol, 1996; 15(2): 101-5.

[58] Aboussouan LS, Respiratory disorders in neurologic diseases. Cleveland Clinic Journal of Medicine, 2005; 72: 511 - 520.
[59] Katz SL, Assessment of Sleep-Disordered Breathing in Pediatric Neuromuscular Diseases, Pediatrics, 2009; 123: S222 - S225.
[60] Landon C, AMBULATORY PHYSIOLOGIC MONITORING IN HOME ASSESSMENT OF NEUROMUSCULAR DISEASE, Chest Meeting Abstracts, 2006; 130: 238S - 239S.
[61] Bach JR, Gonçalves MR, Noninvasive ventilation or paradigm paralysis?, Eur. Respir. J., 2004; 23: 651.
[62] Birnbaum S, Pulse Oximetry: Identifying Its Applications, Coding, and Reimbursement, Chest, 2009; 135: 838 - 841.
[63] Bourke SC, Bullock RE, Williams TL, Shaw PJ, Gibson GJ, Noninvasive ventilation in ALS: Indications and effect on quality of life, Neurology, 2003; 61: 171 - 177.
[64] Bourke SC, Gibson GJ, Sleep and breathing in neuromuscular disease, Eur. Respir. J., 2002; 19: 1194 - 1201.
[65] Bourke SC, Tomlinson M, Williams TL, Bullock RE, Shaw PJ, Gibson GJ, Effects of non-invasive ventilation on survival and quality of life in patients with amyotrophic lateral sclerosis: a randomized controlled trial. Lancet Neurol, 2006; 5(2): 140-7.
[66] Farrero E, Prats E, Povedano M, Martinez-Matos JA, Manresa F, Escarrabill J, Survival in Amyotrophic Lateral Sclerosis With Home Mechanical Ventilation: The Impact of Systematic Respiratory Assessment and Bulbar Involvement, Chest, 2005; 127: 2132 - 2138.
[67] Mustfa N, Walsh E, Bryant V, Lyall RA, Addington-Hall A, Goldstein LH, Donaldson N, Polkey MI, Moxham J, Leigh PN, The effect of noninvasive ventilation on ALS patients and their caregivers, Neurology, 2006; 66: 1211 - 1217.
[68] Ambrosino N, Carpenè N, Gherardi M, Chronic respiratory care for neuromuscular diseases in adults, Eur. Respir. J., 2009; 34: 444 - 451.
[69] Tabachnik E, Muller NL, Bryan AC, Levison H, Changes in ventilation and chest wall mechanics during sleep in normal adolescents,J Appl Physiol, 1981; 51: 557 - 564.
[70] Lyall RA, Donaldson N, Polkey MI, Leigh PN, Moxham J, Respiratory muscle strength and ventilatory failure in amyotrophic lateral sclerosis, Brain, 2001; 124: 2000 - 2013.
[71] Hadjikoutis S, Wiles CM, Venous serum chloride and bicarbonate measurements in the evaluation of respiratory function in motor neuron disease, QJM, 2001; 94: 491 - 495.
[72] Santos C, Braghiroli A, Mazzini L, Pratesi R, Oliveira LV, Mora G, Sleep-related breathing disorders in amyotrophic lateral sclerosis. Monaldi Arch Chest Dis, 2003; 59(2): 160-5.
[73] Arnulf I, Similowski T, Salachas F, Garma L, Mehiri S, Attali V, Behin-Bellhesen V, meininger V, Derenne JP, Sleep Disorders and Diaphragmatic Function in Patients with Amyotrophic Lateral Sclerosis, Am. J. Respir. Crit. Care Med., 2000; 161: 849 - 856.
[74] Takekawa H, Kubo J, Miyamoto T, Miyamoto M, Hirata K, Amyotrophic lateral sclerosis associated with insomnia and the aggravation of sleep-disordered breathing. Psychiatry Clin Neurosci, 2001; 55(3): 263-4.
[75] Kimura K, Tachibana N, Kimura J, Shibasaki H, Sleep-disordered breathing at an early stage of amyotrophic lateral sclerosis. J Neurol Sci, 1999; 164(1): 37-43.
[76] Ferguson KA, Ahmad D, George CFP, Strong MJ, Sleep-Disordered Breathing in Amyotrophic Lateral Sclerosis, Chest, 1996; 110: 664 - 669.

[77] David WS, Bundlie SR, Mahdavi Z, Polysomnographic studies in amyotrophic lateral sclerosis. J Neurol Sci, 1997; 152 Suppl 1: S29-35.

[78] Bourke SC, Gibson GJ, Sleep and breathing in neuromuscular disease, Eur. Respir. J., 2002; 19: 1194 - 1201.

[79] Bourke SC, Tomlinson M, Williams TL, Bullock RE, Shaw PJ, Gibson GJ, Effects of non-invasive ventilation on survival and quality of life in patients with amyotrophic lateral sclerosis: a randomised controlled trial. Lancet Neurol, 2006; 5(2): 140-7.

[80] Ozsancak A, D'Ambrosio C, Hill NS, Nocturnal Noninvasive Ventilation, Chest, 2008; 133: 1275 - 1286.

[81] Barbe F, Quera-Salva MA, McCann C, Gajdos P, Raphael JC, de Lattre J, Agusti AG, Sleep-related respiratory disturbances in patients with Duchenne muscular dystrophy, Eur. Respir. J., 1994; 7: 1403 - 1408.

[82] Smith PE, Edwards RH, Calverley PM , Ventilation and breathing pattern during sleep in Duchenne muscular dystrophy. Chest, 1989; 96: 1346 - 1351.

[83] Suresh S, Wales P, Dakin C, Harris MA, Cooper DG, Sleep-related breathing disorder in Duchenne muscular dystrophy: disease spectrum in the paediatric population. J Paediatr Child Health, 2005; 41(9-10): 500-3.

[84] Kirk VG, Flemons WW, Adams C, Rimmer KP, Montgomery MD, Sleep-disordered breathing in Duchenne muscular dystrophy: a preliminary study of the role of portable monitoring. Pediatr Pulmonol, 2000; 29(2): 135-40.

[85] Della Marca G, Frusciante R, Dittoni S, Vollono C, Buccarella C, Iannaccone E, Rossi M, Scarano E, Pirronti T, Cianfoni A, Mazza S, Tonali PA, Ricci E, Sleep disordered breathing in facioscapulohumeral muscular dystrophy. J Neurol Sci, 2009; 285(1-2): 54-8.

[86] Rowland LP, 11th ed Merritt`s Neurology, 2005, Lippincot, Williams&Wilkins

[87] Finnimore AJ, Jackson RV, Morton A, Lynch E, Sleep hypoxia in myotonic dystrophy and its correlation with awake respiratory function. Thorax, 1994; 49: 66 - 70.

[88] Kiyan E, Okumus G, Cuhadaroglu C, Deymeer F, Sleep apnea in adult myotonic dystrophy patients who have no excessive daytime sleepiness. Sleep Breath, May 2009.

[89] Labanowski M, Schmidt-Nowara W, Guilleminault C, Sleep and neuromuscular disease: Frequency of sleep-disordered breathing in a neuromuscular disease clinic population, Neurology, 1996; 47: 1173 - 1180.

[90] Laberge L, Bégin P, Dauvilliers Y, Beaudry M, Laforte M, Jean S, Mathieu J, polysomnographic study of daytime sleepiness in myotonic dystrophy type 1, J. Neurol. Neurosurg. Psychiatry, 2009; 80: 642 - 646.

[91] Ono S, Takahashi K, Jinnai K, Kanda F, Fukuoka Y, Kurisaki H, Mitake S, Inagaki T, Yamano T, Nagao K, Loss of serotonin-containing neurons in the raphe of patients with myotonic dystrophy: A quantitative immunohistochemical study and relation to hypersomnia, Neurology, 1998; 50: 535 - 538.

[92] Martinez-Rodriguez JE, Lin L, Iranzo A, Genis D, Marti MJ, Santamaria J, Mignot E, Decreased hypocretin-1 (Orexin-A) levels in the cerebrospinal fluid of patients with myotonic dystrophy and excessive daytime sleepiness. Sleep, 2003; 26(3): 287-90.

[93] Quera-Salva MA, Guilleminault, S, Chevret C, Troche G, Fromageot C, Crowe McCann C, R Stoos, de Lattre J, Raphael JC, Gajdos P, Breathing disorders during sleep in myasthenia gravis, Ann Neurol, 1992; 31(1): 86-92.

[94] Manni R, Piccolo G, Sartori I, Castelnovo G, Raiola E, Lombardi M, Cerveri I, Fanfulla F, Tartara A, Breathing during sleep in myasthenia gravis. Ital J Neurol Sci, 1995; 16(9): 589-94.
[95] Amino A, Shiozawa Z, Nagasaka T, Shindo K, Ohashi K, Tsunoda S, Shintani S, Sleep apnoea in well-controlled myasthenia gravis and the effect of thymectomy. J Neurol, 1998; 245(2): 77-80.
[96] Nicolle MW, Rask S, Koopman WJ, C.F.P. George, J. Adams, Wiebe S, Sleep apnea in patients with myasthenia gravis, Neurology, 2006; 67: 140 - 142
[97] Prudlo J, Koenig J, Ermert S, Juhasz J, Sleep disordered breathing in medically stable patients with myasthenia gravis. Eur J Neurol, 2007; 14(3): 321-6.
[98] Wierzba-Bobrowicz T, Lewandowska E, Lugowska A, Rola R, Stepien T, Ryglewicz D, Pasennik E, Adult glycogenosis type II (Pompe's disease): morphological abnormalities in muscle and skin biopsies compared with acid alpha-glucosidase activity. Folia Neuropathol, 2007; 45(4): 179-86.
[99] Lewandowska E, Wierzba-Bobrowicz T, Rola R, Modzelewska J, Stepien T, Lugowska A, Pasennik E, Ryglewicz D, Pathology of skeletal muscle cells in adult-onset glycogenosis type II (Pompe disease): ultrastructural study. Folia Neuropathol, 2008; 46(2): 123-33.
[100] Bembi B, Cerini E, Danesino C, Donati MA, Gasperini S, Morandi L, Musumeci O, Parenti G, Ravaglia S, Seidita F, Toscano A, Vianello A, Management and treatment of glycogenosis type II, Neurology, 2008; 71: S12 - S36.
[101] Mellies U, Ragette R, C. Schwake, M. Baethmann, T. Voit, and H. Teschler Sleep-disordered breathing and respiratory failure in acid maltase deficiency, Neurology, 2001; 57: 1290 – 1295
[102] Naegele B, Thouvard V, Pepin JL, Levy P, Bonnet C, Perret JE, Pellat J, Feuerstein C, Deficits of cognitive executive functions in patients with sleep apnea syndrome. Sleep, 1995; 18(1): 43-52.
[103] Alchanatis M, N Zias, N Deligiorgis, A Amfilochiou, G Dionellis, and D Orphanidou Sleep apnea-related cognitive deficits and intelligence: an implication of cognitive reserve theory. J Sleep Res, 2005; 14(1): 69-75.
[104] Alchanatis M, Deligiorgis N, Zias N, Amfilochiou A, Gotsis E, Karakatsani A, Papadimitriou A, Frontal brain lobe impairment in obstructive sleep apnoea: a proton MR spectroscopy study, Eur. Respir. J., 2004; 24: 980 - 986.
[105] Gibson GE, Peterson C, Jenden DJ, Brain acetylcholine synthesis declines with senescence, Science, 1981; 213: 674 - 676.
[106] Shimada M, Alteration of acetylcholine synthesis in mouse brain cortex in mild hypoxic hypoxia. J Neural Transm, 1981; 50(2-4): 233-45.
[107] Kamba M, Suto Y, Ohta Y, Inoue Y, Matsuda E, Cerebral Metabolism in Sleep Apnea . Evaluation by Magnetic Resonance Spectroscopy, Am. J. Respir. Crit. Care Med., 1997; 156: 296 - 298.
[108] Jordan W, Hagedohm J, Wiltfang J, Laier-Groeneveld G, Tumani H, Rodenbeck A, Rüther E, Hajak G, Biochemical markers of cerebrovascular injury in sleep apnoea syndrome, Eur. Respir. J., 2002; 20: 158 - 164.
[109] Svatikova A, Wolk R, Magera MJ, Shamsuzzaman AS, Phillips BG, Somers VK, Plasma homocysteine in obstructive sleep apnoea, Eur. Heart J., 2004; 25: 1325 - 1329.
[110] Kamba M, Inoue Y, Higami S, Suto Y, Ogawa T, Chen W, Cerebral metabolic impairment in patients with obstructive sleep apnoea: an independent association

of obstructive sleep apnoea with white matter change, J. Neurol. Neurosurg. Psychiatry, 2001; 71: 334 - 339.

[111] Macey KE, Macey PM, Woo MA, Henderson LA, Frysinger RC, Harper RK, Alger JR, Yan-Go F, and RM Harper, Inspiratory loading elicits aberrant fMRI signal changes in obstructive sleep apnea. Respir Physiol Neurobiol, 2006; 151(1): 44-60.

[112] O'Donoghue FJ, Briellmann RS, Rochford PD, Abbott DF, Pell GS, Chan CHP, Natalie Tarquinio, Graeme D. Jackson, and Robert J. Pierce Cerebral Structural Changes in Severe Obstructive Sleep Apnea, Am. J. Respir. Crit. Care Med., 2005; 171: 1185 - 1190.

[113] Kadotani H, Kadotani T, Young T, Peppard PE, Finn L, Colrain IM, Murphy GM Jr, Mignot E, Association Between Apolipoprotein E €4 and Sleep-Disordered Breathing in Adults, JAMA, 2001; 285: 2888 - 2890.

[114] Gottlieb DJ, DeStefano AL, Foley DJ, Mignot E, Redline S, Givelber RJ, Young T, APOE €4 is associated with obstructive sleep apnea/hypopnea: The Sleep Heart Health Study, Neurology, 2004; 63: 664 - 668.

[115] Feuerstein C, Naegele B, Pepin JL, Levy P, Frontal lobe-related cognitive functions in patients with sleep apnea syndrome before and after treatment. Acta Neurol Belg, 1997; 97(2): 96-107.

[116] Bliwise DL, Sleep apnea, APOE4 and Alzheimer's disease 20 years and counting?, J Psychosom Res, 2002; 53(1): 539-46.

[117] Zimmerman ME, Todd Arnedt J, Stanchina M, Millman RP, Aloia MS, Normalization of Memory Performance and Positive Airway Pressure Adherence in Memory-Impaired Patients With Obstructive Sleep Apnea, Chest, 2006; 130: 1772 - 1778.

[118] Moraes W, Poyares D, Sukys-Claudino L, Guilleminault C, Tufik S, Donepezil Improves Obstructive Sleep Apnea in Alzheimer Disease: A Double-Blind, Placebo-Controlled Study, Chest, 2008; 133: 677 - 683.

[119] Bliwise DL, Yesavage JA, Tinklenberg JR, Dement WC, Sleep apnea in Alzheimer's disease. Neurobiol Aging, 1989; 10(4): 343-6.

[120] Hoch CC, Reynolds CF 3rd, Kupfer DJ, Houck PR, Berman SR, JA Stack, Sleep-disordered breathing in normal and pathologic aging. J Clin Psychiatry, 1986; 47(10): 499-503.

[121] Reynolds CF 3rd, Kupfer DJ, Taska LS, Hoch CC, Sewitch DE, Restifo K, Spiker DG, Zimmer B, Marin RS, Nelson J, Sleep apnea in Alzheimer's dementia: correlation with mental deterioration. J Clin Psychiatry, 1985; 46(7): 257-61.

[122] Matthews KD, Richter RW, Binswanger's disease: its association with hypertension and obstructive sleep apnea. J Okla State Med Assoc, 2003; 96(6): 265-8; quiz 269-70.

[123] Dhawan V, Healy DG, Pal S, Ray Chaudhuri R, Sleep-related problems of Parkinson's disease, Age Ageing, 2006; 35: 220 - 228.

[124] Postuma RB, Gagnon JF, Vendette M, JY Montplaisir Idiopathic REM sleep behavior disorder in the transition to degenerative disease. Mov Disord, 2009; 24(15): 2225-32.

[125] Diederich NJ, Vaillant M, Leischen M, Mancuso G, Golinval S, Nati R, Schlesser M, Sleep apnea syndrome in Parkinson's disease. A case-control study in 49 patients. Mov Disord, 2005; 20(11): 1413-8.

[126] Jahan I, Hauser RA, Sullivan KL, Miller A, Zesiewicz TA, Sleep disorders in Parkinson's disease., Neuropsychiatr Dis Treat, 2009; 5: 535-40.

[127] Young A, Home M, Churchward T, Freezer N, Holmes P, Ho M, Comparison of sleep disturbance in mild versus severe Parkinson's disease.Sleep, 2002; 25(5): 573-7.

[128] Maria B, Sophia S, Michalis M, Charalampos L, Andreas P, John ME, Nikolaos SM Sleep breathing disorders in patients with idiopathic Parkinson's disease. Respir Med, 2003; 97(10): 1151-7.

[129] Monaca C, Duhamel A, Jacquesson JM, Ozsancak C, Destee A, Guieu JD, Defebvre L, Derambure P, Vigilance troubles in Parkinson's disease: a subjective and objective polysomnographic study. Sleep Med, 2006; 7(5): 448-53.

[130] Gilman S, Chervin RD, Koeppe RA, Consens FB, Little R, An H, Junck L, Heumann M, Obstructive sleep apnea is related to a thalamic cholinergic deficit in MSA, Neurology, 2003; 61: 35 - 39.

[131] Munschauer FE, Loh L, Bannister R, Newsom-Davis J, Abnormal respiration and sudden death during sleep in multiple system atrophy with autonomie failure, Neurology, 1990; 40: 677.

[132] Glass GA, Josephs KA, Ahlskog JE, Respiratory Insufficiency as the Primary Presenting Symptom of Multiple-System Atrophy, Arch Neurol, 2006; 63: 978 - 981.

[133] Gilman S, Chervin RD, Koeppe RA, Consens FB, Little R, An H, Junck L, Heumann M, Obstructive sleep apnea is related to a thalamic cholinergic deficit in MSA, Neurology, 2003; 61: 35 - 39.

[134] Benarroch EE, Schmeichel AM, Low PA, Parisi JE, Depletion of putative chemosensitive respiratory neurons in the ventral medullary surface in multiple system atrophy, Brain, 2007; 130: 469 - 475.

[135] Benarroch EE, Schmeichel AM, Dugger BN, Sandroni P, Parisi JE, Low PA, Dopamine cell loss in the periaqueductal gray in multiple system atrophy and Lewy body dementia,Neurology, 2009; 73: 106 - 112.

[136] Guilleminault C, Briskin JG, Greenfield MS, Silvestri R, The impact of autonomic nervous system dysfunction on breathing during sleep. Sleep, Sep 1981; 4(3): 263-78.

[137] Weston MC, Stornetta RL, Guyenet PG, Glutamatergic neuronal projections from the marginal layer of the rostral ventral medulla to the respiratory centers in rats. J Comp Neurol, 2004; 473(1): 73-85.

[138] Gigli GL, Calia E, Marciani MG, Mazza S, Mennuni G, Diomedi M, Terzano MG, Janz D, Sleep microstructure and EEG epileptiform activity in patients with juvenile myoclonic epilepsy. Epilepsia, 1992; 33(5): 799-804.

[139] Bonakis A, Koutroumanidis M, Epileptic discharges and phasic sleep phenomena in patients with juvenile myoclonic epilepsy, Epilepsia, 2009; 50(11): 2434-45.

[140] Manni R, Terzaghi M, REM behavior disorder associated with epileptic seizures, Neurology, 2005; 64: 883 - 884.

[141] Bateman LM, Li CS, Seyal M, Ictal hypoxemia in localization-related epilepsy: analysis of incidence, severity and risk factors, Brain, 2008; 131: 3239 - 3245.

[142] Seyal M, Bateman M, Ictal apnea linked to contralateral spread of temporal lobe seizures: Intracranial EEG recordings in refractory temporal lobe epilepsy. Epilepsia, 2009.

[143] Nashef L, Hindocha N, Makoff A, Risk factors in sudden death in epilepsy (SUDEP): the quest for mechanisms. Epilepsia, 2007; 48(5): 859-71.

[144] So E, What is known about the mechanisms underlying SUDEP?, Epilepsia, 2008; 49 Suppl 9: 93-8.

[145] Jehi L, Najm IM, Sudden unexpected death in epilepsy: impact, mechanisms, and prevention. Cleveland Clinic Journal of Medicine, 2008; 75: S66.

[146] Pezzella M, Striano P, Ciampa C, Errichiello L, Penza P, Striano S, Severe pulmonary congestion in a near miss at the first seizure: further evidence for respiratory dysfunction in sudden unexpected death in epilepsy. Epilepsy Behav, 2009; 14(4): 701-2.

[147] So E, Sam MC, Lagerlund TL, Postictal central apnea as a cause of SUDEP: evidence from near-SUDEP incident. Epilepsia, 2000; 41(11): 1494-7.

[148] Trotti LM, Bliwise DL, Sleep apnea as a transient, post-ictal event: report of a case, Epilepsy Res, 2009; 85(2-3): 325-8.

[149] Dyken ME, Yamada T, Glenn CL, Berger HA, Obstructive sleep apnea associated with cerebral hypoxemia and death, Neurology, 2004; 62: 491 - 493.

[150] Johnston SC, Siedenberg R, Min JK, Jerome EH, Laxer KD, Central apnea and acute cardiac ischemia in a sheep model of epileptic sudden death. Ann Neurol, 1997; 42(4): 588-94.

[151] Malow BA, Gail A. Fromes, and Michael S. Aldrich Usefulness of polysomnography in epilepsy patients, Neurology, 1997; 48: 1389 - 1394.

[152] Malow BA, Levy K, Maturen K, Bowes R, Obstructive sleep apnea is common in medically refractory epilepsy patients, Neurology, 2000; 55: 1002 - 1007.

[153] Malow BA, Weatherwax KJ, Chervin RD, Hoban TF, Marzec ML, Martin C, Binns LA; Identification and treatment of obstructive sleep apnea in adults and children with epilepsy: a prospective pilot study.Sleep Med, 2003; 4(6): 509-15.

[154] Beran RG, Plunkett MJ, Holland GJ, Interface of epilepsy and sleep disorders.Seizure, 1999; 8(2): 97-102.

[155] Weatherwax KJ, Lin X, Marzec ML, Malow BA, Obstructive sleep apnea in epilepsy patients: the Sleep Apnea scale of the Sleep Disorders Questionnaire (SA-SDQ) is a useful screening instrument for obstructive sleep apnea in a disease-specific population. Sleep Med, 2003; 4(6): 517-21.

[156] Hollinger P, Khatami R, Gugger M, Hess CW, Bassetti CL, Epilepsy and obstructive sleep apnea. Eur Neurol, 2006; 55(2): 74-9.

[157] Chihorek AM, Abou-Khalil B, and Beth A. Malow Obstructive sleep apnea is associated with seizure occurrence in older adults with epilepsy, Neurology, 2007; 69: 1823 - 1827.

[158] Hollinger P, Khatami R, Gugger M, Hess CW, Bassetti CL, Epilepsy and obstructive sleep apnea. Eur Neurol, 2006; 55(2): 74-9.

[159] Malow BA, Foldvary-Schaefer N, Vaughn BV, Selwa LM, Chervin RD, Weatherwax KJ, Wang L, and Y. Song Treating obstructive sleep apnea in adults with epilepsy: A randomized pilot trial, Neurology, 2008; 71: 572 - 577.

[160] Somjen GG, Mechanisms of Spreading Depression and Hypoxic Spreading Depression-Like Depolarization, Physiol Rev, 2001; 81: 1065 – 1096

[161] Rola R, Szulczyk P, Kinetic properties of voltage-gated Na+ currents in rat muscular sympathetic neurons with and without adenosine triphosphate and guanosine triphosphate in intracellular solution. Neurosci Lett, 2004; 359(1-2): 53-6.

[162] Földvary-Schaefer N, Stephenson L, Bingaman W, Resolution of obstructive sleep apnea with epilepsy surgery? Expanding the relationship between sleep and epilepsy. Epilepsia, 2008; 49(8): 1457-9.

[163] Holmes MD, Chang M, Kapur V, Sleep apnea and excessive daytime somnolence induced by vagal nerve stimulation, Neurology, 2003; 61: 1126 - 1129.

9

The Effects of Sleep-Related Breathing Disorders on Waking Performance

A. Büttner(-Teleaga)[1,2]
[1]*Woosuk University, Samnye-up, Wanju-gun, Jeonbuk-do,*
[2]*University of Witten-Herdecke, Witten,*
[1]*South Korea*
[2]*Germany*

1. Introduction

Sleep is a necessary and reversible behavioural state of perception, cognition, psyche and physical conditions. Abnormal sleep behaviours may include e.g. difficulties in falling asleep, breathing difficulties such as different kinds of apneas, sleep paralysis, hypnagogic hallucinations, sleep onset-REM, leg movements, sleepwalking, sleep talking, tooth grinding and other physical activities. These anomalies involving sleep processes also include sleep itself, dream imagery or muscle weakness.

Within sleep there are two separate states, non-rapid eye movement (NREM) and rapid eyes movement (REM). REM sleep is defined by EEG activation, muscle atony, and episodic bursts of rapid eye movement. NREM (non-REM) sleep is subdivided into four stages (stages 1, 2, 3 and 4 - Rechtschaffen & Kales) or three stages (N1, N2 and N3 - AASM), which are defined by the electroencephalogram (EEG). The NREM stages are parallel to the depth of sleep continuum (lowest in stage 1 and highest in stage 4 sleep).

NREM sleep and REM sleep continue to alternate through the night in cyclically. REM sleep episodes become longer across the night, stages 3 and 4 become shorter across the night.

Sleep disorders have an impact on the structure and distribution of sleep. A distinction is important in diagnosis and in the choice of treatments. There are three very important sleep disorders: Insomnia, Narcolepsy and Sleep Apnea Syndrome.

Altogether, in Western Europe already suffer more than 10 % of the population from *Sleep-Awake-Disturbances* which has to be treated urgently; 800,000 from Sleep Apnea Syndromes and 25,000 from Narcolepsy (PETER et al. 1995).

1. *Insomnia* is a sleeplessness and includes a decreased total sleep time, a poor sleep efficiency too little and a poor sleep quality caused by one or more of the following: trouble falling asleep (delayed sleep latency), waking up a lot during the night with trouble returning to sleep, waking up too early in the morning, and/or having un-refreshing sleep/not feeling well rested (even after sleeping 7 to 8 hours at night). Under this criterion the frequency is in the western industrial countries between 20-30 % in which about 10-15 % suffer under a very severe illness and 40 % of all depressions may be preceded by insomnia first.
2. *Narcolepsy* is a genetic disorder and characterized by sleep onset REM sleep, hypnagogic hallucinations, sleep paralysis, cataplexy and excessive daytime sleepiness.

The exact prevalence of the general population is unknown. Great differences exist in its appearance frequency. So the frequency of Japan is 0.16 % and of Israel 0.0002 %. Central Europe (0.006 %) and the USA (0.06-0.1 %) are located in the middle.

3. *Sleep Apnea Syndromes* (SAS) are common disorders, which are characterized by repeated oropharyngeal occlusions occurring during the sleep time (sleep-related breathing problems, intermittent hypoxemia) and may be associated with suppression of SWS sleep (disrupted and fragmentized sleep architecture). Due to intermittent hypoxemia and disrupted sleep architecture, SAS leads to impaired daytime functioning in various (neuro)psychological and affective domains and has been associated with increased morbidity and mortality, principally from adipositas, cardiovascular and neurological diseases.

   The prevalence of moderate SAS (AHI >15/h) is 9% in male and 4% in female, respectively. 25-30 % Sleep Apnea Syndromes were described at patients with hypertension and 35-45 % with patients with on the left heart-failure. The SAS frequency increases with an advancing age and reaches their peak at the age from 50 to 70 years. 80% of the patients suffer under excessive daytime sleepiness and a reduced sustained attention. Resulting from this it comes to performance losses both professional and in the ability to drive motor vehicles.

Fragmentation of sleep and *increased frequency of arousals* occur in association with this three disorders and a number of other sleep disorders as well as with medical disorders involving physical pain or discomfort.

In this chapter, the author will describe neuropsychological dysfunctions/courses and neuropsychiatric syndromes due sleep disorders which were characterized by

1. excessive daytime sleepiness
2. attention deficit,
3. memory dysfunction,
4. executive dysfunction,
5. driving difficulties,
6. motivation and emotional deficits,
7. psychiatric consequences (e.g. depression, anxiety) and
8. lack of ability to recognize the effects of behaviour.

There are wide varieties of difficulties in assessment, treatment and rehabilitation for cognitive impairment, psychiatric disorders and behavioural disability after sleep disorders.

In our studies we used neuropsychological and neuropsychiatric methods in different patient groups in a sleep laboratory. Over the past five years we have been testing and treating more than 2000 patients with different sleep disorders and more than 5000 neurological patients.

During admission to the clinic, all patients were selected according to their clinical diagnosis (ICD-10) and were examined neurologically, (neuro)psychologically, psychiatrically and medically. The test persons must not suffer from any severe psychiatric disorders. The study was carried out involving randomly selected patients with sleep disorders.

2. Excessive daytime sleepiness in patients with Sleep Apnea Syndrome

2.1 State of research

2.1.1 Sleep Apnea Syndromes and neuropsychological disorders

In addition to nocturnal Sleep Apnea Syndrome symptoms there are a lot of daytime symptoms. It is assumed that the reduced sleep quality, arising out of deep sleep or REM-suppression, resulting in increased nocturnal arousal responses, or constantly occurring waking or a reduced relaxation function (Weeß et al. 1998a/b) and cognitive damage caused by intermittent hypoxia (Montplaisir et al. 1992). As the main symptom is excessive daytime sleepiness (EDS) is considered.

It is also assumed that the OSAS accompanying Insomnia and sleepiness influence cognitive functions (Jennum et al. 1993). As reported by Schwarzenberger et al. (1987) that patients with EDS have complaints and problems in situations of physical rest and during prolonged monotonous concentration tasks. A study by Kales (1985) showed that 76% of OSAS patients have cognitive deficits in the areas of thinking, learning ability, memory, communication and the ability to learn new information. Naëgelé et al. (1995) were able to establish in Sleep Apnea Syndrome patients that they were reduced at executive functions when these tasks involve the acquisition of information to memory processing. Another study by Cassel et al. (1995) showed that Sleep Apnea Syndrome patients have a reduced non-verbal performance and processing speed. Regarding the central nervous system activation (*alertness*), selective attention and sustained attention in Sleep Apnea Syndrome patients Kotterba et al. (1998) found, that they were impaired, and that they have a reduced vigilance (Barbè et al. 1998).

The cause of cognitive and neuropsychological deficits in the EDS itself, the sleep fragmentation and arousals and nocturnal hypoxemia are discussed (Findley et al. 1986, Greenberg et al. 1987, Guilleminault et al. 1988, Colt et al, 1991, Bédard et al. 1991, Roehrs et al. 1995).

2.1.2 Causes of neuropsychological deficits (Büttner 2001, 2009)

Two concepts play a central role, first, the hypoxia and the other the disturbed sleep architecture in the causes of the neuropsychological and/or cognitive deficits in Sleep Apnea Syndrome patients.

Both factors appear usually occur together, so that it is hardly possible to separate the two. Several studies confirm the link between *nocturnal oxygen desaturation* and neuropsychological deficits. Greenberg et al. (1987) showed, for example, that the nocturnal hypoxia is the cause of the neuropsychological deficits and daytime sleepiness. In another study conducted by Findley et al. (1986) showed that there is a correlation between hypoxia during sleep and wakefulness with the degree of cognitive impairment, but not between sleep fragmentation and the cognitive functions. In a study of Kotterba et al. (1998), various neuropsychological parameters correlate with the degree of hypoxia, but not with the arousal index and AHI. Montplaisir et al. (1992) describe the nocturnal hypoxia as the best predictor for both daytime alertness as well as daytime sleepiness.

For other investigators, the cause of the neuropsychological deficits such as those of daytime sleepiness exist in the *disruption of sleep patterns* or *sleep fragmentation*, accompanied by a reduction in the proportion of REM and slow wave sleep. According to Bonnet et al. (1985) healthy persons' sleep fragmentation leads to neuropsychological impairment. Other researchers such as Telakivi et al. (1988) and Guilleminault et al. (1988) find that sleep fragmentation has an important impact on neuropsychological deficits. This allowed Guilleminault et al. (1988) to conclude in a study that the sleep fragmentation would be the best predictor of the occurrence of daytime fatigue is, and that there is no relationship between daytime sleepiness and respiratory parameters such as RDI or oxygen desaturations. This could confirm also by Colt et al. (1991) in a study. Nocturnal hypoxias were induced during a night under nCPAP therapy and, no effect on daytime sleepiness could be found. So it was adopted by this study that the day's fatigue does not caused by a decrease of intermittent nocturnal oxygen saturation, but rather by the sleep fragmentation. Bédard et al. (1991) suggested it was an *interaction of both factors*; both sleep fragmentation and nocturnal hypoxia were of great importance in the emergence of decreased vigilance or neuropsychological deficits, with the hypoxia seemingly playing a larger role in severe cases. In addition, the *daytime sleepiness* itself is responsible for the cognitive deficits (Roehrs et al. 1995).

Other assumptions are that neither the disturbed sleep architecture nor nocturnal hypoxias play a role for the neuropsychological deficits in OSAS. Thus Ingram et al. (1994) showed that there are no differences in vigilance between OSAS patients and normal subjects. The reduction of vigilance could be determined by age. Research of Kotterba et al. (1998) and Büttner et al. (2004b) were able to contradict these suggestions, as they found differences of vigilance between OSAS patients and healthy individuals, but no age differences. Severity of OSAS, as measured by the AHI or RDI, or nCPAP compliance may also play a role (Cassel et al. 1989, Engleman et al. 1993, John (et al.) 1991, 1992, 1993).

2.1.3 Daytime sleepiness, fall asleep and driving performance (Büttner 2001, 2009)

The ability to drive safely and without accident needs sustained attention and alertness (Guilleminault et al. 1978, Bradley et al. 1985, Podszus et al. 1986, Findley et al. 1988a/b, 1989b, 1990, 1991, 1995, He et al. 1988, Mitler et al. 1988, Lamphere et al. 1989, Roehrs et al. 1989, Bédard et al. 1991, Cassel et al. 1991a/b, 1993, 1996, Kribbs et al. 1993a/b, ATS 1994, Martin et al. 1996, Gerdesmeyer et al. 1997, Krieger et al. 1997, Randerath et al. 1997, 1998, Weeß 1997, Weeß et al. 1998a/b).

Increased daytime sleepiness is one of the most common causes of road accidents. Driver fatigue is the cause in up to 25% of highway accidents (Langlois et al. 1985, Pack et al. 1994, Horne et al. 1995). A study of 67 671 non-alcohol-related car accidents in France in the years 1994-1998 showed that the risk of accidents involving fatalities or serious injuries in fatigue-related accidents is increased as compared to non-fatigue-related accidents significantly (Philip 2000). An analysis of fatal accidents on highways in Bavaria in 1991 showed that 49 of 204 accidents (24%) caused by falling asleep at the wheel (Langwieder et al. 1994). Obstructive Sleep Apnea Syndrome is again one of the most common causes of daytime sleepiness is increased (American Thoracic Society 1994, McNicholas, 1999).

Reliable data on sleepiness-related causes of accidents due to the German data protection regulations is not available and caused on it the published data's are very inconsistent: According to Seko et al. (1986) 45% of all fatal road accidents were caused by falling asleep at the wheel or a micro-sleep, but declared by the Federal Statistical Office at Wiesbaden (1988) only 0.5% of all traffic accidents (Seko et al. 1986, Federal Statistical Office Wiesbaden 1988, Cassel et al. 1993). A study of Zulley et al. showed that 38% in all traffic accidents on Bavarian highways were due vigilance reduction and 24% of all serious accidents (Zulley et al. 1995).

The sleep-related vigilance and sustained attention losses were intensified, especially exacerbated by the effects of biological rhythms (Hildebrandt et al. 1974, Hildebrandt 1976, Mitler 1991, Cassel et al. 1991c, 1993, Zulley 1995).

As early as 1955 Prokop and Prokop discussed regarding traffic safety and the importance of fatigue and falling asleep, but without to discuss the sleep-related aspects or causes (Prokop & Prokop 1955, Cassel et al. 1993). At first in 1978 Guilleminault et al. showed a possible increased risk for patients with sleep-disordered breathing (Guilleminault et al. 1978, Cassel et al. 1991a/b).

George et al. (1987) took up this assumption and investigated the accident probability of 27 suspected OSAS patients. In 93% of patients were entered injuries in the accident register of *Motor Vehicle Branch* of Manitoba (Canada), but only 54% of the control group participants. Unfortunately, in seven patients, the polysomnographic confirmation of the diagnosis and the information on the period of specified accidents are missing (George et al. 1987, Cassel et al. 1991a/b, Weeß 1997, Weeß et al. 1998 a/b). Findley et al. (1988b) found that 29 OSAS patients (AHI> 5) a three-fold increased probability of accidents compared to all license holders of Virginia (USA), and even a seven-fold increased compared to a control group (n = 35). However, Findley et al. didn't give the information whether the OSAS diagnosis was already known in the survey (Findley et al. 1988b, Cassel et al. 1991a/b, Weeß 1997, Weeß et al. 1998 a/b). Later studies and studies by Cassel et al. (1991a/b, 1996), the ATS (1994) and Krieger et al. (1997) confirmed these findings. Thus, patients with Sleep Apnea Syndrome seem increasingly to suffer from severe fatigue and falling asleep while driving (see also George et al. 1987, 1996b, Findley et al. 1988b). With increasing impairment of those affected persons by the symptoms of Obstructive Sleep Apnea are also accumulated self-inflicted, sustained attention-related injuries (Cassel et al. 1991a/b, 1996, ATS 1994, Kruger et al. 1997).
According to Young et al. (1997), the relative risk of an accident within five years, causing increased for men with sleep-related breathing disorders by factor of 3. Several studies show a minimum of a 2-fold to 3-fold, up to 7-fold increased risk of accidents (George et al. 1987, 1999, Findley et al. 1988, 2000, Horne & Reyner 1995, Wu & Yan-Go 1996, Young et al. 1997, Barbé et al. 1998, Terán-Santos et al. 1999, Horstmann et al. 2000, LLoberes et al. 2000, Sharma & Sharma 2008). For example, George et al. (1999) investigated the relationship between accident rates and the number of traffic offenses in OSAS patients, with the result that the frequency of accidents and the number of traffic violations during a period of five years was significantly higher compared to a control group.
A special group in this context represent professional drivers, bus and truck drivers, because they spend a lot of professional time on the road and also with some larger vehicles usually dangerous cargo or other people, so that probably occur in an accident caused considerable damage and injury. These people have to suffer through their work and the associated lifestyle at increased risk of interference with OSAS. Thus for example truck drivers have a very irregular sleep-wake rhythm (Stradling 1989, Stoohs et al. 1995). In 1994 Stoohs et al. researched the influence of sleep-disordered breathing (SDB) and obesity among commercial drivers of large trucks. Drivers with SDB cause twice as many accidents per 1000 driven miles, than that without SDB, and obesity, the accident rate still increased. Accidents caused by overtiredness-related un-roadworthy and related offenses are likely among professional drivers having accepted a level that is comparable to the drunken crime (Meyer 1990).
The diagnosis of central nervous system stimulation as well as the diagnosis of daytime sleepiness has therefore central importance in the sleep medical field. Thus, the daytime sleepiness is on the one hand understood as an important symptom of non-restorative sleep, but on the other hand can also be closed due to their expression on the severity of this sleep disorder. Ultimately, their diagnostic evaluation is also an important criterion for therapy evaluation.
The sleepiness-related medical history or diagnosis is used to assess the clinical and social impact of daytime sleepiness. In particular, the severity and the social and medical risk will be assessed. It can also be used as parameters of the differential diagnosis of fatigue. This anamnesis can be supported by the use of orienting processes or by the method of screening.

It is used especially in the assessment of type and of frequency about the tendency to fall asleep, micro-sleep episodes and monotony intolerance at work (especially in monitoring activities) and to capture the possibility of active participation in road traffic and other social situations (Walsleben 1992, Weeß 2011).

The *Epworth Sleepiness Scale* (ESS), the *Stanford Sleepiness Scale* (SSS), the *Multiple Sleep Latency Test* (MSLT) and the *Maintenance Wakefulness Test* (MWT) are among the methods that are most widely used for the investigation of daytime sleepiness in sleep disorders. The ESS reflects the global and subjective severity of daytime sleepiness in eight different situations and activities of daily living. The SSS is, however, to capture subjective circadian fluctuations of daytime sleepiness. To objective capture electrophysiological and standardized tests are often, such as the MSLT and the MWT used to determine the degree of alertness on the basis of tonic activation.

If, on the basis of questionnaire data and medical history of sleeping on the basis of suspicion that a pathological daytime sleepiness (Table 1) exists, then objective analysis methods can be used to measure sleepiness-related functions.

Central nervous system activation
Vigilance
Selected Attention
Divided Attention

Table 1. Sleepiness functions

2.2 Epworth Sleepiness Scale (ESS)

The Epworth Sleepiness Scale (ESS) of Johns (1991) is very often used as a screening method for detecting the global daytime sleepiness and fall asleep in sleep disorders, especially used in hypersomnias. It is asked retrospectively, how high is the probability to fall asleep in eight everyday situations. The scale has a 4-step response format, in which values between 0 and 3 (0 = never to 3 = strongly agree) must be marked and results are added up a total maximum value of 24.

Following Johns (1991, 1992, Johns & Hocking 1997) a cut-off value $\geq$ 11 indicates a pathological daytime sleepiness. Standardization studies for the German-speaking countries were presented by Büttner et al. (2004c) and Sauter and colleagues (2007). The study found that 85% of healthy persons achieved a total value < 10, which corresponds to the calculated cut-off values in other studies (Johns 1991, Johns & Hocking 1997). The test-retest reliability of the ESS was calculated by Johns (1994) and based on a survey after five months in 87 healthy medical students. It was r_{tt} = .82 (p <.001), even the quality of internal consistency was confirmed (Cronbach's alpha = .88 (p <.001).

The ESS has in spite of it being subjective and a global assessment of daytime sleepiness (Johns 2000) has a very good validity. At a cut-off value > 10 it shows a high sensitivity of 93.5% and - high specificity 98.4%. The ESS is thus a highly reliable and valid procedure. The short implementation time and simple evaluation makes it very economical and cost effective. In addition, it can also be used for measuring the effectiveness of nCPAP therapy.

Nevertheless the ESS does not lend itself to capture gradually different levels of sleepiness (Sangal et al. 1997b) and that four of the eight items have very low selectivity (Rühle et al. 2005).

2.3 Stanford Sleepiness Scale (SSS)

The Stanford Sleepiness Scale (SSS) of Hoddes et al. (1973) is a scale on which momentary alertness can be assessed on a grading of 1 to 7 and thus serves to assess the circadian variations in daytime sleepiness. The scale describes gradual gradations of awareness; it varies between very alert and drowsy conditions. The alertness descriptions are also described, each with typical sensations (e.g. *some slack, slows, woozy*) characterized. Studies on the sensitivity of the scale showed that ratings in 15-minute intervals represent discrete changes in the degree of alertness. According to the response ratings point values are assigned for each time interval, which are then summated.

2.4 Multiple Sleep Latency Test (MSLT)

The Multiple Sleep Latency Test by Carskadon and Dement (1977) recorded the sleep latency lying down and is recommended for the investigation of daytime sleepiness in OSAS patients in the ICSD-2. The MSLT is based on the assumption that a strong physiological sleepiness can reduce the sleep latency (Arand et al. 2005).

For a long time the MSLT has been considered a gold standard for the investigation of daytime sleepiness (Carskadon et al. 1986). The MSLT (as well as the Maintenance of Wakefulness Test (MWT)) is often used to determine the alertness with expert's investigations, e.g. to assess the driving ability (Poceta et al. 1992). Five times a day electrophysiological recordings (C3/A2, C4/A1, EOG, EMG) are performed in 2-hour intervals. The first time of measurement should be from 1.5 to 3 hours after waking. The patient lies in a darkened room and is asked to fall asleep. During the test procedure, the patient is monitored with a video recording.

A pathological fall asleep exists, when the medium sleep latency is < 5 minutes (Richardson et al. 1982). The gray area is between 5-10 minutes and > 10-20 minutes is a normal finding. But are also divergent standard values of 5-8 minutes; thereby establishing of normal values is equivalent to a kind of "rule of thumb" (Guilleminault et al. 1994, van den Hoed et al. 1981, Johns 2000). Although the MSLT perform and should be evaluated strictly according to objective criteria and standardized, it seems to have low implementation objectivity, because the results of individual tests vary greatly (Danker-Hopfe et al. 2006). As other reasons for the inconsistent individual test results Thorpy (1992) describes the different day times and measuring times and not objectified sleep deprivation and sedative or stimulating effects of drugs. In spite of these influences, however satisfactory test-retest reliabilities of $r_{tt} = .65$ to .97 (van den Hoed et al. 1981, Zwyghuizen-Doorenbos et al. 1998) have been found.

Another problem of MSLT is the limited external generalization of daytime sleepiness in everyday situations (Johns 1994). The assumption that the MSLT describe daytime sleepiness - as reflection of everyday life - Johns (2000) keeps being wrong. As a predictor of MSLT is therefore not own, regardless how strict standards and criteria were met. In considering of the relationship between ESS and MSLT are unsatisfactory correlation of $r = .27$ ($p < .001$) or on those that are not significant (Mitler et al 1998.). Reasons for the inconsistent correlations are different: Either there are satisfactory (significant) correlations when all patients fell asleep in all MSLT times or when the patients rarely slept or not fell asleep (Chua et al. 1998).

2.5 Maintenance of Wakefulness Test (MWT)

The Maintenance of Wakefulness Test of Poceta et al. (1992) examines the ability to stay awake in a sleep-inducing situation. The patient sits in a darkened room on a comfortable chair or on the bed and will be asked to refrain movements (e.g., grimacing, shaking), which may prevent falling asleep to refrain (Hartse et al. 1982, Mitler et al. 1982). Three to four times a day electrophysiological recordings (C3/A2, C4/A1, EOG and EMG) are recorded in 2-hour intervals of 20 minutes. The earliest start of the first test procedure should be scheduled two hours after waking. As with the MSLT test history is filmed with a video camera. Evaluated will be the sleep latency from the moment "light off" until the onset of the first two epochs of sleep stage 1 or 2.

In various standardization studies, inconsistent cut-off values were found from 13.5 to 18 minutes (Banks et al. 2004, Rühle 2005). Reasons for the different standard values according to Shreter et al. (2006) are that the test exercises have a significant influence on occasion staying awake in the test situation. So they provided proof that the sleep latency on the MWT was deliberately suppressed because the OSAS patients were afraid to get the license revoked. In considering the relationship between the MWT and ESS were calculated a satisfactory correlation of $r = .48$ ($p < .001$), with the common variance of the two devices was only 23% (Sangal et al. 1997b).

2.6 Pupillography (Fig. 1)

The Pupillograph Sleepiness Test (PST) from Amtech (Weinheim) reflects the fatigue waves of the pupil described by Löwenstein. Normally, the pupil size will be constant in normal central nervous system activation in the dark for a long time. However, occur with increased daytime sleepiness after a few minutes spontaneous fluctuations (oscillations) on the pupil, which are recorded with infrared videography. Cause of fluctuations in pupil size is a mechanism of the autonomic nervous system. With reduced central nervous system activating two divisions acting simultaneously, which inhibit the Edinger-Westphal nucleus. This leads to instability of the central sympathetic activation and consequently fluctuating in an inhibition of parasympathetic activity and the Edinger-Westphal nucleus (Löwenstein et al. 1963, Yoss et al. 1970).

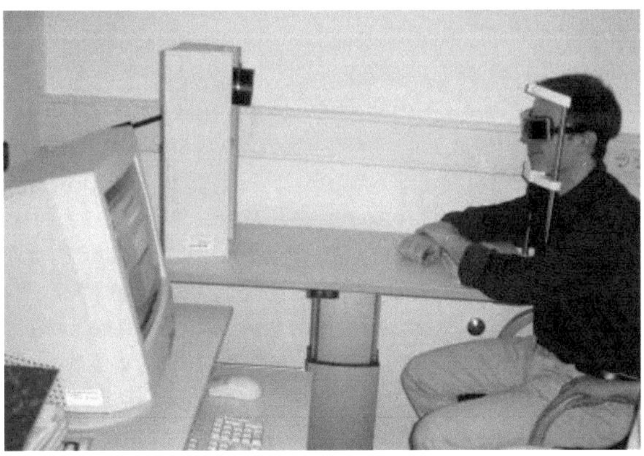

Fig. 1. Experimental setup for the pupillography. The patient wears an infrared protective goggle, has propped his chin on a device and looks toward the infrared camera.

Evaluation

The average Pupil Unrest Index (PUI) is the average pupil size fluctuations in millimetres per second over a period of 11 minutes. Higher PUI values indicate a clinically significant daytime sleepiness in (Table 2). In a normal population (n = 349) between 20 and 60 years, was found a mean value for ln PUI of 1.50 ± 0.39 mm/min. Thus, abnormal values are obtained from ln PUI > 1.89 and pathological values from ln PUI > 2.28. The cut-off value of > 6.64 was found for 84.1% of a healthy sample (Wilhelm et al 2001), which was established that this is independent of gender and age (r = .85 to .94). The PUI correlated low, but significantly with the subjective estimates of daytime sleepiness in SSS (r = .29, p < .010). The implementation objectivity and evaluation objectivity seem to be sufficiently given, because the change in pupil size can be deliberately manipulated. The reliability was tested in healthy control subjects and is satisfactory (r = .64, p < .001) (Weeß et al. 2000).

Value range	Mean-2SD	Mean-SD	Mean	Mean+SD	Mean+2SD
ln PUI (mm/min)	0.73	1.11	1.50	1.89	2.28
Percentile	2.3%	15.9%	50.0%	84.1%	97.7%
PUI (mm/min)	2.07	3.05	4.50	6.64	9.80

Table 2. Percentile of the normal reference range for ln PUI and PUI

2.7 Reading test (Fig. 2)

In the first version of the *Reading test*, it was up to the patients and healthy controls, to select a passage according to their interests. Therefore, it was possible that the individual level of activation of OSAS patients may have influenced the excitement level of the books. For this reason, the story "One day, maybe one night" by Arnold Stadler (2003) was selected. This is a retrospective narrative. Due to the low excitement level of the narrative it was assumed that the degree of tonic activation would remain constant.

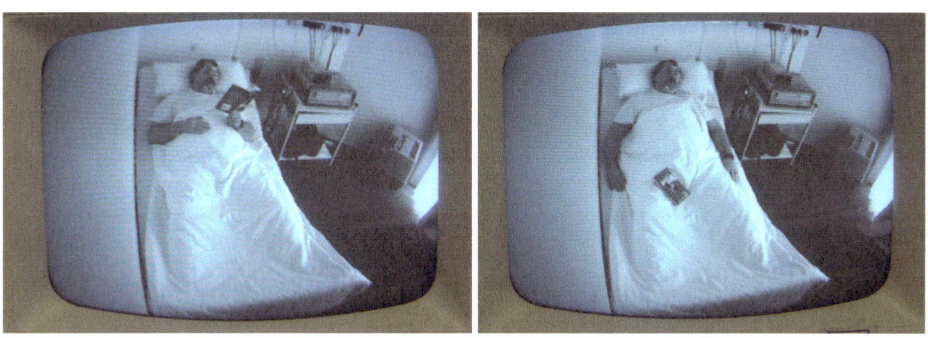

A B

Fig. 2. In 2A is seen as the patient reads in a semi-recumbent position, the modified form of the story "One day, maybe one night" by Arnold Stadler (Fischer paperback 2003). In the face of the electrodes are glued EOG, EEG and the EMG and its right to recognize a polysomnography. In **2B**, the patient is asleep and the book has resigned.

The text was justified, typed in the font "Times New Roman" and the size 12. The pages were not numbered and included 36 lines with 11 cm length. A lamp (40 watts) was used for lighting, placed at a distance of one meter above the patient's head. At the beginning of the *Reading test*, the patient was informed by a verbal instruction, to read the text as possible in the normal reading speed and without interruptions. Patients were asked to keep the book at a distance of 40 cm. Lack of vision and of reading ability has been excluded by spontaneous, aloud reading of few sentences, if the patient was able to read 3-5 sentences correctly and fluently. About the intention and the period of reading, the patients were not informed in order to allay apprehensions and expectations.

Evaluation

The reading movements are simultaneous eye movements, which are characterized by either internal or external amplitude deflections in the EOG. It occurs while reading a specific rhythm EOG, as the eyes "jump" at the end of the line to the next line start. The reading movements can be distinguishing well visually by small and big eye movements (Fig. 3). All reading movements were counted that occurred after a minimum interval of 3 seconds.

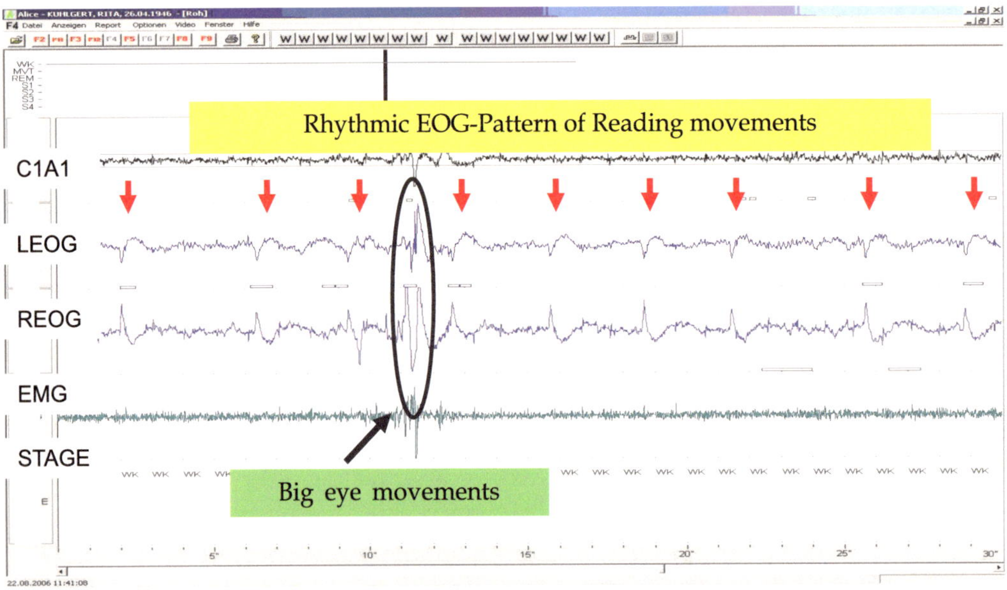

Fig. 3. On display are the reading movements of the left and right eye (LEOG and REOG) as a rhythmic, blue wave pattern. The reading movements occur during reading, when the eyes "jump" at the line end of the text (right) to line beginning (left). Large eye movements (e.g. view movements) are characterized by large amplitude fluctuations.

In the present study, the following variables were used and calculated: the average, the highest and the lowest reading frequency (read line per epoch), sleep latency (in minutes) and the number of read pages.

Results

The average reading rate of the patients (n = 75) was 7.0 +/- 3.5 lines per epoch. In healthy volunteers (n = 16) it was 9.4 +/- 4.0 lines per epoch. All healthy subjects were evaluated for daytime sleepiness than normal, since neither sleep onset tendencies nor decreasing reading frequencies were observed. In 32 of the 70 OSAS patients (45.5%), however, sleep latency was found within 60 minutes. Also the reading frequency decreased over time. Rühle and colleagues calculated for the first time, the sensitivity and specificity of the *Reading test*, finding a cut-off value of greater than 11 for a pathological daytime sleepiness (Rühle et al. 2007). The standardized *Reading test* achieved a sensitivity of 76.2% and a specificity of 66.7% (Erle et al. 2009).

2.8 Conclusion

2.8.1 Effect size analysis of the Epworth Sleepiness Scale

Rühle and colleagues (2005) researched into an effect size analysis of the ESS the question, if daytime sleepiness could be investigated through a situation. Therefore, the authors analyzed the effect sizes of the eight items. From methodological considerations, it was reasonable to imagine, to come across items with good to very good discriminatory power, because the ESS has a good to very good reliability and validity.
In the study, which took place in the sleep laboratory of the Helios Clinic in Hagen-Ambrock, 209 male OSAS patients and 164 healthy subjects participated. To calculate the effect sizes for each item the difference between of the two item means (of patients and healthy subjects) was divided by the standard deviation of the normal population. Rühle et al. received low to very good effect sizes (ES) between 0.19 to 1.50 The best effect sizes were found for the situation "in reading" (ES = 1.50), "watching TV" (ES = .90), "sit and be passive" (ES = .85) and for "traffic-related stopping" (ES = .61). Similarly, there was an increased mean effect size of ES = .88 for the four selected items, compared to a mean effect size of ES = .68 for the total scale. Some situations of ESS was associated with both healthy subjects and OSAS patients with a high propensity for sleep, e.g. to "lie down to rest" (ES = .19), as a "passenger" (ES = .22) and "talk with someone sitting" (ES = .24). For the development of everyday life and job-related tests - as it had been suggested by Johns (2000), the reading activity was an important characterisation of daytime sleepiness, because it discriminates at the best between OSAS patients and healthy individuals in comparison to the other ESS items.

2.8.2 MSLT and MWT criticism

Although MWT and MSLT are often used in practice, since years there is the assumption that its operationalization does not correspond to the tonic activation. Johns (1998) excludes that the MSLT is suitable as a predictor of daytime sleepiness in everyday situations, regardless how strict are implementation and evaluation standards. Although have the sleep latency on both tests satisfactory correlations as Sangal and colleagues (1992, 1997a) showed in subjects with various sleep disorders ($r = .41$, $p < .001$) and in Narcolepsy patients ($r = .52$, $p < .001$). However, the tests clarify maximum of 20-25% of common variance, indicating that the test methods measure different constructs of daytime sleepiness. Reasons for the average correlations according to Sangal et al. (1992) are that patients with pathological MSLT values were able to stay awake in the MWT, while others who fell asleep in the MWT were able to stay awake in the MSLT.
In addition, Johns described measurement error as reasons for the variability of individual test results. It argues that the measurements are depended on the situation character, internal attitude and physical condition of the patient. Kotterba and colleagues (2007) reported that the sleep latency of the MSLT corresponds to the individual property to switch off quickly. In the opinion of John (2000) was the MLST least suitable and is no longer regarded as the gold standard.
In handling the tests are very time-consuming and labour intensive (because of multiple tests during the day) as well as it is uneconomical. This would be calling in question the use of the method (Danker-Hopfe et al. 2006, Johns 2000). Because the claim of a standardized implementation and evaluation it could also be performed only by professionally-equipped sleep laboratories (Randerath 1997). Daytime sleepiness can be measured more easily and possibly more effectively with the ESS (Johns 2000).

2.8.3 Summary and outlook

Although the MSLT and MWT have been used frequently, in many studies was found evidence that the reliability and validity of the procedures are unsatisfactory. In addition, the two test methods don't correspond to any real life situation (Johns, 2000). Even if it is objective and standardized measuring instruments, have been repeatedly confirmed weaknesses in the implementing objectivity of the individual tests as well as their generalization ability (Danker-Hopfe et al. 2006). John's criticism is that the reliability and validity verification of MWT and MSLT were not gone in any way according to objective and standardized criteria. The ESS compared to the MSLT and MWT has good reliability and validation criteria, sensitivity and specificity measures. Its only drawback lies in the fact that the subjective assessments are based on individual perception and trust and the honesty of the patient.

Johns (2000) emphasizes the need to find an objective test, such as the ESS is valid and able to quantify the alertness in various everyday situations. Such a test would represent a true gold standard. Result of this strong criticism and of the clinical relevance of developing a new measuring method, Rühle et al. (2005) analyzed the effect sizes of the ESS. They pursued the goal, to detect the daytime sleepiness of life situation as objective, reliable and valid as possible. The analysis of the ESS and its implications led to the experimental derivation, design and construction of the *Reading test* (pilot study: Rühle et al. 2007, main study: Erle et al. 2009).

2.8.4 Conclusion of the reading test

Both the pilot study and the main study, the alertness impairments in OSAS patients with the reading activity, a simple spiritual activity were operationalized. In contrast to the MSLT and MWT daytime sleepiness was not measured in an experimental laboratory situation, but in an everyday clinical situation. The *Reading Test* is suitable for the determination of daytime sleepiness, because it probably produces a low level of attention. The reading activity will be documented and monitored continuously by EOG. Therefore, the non-reading phases can be observed, e.g. at the beginning of sleep, movement and looking around of the patient. In addition, the behaviour spectrum of patients are also detected in the EMG, as unwanted movements (facial grimacing and head movements), which can prevent sleep. This aspect would be particularly relevant in experiments.

3. Vigilance and attention in patients with Sleep Apnea Syndrome

3.1 State of research (Fig. 4)

Attention underlies performance of intellectual and everyday tasks. Depending on requirement character, novelty, intensity and level of activity, different components of attention are required.

The central nervous system activation (*alertness*) reflects the degree of general alertness and represents a kind of basic activation and general responsiveness. It is unconscious, and affected by the autonomic nervous system and the physiological diurnal state of the organism. Two variants of the central nervous system activation are described. The *tonic activation* is the stable level of attention over a long period of time. A disruption in tonic activation is manifested by a slowing of cognitive and motor processes. The tonic activation can be measured with the Multiple Sleep Latency Test *MSLT* (Carskadon & Dement 1977, Carskadon et al. 1986), the Maintenance of Wakefulness Test *MWT* (Poceta et al. 1992) or the

Pupillography (company Amtech, Weinheim, Wilhelm et al. 1998, 2001). A newer method to quantify the tonic activation is the *Reading test* (Erle et al. 2009).
The *phasic activation* is manifested in stimulus situations, in which short-term increases of the activation in the resting state are required. Limitations of the phasic activation can result in delayed reaction rapidities up to omitted reactions. The phasic activation may be tested for example in the kind of reaction time measurements, e.g. with the test battery of Zimmermann and Fimm (TAP / 1994), event-related EEG deductions or on the basis of the heartbeat rate or skin conductivity.

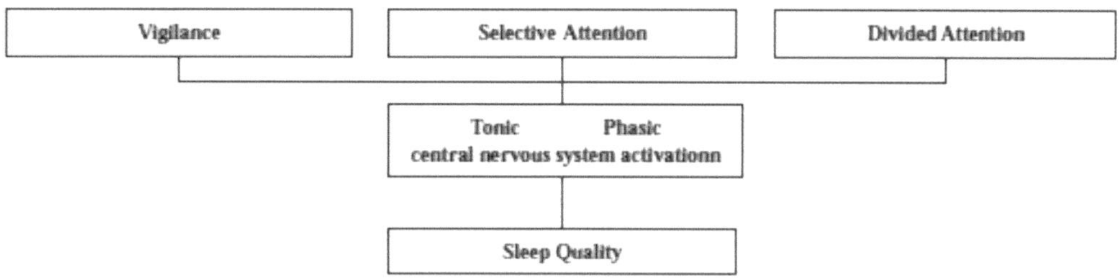

Fig. 4. Proposed relationship between sleep quality and sleepiness-related restrictions during the day

Sustained attention is the ability to direct attention over a long period to one or more randomly occurring stimuli and to respond to minimal stimuli changes (Davies, Jones and Taylor 1984). *Vigilance,* which is a variant of sustained attention, requires long-term attention performance in minimally and irregularly occurring stimuli. As reliable indicators false (i.e. incorrectly or delayed) and omitted responses as well as reaction times can be measured as an expression of sustained attention and vigilance. Furthermore, particularly in the field of sleep medicine the *Clock Test* by Mackworth (1948), modified by Quatember and Maly (Sturm und Büssing, 1993), and the *vigilance test "Carda"* by Randerath et al. (1997, 2000) and Gerdesmeyer et al. (1997) and the *sustained attention test "Carsim"* by Büttner et al. (2000a/b, 2001) have been used to test the vigilance and sustained attention.
Selective attention is also the ability to focus on specific relevant stimuli and to suppress simultaneously occurring irrelevant stimuli. The kind of attention function can be investigated by choice-reaction tasks or orienting responses, e.g. based on the subtest "*Selective attention*" to the *TAP*[1].
Divided attention describes the capacity for serial and parallel information processing and the flexibility of selecting to switch back and forth at least two different sources of information (Sturm and Zimmermann 2000). Relevant stimuli can each occur in one or two sources of information to which the person have to respond as quickly as possible. Divided attention can be measured with dual-task activities (e.g. using the subtest "*Divided attention*" of the *TAP*).
As with many sleep-related disorders, such as hypersomnias and dyssomnias, the victims suffer from, in addition to their nocturnal symptoms, increased daytime sleepiness and the tendency to fall asleep (Büttner et al. 2004b). These difficulties are in turn associated with attention-related deficits and limitations (including Gerdesmeyer et al. 1997, Müller et al. 1997, Randerath et al. 1997, 1998, Weeß 1997, Weeß et al. 1998a/b, Büttner et al. 2003b, 2004b).

---

[1] TAP = German: **T**estbatterie zur **A**ufmerksamkeits**p**rüfung; English translation: Test battery for Attentional Performance

Consequence of this reduced performance include an increased risk of accidents at work and in traffic and thus a higher socio-medical risk (e.g. Bradley et al. 1985, Podszus et al. In 1986, He et al. 1988, Mitler et al. 1988, Lamphere et al. 1989, Roehrs et al. 1989, Bédard et al. 1991, Kribbs et al. 1993a/b, Gerdesmeyer et al. 1997, Randerath et al. 1997, 1998, Weeß 1997, Weeß et al. 1998a/b, Büttner et al. 2000a/b, Büttner 2001).

To explore the difficult relationship between sleep, daytime fatigue and physical and mental performance is based mainly on three conditions (Johnson 1982, Weeß 1997, Weeß et al. 1998a/b). Thus, the three mentioned above parameters will be affecting through a variety of other variables, for example by the motivation of the healthy subjects or patients, or the daily and weekly rhythm. Furthermore, daytime fatigue and performance as well as their underlying attention-related processes are complex constructs. This analysis will be complicated also by the lack of standard term uses in the medical and psychological literature (Johnson 1982, Weeß 1997, Weeß et al. 1998a/b).

There are, both in the medical and especially in sleep medicine research, a number of different research approaches and definitions regarding the attention and attention-driven processes (Rützel 1977, Rapp 1982, Brickenkamp & Karl 1986, Posner & Rafal, 1987, Säring 1988, Posner & Petersen, 1990, Posner 1995), which accentuate different characteristics and aspects of the daytime performance (James 1890, Head 1926, Mackworth JF 1956, Mackworth N 1958, Schmidtke 1965, Norman 1973, Bäumler 1974, Harnatt 1975, Rützel 1977, Brickenkamp & Karl 1986, Posner & Rafal, 1987, Säring 1988, Posner & Petersen, 1990, Rollet 1993, Schmöttke & Wiedl 1993).

Currently, in the sleep medicine literature, mainly the concept of Posner and Rafal (1987) will be used (Keller et al. 1993, Weeß 1997, Weeß et al. 1998a/b).

Also problematic are the very diverse conducted empirical analysis of attention and its components and the varying quality of the validation test procedures and instruments. Thus, inter alia vigilance covered by inappropriate (Stephan et al. 1991), too complex (Bédard et al. 1993) or timely too short (Bédard et al. 1991, 1993) test requirements (Weeß 1997, Weeß et al. 1998a/b).

To capture the tendency to fall asleep in Obstructive Sleep Apnea is conducted usually by the MSLT (Multiple Sleep Latency Test) (Poceta et al. 1992), because it correlated most strongly with the subjective state/mood of OSAS. However, through it the attention and vigilance will be detected only indirectly (Denzel et al. 1993).

For this purpose researched Denzel et al. (1993) for more suitable methods and examined in this context, two computerized neuropsychological test procedures, a vigilance and a attention test, in which the attention test was checked under three experimental conditions (visual, auditory, combined). In both the dual-task-task as well as the vigilance testing was found significant differences before and after nCPAP therapy (Denzel et al. 1993).

Similar results - i.e. a significant improvement of vigilance under nCPAP - were found already by Kesper-Schwarzenberger et al. (1991), Cassel et al. (1991) and George et al. (1997; *DADT*)

As important criteria was found the standardization of experimental conditions (Horn et al. 1983, Denzel et al. 1993) and the design of the experimental setup (the author). Thus showed, inter alia, that an immediate auditory feedback about the correctness improved the occurred reactions improved the motivation of the patients, thereby obscuring the effects of sleep deprivation and their resulting poor performance (Wilkinson 1961, Steyvers & Gaillard 1993, Weeß 1997, Weeß et al. 1998a/b).

3.2 Vigilance test *Carda* (Fig. 5)

The Ambrock vigilance test "Carda" by Randerath et al. (1997) recorded the vigilance performance over a period of 30 minutes. The patient sits in a semi-darkened room in front of a black computer screen and look at the picture of a street with a running road median and the lateral lane boundaries. They are asked to respond within one second of a with a computer keyboard button on stimuli (white flashing rectangles), which occur in time and space for 20 ms randomly. In each 10-minute interval 100 stimuli appearing, in the total period 300 will be shown. After a brief instruction and a short practice the test is started via a menu driven DOS computer program.

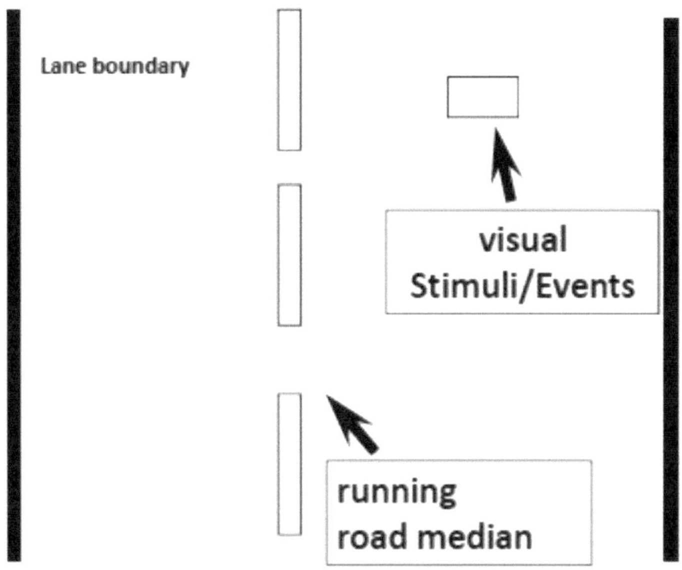

Fig. 5. Driving Simulator *Carda* by Gerdesmeyer et al. 1997, Randerath et al. 1997, 1998

Evaluation

Right and false reactions are calculated in relation to the presented events (in percentage), the latter being registered as an error. The unfounded (delayed) reactions are given in absolute numbers. The age-and gender-independent cut-off value for the error is 5.75% (SD = 11.3%) after a standardization study with healthy volunteers of Randerath and colleagues (2000). For the unfounded responses and response times are currently no cut-off values. Measurements for the reliability and validity are pending.

3.3 Sustained attention test *Carsim* (Fig. 6)

The Ambrock sustained attention test "Carsim" by Büttner et al. (2000a/b, 2001) recorded its performance over a period of 30 minutes. The image with a road median and lane boundary is simulated polychrome. On the right side of the road obstacles (in the kind of no entry signs) can be presented, which are only briefly visible in each case (e.g. for 200 ms). Their appearance is timely random, in which a fixed number of events can be adjusted with a 5-minute section. The patient now has the task to keep up with the help of a steering wheel in his lane the ideal track (*tracking*) and by using of two buttons (both same function), which are located on the steering console, to respond on appearing obstacles (*visual search*).

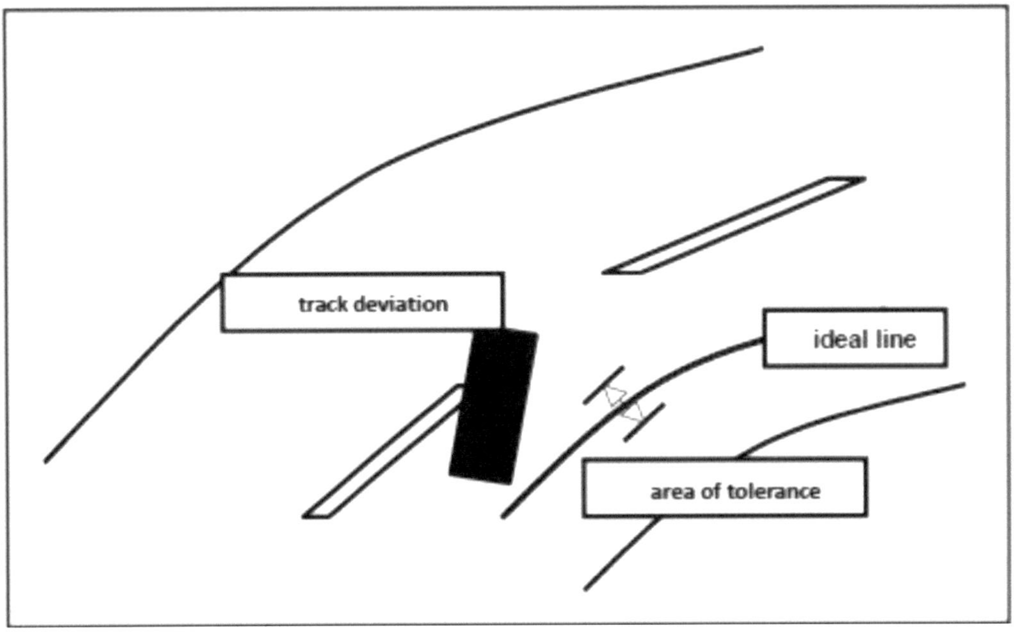

Fig. 6. Driving Simulator *Carsim* by Büttner et al. 1999, 2000

Evaluation

Depending on the steering wheel movements, the position of the vehicle on the road will be recalculated and visualized on-line. The program records the time deviation from the ideal line (*tolerance deviation time*) and of the lane (*tracking deviation time*) and the right, the missing, the unfounded reactions and the reaction time (Büttner et al. 2000a/b, Büttner 2001). Tolerance or track deviation is the number of tracking errors, which in absolute terms described, exceeds the tolerance and lane width in the test. By converting the number of pixels we obtain the time in seconds, which was driven outside the tolerance range or beyond the roadway.

Standardization and quality criteria

The average error of the tracking deviation time was 2.3 ± 4.5 s in the calibration sample, the limit of the track deviations of healthy persons in a 95% confidence interval was < 13.2 s, 98% of healthy individuals have had values between 0 to 150 track deviations. The mean error of tolerance deviation time was 96.0 ± 177.0 s in the healthy person's, the limit of tolerance deviations of the calibration sample in a 95% CI was < 450.4 s (Büttner et al. 2000a/b, Büttner 2001).

The verification of the *reliability* using the *Cronbach alpha* was for the tracking component r = .9785, for the visual search r = .9666 and for the reaction time = .8943. The verification of the *test-retest reliability* (after 3 days) was for the tracking component r_{tt} = .9855, for the visual search r_{tt} = .9447 and for the reaction time r_{tt} = .9211 (Büttner et al. 2000a/b, Büttner 2001).

3.4 Sustained attention test *Quatember & Maly* (Fig. 7)

With the computerized sustained attention "Clock test" of Quatember and Maly (Wiener Testsystem TM, Schufried, Austria 1994; modified for Task force *Vigilance* and *SIESTA group* of DGSM[2]) the sustained attention will be evaluated under monotone conditions and the processing diligence will be measured in the kind of errors and reaction times over a period of 60 minutes. There are two types of errors: missed and incorrect (delayed) responses reactions. Patients are instructed to press a key on the computer keyboard when the "moving point" in a points circle one point skips. At the beginning of the test will be started shortly to introduce the circular arrangement of points. During implementation, the patients sit in a relaxed position ca. 60-80 cm in front of the screen in a semi-darkened room.

Evaluation

The average reaction rate (in milliseconds), the degree of right, incorrect and omitted responses were recorded at Q&M-sustained attention test.Danker-Hopfe, Sauter and Popp (2006) determined in a standardization study with healthy volunteers cut-off values of more than 3 for omitted responses, more than 4 for incorrect responses and longer than 498 milliseconds for the response times of subjects. Standard values for OSAS patients are not yet available.

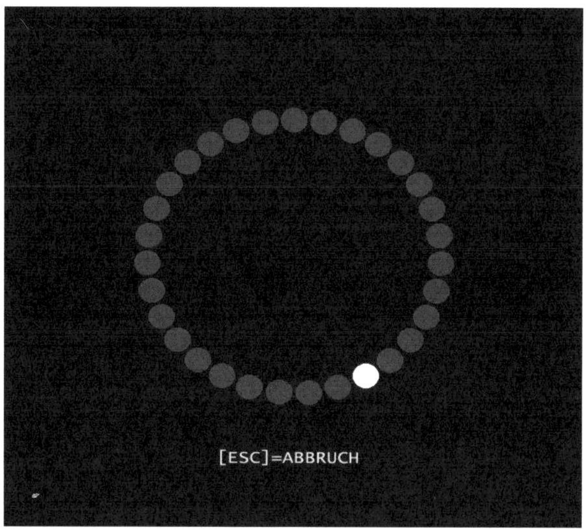

Fig. 7. Sustained attention test by Quatember and Maly (1994)

3.5 Conclusion

The driving simulator *Carda*, similar to the test developed by Findley, does not fulfil the requirements that are important on a real tracking test. It is rather a reaction test, which describes the attention and the vigilance.

Krieger et al. (1997) were able to demonstrate by means of questionnaires that the accident rate in OSAS patients was often caused by sleepiness and that both the rate of accidents and

[2] DGSM = Deutsche Gesellschaft für Schlafforschung und Schlafmedizin (engl.: German Society of Sleep Research and Sleep Medicine)

nearly accidents could be reduced with nCPAP therapy. A test for assessment of accident risk would therefore be helpful.
Findley was found a correlation between the number of accidents and the error rate in a driving simulator test using *Steer Clear* and data's of *Accidents Authority* Virginia/USA. He also had verified a certain connection between accident rate and Sleep Apnea Syndrome and a dependence on the severity of the disease (Findley et al. 1989, 1995, 1999, 2000). Tests of this kind should be used only with great caution on the question of driving ability, because it detected only a few aspects.
Due to the simple construction *Steer Clear* and *Carda* offer also some advantages, because the technical effort is relatively low and even restricted patients can understand the task very well. However, the tests can only evaluate the response to nCPAP treatment in cases with much higher error rate and can control it course.

	Carda	**Carsim**
Monotony	(+)	+++
Continuity	-	++
Interactivity	-	+++
Usability	+++	++

Table 3. Design and properties of the two simulation programs

The severity of sleepiness, as assessed by the ESS, didn't correlate with the results of driving simulators. Sleepiness/drowsiness describes the degree of alertnes and will be influenced by central nervous system activation (Weeß et al. 2000). Because the test situation, the sleepiness is often compensated in moderate limitations (ESS < 13) - in our patients, the ESS score was on average = 11.0 - so that the error rate or track deviation showed no relevant dependence. However, in OSAS patients with profound sleepiness (ESS score > 13) a higher number of errors were found in *Carda* reached a higher (Randerath et al. 2000). Under the testing with *Carsim*, the number of patients who have had a pathological deviation is much higher. The complex task of interactive driving simulation recorded thus patients with reduced performance, special with difficulties in the divided attention and interactive activities. This could be proven, to persons whose driving performance was checked after alcohol administration with a driving simulator. In OSAS capacity was similar limited to persons with a blood alcohol of 95 ± 25 mg/dl (George et al. 1996a).
Studies, which correlate the laboratory results of tracking tests with the real frequency of accidents, are still missing. It would be therefore desirable to obtain objective data on road authorities to characterize better any risk patients with this sensitive instrument. A tracking-driving simulator has a higher reality character than a reaction test, because it realized better the task, i.e. the reflection of driving situation (George 2000). Yet here, too, it is important to be sceptical about its evidence power, because the driving performance is dependent of many factors (e.g. responsible acting), which cannot be detected alone by simulation tests. A driving simulator test should be used only as one of several components in the complex assessment of driving ability.
The interactive driving simulator test *Carsim*, designed by the Ambrock task force, can also be used for further questions: In OSAS patients may be improve due to different treatment modalities several sub-components of attention (such as selective attention, divided

attention, sustained attention, processing speed) (Büttner et al. 2000a/b, Büttner 2001). An interactive driving simulator should reflect several of these changes and should be a more suitable instrument, because tracking tasks reflect more components of the limited capabilities in comparison to reaction tests (*Carda*).
We could demonstrate that an interactive driving simulator (e.g. *Carsim*) describes the disorder of OSAS patients more sensitive. It is used, therefore, specifically in clinical trials for the assessment of treatment effects to attention increase (e.g., nCPAP or theophylline (Büttner et al. 1999 or 2003a, 2004a)).Due the easy use also *Carda* will continue to be a suitable method to detect neuropsychological disorders and demonstrate treatment effects in clinical routine.

4. Memory processes in patients with Sleep Apnea Syndrome

4.1 State of research

Jenkins & Dallenbach (1924) could show for the first time that learning tasks which are presented before sleep could be keep better than tasks that are presented before wakefulness. This was confirmed in other studies (Hennevin et al. 1995, Smith 1996). The discovery of REM sleep (Dement & Kleitman 1957) was the start for a more specific research program in which certain stages of sleep each were assigned specific roles for the memory processes. As follow on one hand, REM sleep, was attributed partly memory-favouring effects because of its particular physiological changes, on the other hand, as well as the Slow Wave Sleep (SWS) was attributed the same effects (Hobson & McCarley 1977, Crick 1983, Wilson & McNaughton, 1994, Karni et al. 1994, Squire & Alvarez 1995).
One of the studies on cognitive deficits in the thinking, memory, communication and the ability to learn new information in OSAS patients comes from Kales (1985). In this study 76% of OSAS patients show cognitive deficits in all these areas. A study by Naëgelé et al. (1995) showed that the executive functions, which are important for the acquisition of information during memory processing in OSAS patients, were impaired.
It is assumed that in sleep disorders the often found reduced sleep quality leads, as a result of Slow Wave Sleep or REM suppression, increased nocturnal arousal responses or prolonged awakenings to a reduced recovery function of night sleep (Weeß et al. 1998a/b). According to Jennum et al. (1993), Insomnia and sleepiness affect cognitive functions. Patients with excessive daytime sleepiness complaints have special problems in situations of physical relaxation and during long monotonous concentration tasks (Schwarzenberger-Kesper et al. 1987).
Cassel et al. (1989) were able to detect in Sleep Apnea patients a reduced cognitive performance and a decreased non-verbal processing speed. In this connection they were able to detect a reduced cognitive processing speed on ZVT in OSAS patients. Also Kotterba et al. (1997) detect in 32 of 40 OSAS patients abnormal results on the ZVT. In another study of Kotterba et al. (1998), they found in OSAS patients an impairment of the central nervous system activation (*alertness*), of the selective attention and of the sustained attention. Barbé et al. (1998) verified in Sleep Apnea patients a decreased vigilance.

4.2 Number-connection test (ZVT)

The number-connection test is composed from four number matrices. Each matrix contains 90 unsorted numbers. It must be connected according to the statement by lines from 1 to 90. For estimating the test processing time, the experimenter uses a stopwatch.

The test is used to measure the basal, all intelligence performances underlying, largely milieu independent and genetically related cognitive performance speed. It corresponds with those ability bundles, which in literature will be called as "*liquid*" intelligence, "*perceptual speed*" or "*processing speed*" are. The test has a wide range of applications. It can apply from 8th years up for all age levels; from the special school to high school and universities (for all levels of education). It is very economical and can be use on an individual or group test. For the processing of the tests the subjects require 5 to 10 minutes (Oswald and Roth, 1987).

The high reliability of the test (test-retest reliability between r_{tt} = .84 and r_{tt} = .97[3]; parallel test reliability between r = .95 and r = .98) is largely independent of age and educational level of the subject. The correlations with various intelligence techniques (PSB, HAWIE, IST-70, RAVEN, CFT-3) are between r = .40 and r = .83. For the individual experiments exist currently standards for 8th to 60th years (n > 2,000), standard values for the group version of the ZVT are available for the age range from 9 to 16 years. The mean of the norm sample (16-60 years) is a **T-value** of 50 ± 10.The Sleep Apnea patients achieved before therapy a T-value of **39.82 ± 10.73**, under a only 3-day-CPAP therapy, there was a significant improvement (T-value: **43.08 ± 10.50**) (Büttner et al. 2007).

4.3 Benton Test

The *Benton Visual Retention Test* is one of the best known and most widely used tests of immediate remembering for visual-spatial stimuli. The test consists of three parallel series, each with 10 geometric stimulus cards. The test person or the patient is shown one stimulus card for a short time (10 seconds), the figure of the card is to be draw directly after showing or after a short delay as accurately as possible. Further testing variations allow a shorter presentation time from 5 seconds, direct copying or simply selecting/choosing of a seen template from four alternatives. The *drawing form* allows evaluating, especially in children, the assessment of the draw ability, whereas the *electing/choosing form* evaluates the memory without the drawing component. The German edition follows the fifth American edition of 1992. It contains a simplified scoring system, additional evaluation examples, advanced standard values and a summary with new findings (Benton test at the onset of dementia). The German Benton also contains, in contrast to the U.S., the election form. The numerous new German-published studies for the Benton test were specifically considered. The test is used in adults until an old age and in children older than 7 years (Benton 1974).

Retest reliability for the *drawing form* is r_{tt} = .85[4]. The relationship between *drawing form* and *electing/choosing form* is relatively low (r = .55). There are numerous studies, especially in the

---

[3] This retest reliability has been verified by the authors of the following sources:

1. http://www.google.de/search?q=cache:5m0-sgoxY1AJ:wt.fb3.uni-wuppertal.de/fachschaft/psychologie/studi_hilfen/files/Hauptstudium/Diagnostik/Zahlen-Verbindungs-Test_(ZVT).doc++reliabilit%C3%A4t+zvt+test+&hl=de&lr=lang_de&ie=UTF-8: (r_{tt} = .81) and
2. http://www.testraum.ch/Serie%204/ZVT.htm: (r_{tt} between .81 and .97).

Learning effects of the ZVT may thus be concluded in clinical trials.

[4] This retest reliability has been verified by the authors of the following sources:

1. http://www.testzentrale.de/tests/t0300401.htm: Retest reliability for the *drawing form* was r_{tt} = .85
2. http://www.unifr.ch/ztd/lernsystem/tb/benton.html#Testentwicklung: Retest reliability for the *drawing forms* C, D and E is given as average of r_{tt} = 0.85.

Learning effects of the Benton test may thus be concluded in clinical trials.

evaluation of brain damage.The mean of **correct reproductions** of the 15-44-year old persons was 8 (IQ score of 95-109). In contrast, the mean of the OSAS patients was **6.76** before therapy (IQ score: 70-79), after a 3-day treatment with nCPAP it was **7.84** (IQ score: 80-94).The mean of **error numbers** of 15-39-year-old persons was three (IQ score of 95-104). The error mean of the study patients was **4.46** before therapy (IQ score: 90-94), after 3-day treatment with nCPAP it was **2.66** (IQ score: 105-109) (Büttner et al. 2007).

4.4 Conclusion

As mentioned above, in several studies could be demonstrated neuropsychological and cognitive deficits in OSAS patients (Bédard et al. 1991, Naëgelé et al. 1995, Gresel et al. 1996, Engleman et al. 2000). This allowed finding inter alia differences between healthy subjects and OSAS patients in the assessment of cognitive processing speed and of performance speed (ZVT) (Cassel et al. 1989, Kotterba et al. 1997, Büttner et al. 2007). Also in the Benton test to record the performance of visual memory the OSAS patients showed - compared with healthy subjects - significantly worse results in the number of errors. None significant results were found for the number of correct reproductions. This may have resulted through the sample composition or sample size. On the other hand, it could be that the increased error number and the nearly normal number of correct responses is a criterion or a feature for the detection of neurocognitive deficits in OSAS patients (Büttner et al. 2007).

Conclusion

It can be said that OSAS patients differ from healthy individuals with respect to cognitive skills. These differences can be verified both the memory processes (Benton) and in cognitive processing speed and performance speed (ZVT). These impairments can have serious consequence, if or as long as they remain untreated.

4.4.1 CPAP therapy and its effect

In various studies improved performance under nCPAP therapy have be determined regarding to changes in neuropsychological parameters and/or test performance. Lamphere et al. (1989) could be shown that after one therapy night there was a significant improvement of the attention, which normalized after 14 days of nCPAP. In several studies it could be detected also a reduction in both subjective and objective daytime sleepiness (Montplaisir et al. 1992, Engleman et al. 1993, 1994, Douglas et al. 2000 - according to Schwarzenberg-Kesper et al. (1987) is the improvement of daytime sleepiness an essential motif for a good therapeutic compliance of the patients). Sforza et al. (1995) found after one year of nCPAP treatment an objectively reduced daytime sleepiness, which increased again after a night of therapy interruption. In several studies could be verified also improved further neuropsychological deficits. Kotterba et al. (1998) reported a significant improvement in the simple attention as well as the divided attention, in the cognitive performance and the processing speed. The latter could be replicated also by Büttner et al. (2007). Even an improvement of vigilance or sustained attention, and various cognitive deficits due to the nCPAP therapy was described many times (Denzel et al. 1993, Engleman et al. 1994, Randerath 1997, 2000, Büttner 1999).

Other studies have shown, however, that the cognitive and neuropsychological deficits don't increase or only improving in certain areas, which could indicate an irreversible hypoxic damage of the CNS (Montplaisir et al. 1992, Bédard et al. 1993, Kotterba et al. 1998) and thus point up the importance of early diagnosis and treatment of OSAS underscores.

Conclusion

The difference or the improvement after effective nCPAP therapy suggests the need to use this therapy in OSAS patients, possibly to avoid serious impairment in the memory processes and in cognitive performance or to allow the patient not to suffer under the daytime consequences of Sleep Apnea Syndrome.

5. Summary

In the western and eastern industrial countries, the number of sleep disturbed subjects increased over the time. Undiagnosed and untreated, sleep disorders caused on one hand often by subjective suffering among those affected individuals and on the other hand, due to decreased attention and increased daytime fatigue or daytime sleepiness, to an increased risk of accidents in road traffic and workplace (e.g. Peter et al. 1995, Gerdesmeyer et al. 1997, Randerath et al. 1997, 1998, Büttner et al. 2000a/b).

Sleep Apnea syndromes are common disorders. 1-5% of the population is affected by it (men are about ten times more affected than women). In particular, patients with OSAS suffer in addition to their symptoms often also on a multitude of sequelae, including excessive daytime sleepiness (Büttner et al. 2004e), vigilance decrease (Büttner et al. 2003b, 2004c) and memory disorders (Büttner et al. 2003c/d).

These performance restrictions or impairments affect the affected subjects, both professionally and in their ability to drive motor vehicles (Findley et al. 1988a/b, 1989b, 1990, 1991, 1995, Mitler et al. In 1988, Cassel et al. 1991a/b, 1993, 1996 , ATS 1994, Gerdesmeyer et al. 1997, Krieger et al. 1997, Randerath et al. 1997, 1998, 2000, Weeß 1997, Weeß et al. 1998a/b, Büttner et al. 2000a/b, Büttner 2001). Consequences of this reduced performance are therefore often accidents or nearly accidents by falling asleep at the wheel. However, other cognitive and mental functions and the quality of life can be affected by sleep disorders (Sleep Apnea Syndrome, Insomnia and/or Narcolepsy).

In summary therefore, can be said that sleep disorders and/or sleep diseases are complex disorders which human beings can affect in his totality and in his whole personality. It can therefore affect all physical, mental and spiritual processes. It can lead to lower physical and mental performances; reduce vigilance, impaired attention and concentration. It can affect the quality of life, reduce, limit and/or prevent social contacts and competencies skills, and cause in other psychiatric[5], neurological[6] and organic[7] diseases.

A detailed sleep diagnostics and possibly therapy of previously known sleep disorders and/or sleep diseases is therefore essential to prevent complications and comorbidities, to prevent treatment resistance with respect to other physical and mental diseases and to provide effective medical treatment.

6. References

[1] American Thoracic Society (ATS), Sleep apnea, sleepiness and driving risk, Am J Respir Crit Care Med, 1994; 150: 1464-1473

---

[5] such as depression, anxiety and panic disorders, conduct disorder, personality disorders

[6] such as stroke, cerebral hemorrhage, dementia and Alzheimer's disease

[7] such as hypertension, heart disease / heart infarction

[2] Arand D.L., Bonnet M.H., Hurwitz T., Mitler M.M., Rosa R., Sangal R.B., The clinical use of the MSLT and MWT, Sleep, 2005; 28: 123-144

[3] Banks S., Barnes M., Tarquinio N., Pierce R.J., Lack L.C., McEvoy R.D., Factors associated with Maintenance of Wakefulness Test mean sleep latency in patients with mild to moderate Obstructive Sleep Apnea and normal subjects, Journal of Sleep Research 2004; 13: 71-78

[4] Barbè F., Pericas J., Munoz A., Findley L., Anto J.M., Agusti A.G.N., Automobile Accidents in Patients with Sleep Apnea Syndrome, Am J Respir Crit Care Med, 1998; 158: 18-22

[5] Bäumler G., Mensch und Maschine: Zur Diagnostik der Dauerüberwachungsfähigkeit, Göttingen: Hogrefe-Verlag, 1974

[6] Bèdard M.A., Montplaisir J., Richer F., Malo J., Nocturnal Hypoxemia as a Determinant of Vigilance Impairment in Sleep Apnea Syndrome, Chest, 1991; 100: 367-370

[7] Bédard M.A., Montplaisir J., Richter F., Malo J., Rouleau I., Persistent neuropsychological deficits and vigilance impairment in sleep apnea syndrome after treatment with continuous positive airway pressure (nCPAP), J Clin Exper Neuropsychol, 1993; 15 (2): 330-341

[8] Benton A.L., Der Benton-Test, Bern/Stuttgart: H. Huber-Verlag, 1974

[9] Bonnet M.H., Effect of Sleep Disruption on Sleep, Performance and Mood, Sleep, 1985; 8 (1): 11-19

[10] Bradley T.D., Rutherford R., Grossman R.F., Lue F., Zamel N., Moldofsky H., Phillipson E.A., Role of daytime hypoxemia in the pathogenesis of right heart failure in the obstructive sleep apnea syndrome, Am Rev Respir Dis, 1985; 131: 835-839

[11] Brickenkamp R., Karl G.A., Geräte zur Messung von Aufmerksamkeit, Konzentration und Vigilanz, in: Brickenkamp R., (Hrsg.), Handbuch apperativer Verfahren in der Psychologie, Göttingen: Hogrefe, 1986, 195-211

[12] Büttner A., Randerath W., Rühle K.-H., Therapieverlaufskontrolle der Daueraufmerksamkeit anhand eines neuen Fahrsimulatortests bei OSAS-Patienten, Somnologie, 3 (Suppl.1); 1999: 10

[13] Büttner A., Randerath W., Rühle K.-H., Der Fahrsimulatortest "carsim" zur Erfassung der Vigilanzminderung von SAS-Patienten. Einfluß verschiedener Faktoren auf die Normwerte, Pneumologie, 2000a; 54: 338-344

[14] Büttner A., Randerath W, Rühle K.-H. Normwerte und Gütekriterien eines interaktiven Fahrsimulators ("carsim"), Somnologie, 2000b; 4: 129-136

[15] Büttner A., Die Messung der Daueraufmerksamkeit bei Patienten mit Schlafapnoe-Syndrom mittels Fahrsimulator. Normierung und klinische Überprüfung, Dissertation, Marburg: Tectum-Verlag, 2001

[16] Büttner A., Rühle K.-H., The Therapeutic Effect of Theophylline on Sustained Attention in Patients with Obstructive Sleep Apnea, Somnologie, 2003a; 7: 23-27

[17] Büttner A., Rühle K.-H., Erfassung von Aufmerksamkeits-Defiziten bei Patienten mit obstruktivem Schlafapnoe-Syndrom mit unterschiedlichen Fahrsimulations-Programmen, Pneumologie, 2003b; 57: 722-728

[18] Büttner A., Alnabary R., Rühle K.-H., Gedächtnisprozesse bei obstruktiver Schlafapnoe vor und unter nCPAP, Somnologie, 2003c; 7 (Suppl.1): 62

[19] Büttner A., Alnabary R, Rühle K.-H., Memory processes of obstructive sleep apnoea patients before and under CPAP therapy, Abstractband der IRS + des ISIAN, 2003d; 104-105
[20] Büttner A., Rühle K.-H., The Therapeutic Effect of Theophylline on the Sustained Attention in Patients with Obstructive Sleep Apnoea under nCPAP-therapy, Traffic Injury Prevention, 2004a; Suppl. CD ICADTS: O-25 (1-6)
[21] Büttner A., Rühle K.-H., Vigilance in case of Sleep Apnea Syndrome, Abstractband der ERS + des ISIAN, 2004b; 215
[22] Büttner, A., Schimanski Ch., Galetke W., Rühle K.-H., Normierung Epworth Sleepiness Scale (ESS), Somnologie, 2004c; 8 (Suppl.1): 63
[23] Büttner A., Alnabary R., Rühle, K.-H., Gedächtnisprozesse bei obstruktivem Schlafapnoe-Syndrom vor und unter nCPAP, Nervenheilkunde, 26 (11), 2007, 1018-1026 (CME 1027-1028)
[24] Büttner A., Schimanski C., Galetke W., Rühle K.-H., Ein Fragebogen zur Erfassung der funktionellen Auswirkungen der Tagesschläfrigkeit auf die Lebensqualität beim obstruktiven Schlafapnoe-Syndrom. Functional Outcomes of Sleep Questionnaire (FOSQ), Pneumologie, 2008; 62 (9): 548-552
[25] Büttner A., The Sleep Apnea Syndrome - more as an illness, Nova Science Publishers: New York, 2009
[26] Carskadon M.J., Dement W.C., Sleep tendency: An objective measure of sleep loss, Sleep Research, 1977; 6: 200
[27] Carskadon M.J., Dement W.C., Mitler M.M., Roth T., Westbrook P.R., Keenan S., Guidelines for the Multiple Sleep Latency Test (MSLT): A standard measure of sleepiness, Sleep, 1986; 9: 519-524
[28] Chua L.W.Y., Yu N.C., Golish J.A., Nelson D.R., Perry M.C., Foldvary N., Dinner D.S., Epworth Sleepiness Scale and the Multiple Sleep Latency Test: Dilemma of the elusive link, Sleep, 1998; 21 (Suppl.): 184.
[29] Cassel W., Stephan S., Ploch T., Peter J.H., Psychologische Aspekte schlafbezogener Atemregulationsstörungen, Pneumologie, 1989; 43: 625-629
[30] Cassel W., Ploch T., Sleep apnea accidents: Health risk for healthy people?, in: Peter J.H., Penzel Th., Podszus T., von Wichert P. (Hrsg.), Sleep and Health Risk, Berlin/Heidelberg/New York: Springer-Verlag, 1991a, 279-285
[31] Cassel W., Ploch T., Peter H.J., v. Wichert P., Unfallgefahr von Patienten mit nächtlichen Atmungsstörungen, Pneumologie, 1991b; 45: 271-275
[32] Cassel W., Ploch T., Schlafbezogene Atmungsstörungen: Unfallgefahr als psychosozialer Risikofaktor, in: Hecht K., Engfer A., Peter H.J., Poppei M. (Hrsg.), Schlaf, Gesundheit, Leistungsfähigkeit, Berlin/Heidelberg/NewYork /London/Paris/ Tokyo/Hong-Kong/Barcelona /Budapest: Springer-Verlag, 1993, 233-242
[33] Cassel W., Ploch T., Becker C., Dugnus D., Peter J.H., v. Wichert P., Risk of traffic accidents in patients with sleep-disordered breathing: Reduction with nasal CPAP, Eur Respir J, 1996; 9: 2606-2611
[34] Colt H.G., Haas H., Rich G.B., Hypoxemia vs Sleep Fragmentation as Cause of Excessive Daytime Sleepiness in Obstructive Sleep Apnea, Chest, 1991; 100: 1542-1548
[35] Crick F., Mitchison G., The function of dream sleep, Nature, 1983; 304: 111-114

[36] Danker-Hopfe H., Binder R., Popp R., Sauter C., Büttner A., Böhning W., Weeß H.-G., Erhebung zur Praxis der Durchführung von Multiplen Schlaflatenztests (MSLT) in akkreditierten Schlaflaboren, Somnologie, 2006; 10 (2): 43-52
[37] Davies R.D., Jones D.M., Taylor A., Selective and sustained-attention tasks: Individual and group differences, in: Parasuraman R., Davies D.R. (Hrsg.), Varieties of Attention, Orlando: Academic, 1984, 395-447
[38] Dement W.C., Kleitman, N., Cyclic variations in EEG during sleep and their relations to eye movements, body motility and dreaming, Electroencephalography and Clinical Neurophysiology, 1957; 9: 673-690
[39] Denzel K., Zimmermann P., Rühle K.-H., Quantitative Untersuchungen zur Erfassung der Tagesmüdigkeit, der Vigilanz und der Aufmerksamkeit vor und nach nCPAP-Therapie bei Schlafapnoesyndrom, Pneumologie, 1993; 47: 155-159
[40] Douglas N.J., Engleman H.M., Effects of CPAP on vigilance and related functions in patients with the sleep apnea/hypopnea syndrome, Sleep, 2000; 23 (Suppl. 4): 147-149
[41] Engleman H.M., Cheshire K.E., Deary I.J., Douglas N.J., Daytime sleepiness, cognitive performance and mood after continuous positive airway pressure for thr sleep apnoea/hypopnoea syndrome, Thorax, 1993; 48: 911-914
[42] Engleman H.M., Martin S.E., Deary I.J., Douglas N.J., Effect of continuous positive airway pressure treatment on daytime function in sleep apnoea/hypopnoea syndrome, Lancet, 1994; 343 (8897): 572-725
[43] Engleman H.M., Martin S.E., Kingshott R.N., Douglas N.J., Cognitive function in the sleep apnea/hypopnea syndrome (SAHS), Sleep, 2000; 23 (Suppl. 4): 102-108
[44] Findley L.J., Barth J.T., Powers D.C., Wilhait S.C., Boyd D.G., Suratt P.M., Cognitive Impairment in Patients with Obstructive Sleep Apnea and Associated Hypoxemia, Chest, 1986; 90: 686-690
[45] Findley L.J., Bonnie R.J., Sleep Apnea and Auto Crashes - What is the Doctor to do?, Chest, 1988a; 94: 225-227
[46] Findley L.J., Unverzagt M.E., Suratt P.M., Automobile accidents involving patients with obstructive sleep apnea, Am Rev Respir Dis, 1988b; 138: 337-340
[47] Findley L.J., Fabrizio M.J., Knight H., Norcross B.B., Laforte A.J., Suratt P.M., Driving simulator performance in patients with sleep apnea, Am Rev Respir Dis, 1989a; 140: 529-530
[48] Findley L.J., Fabrizio M.J., Thommi G., Suratt P.M., Severity of sleep apnea and automobile crashes, New England Journal of Medizin, 1989b; 13: 867-868
[49] Findley L.J., Automobile driving in sleep apnea, in: Issa F.G., Suratt P.M., Remmers J.E. (Hrsg.), Sleep and Respiration, Wiley-Liss, Inc., 1990, 337-345
[50] Findley L.J., Weiss J.W., Jabour E.R., Drivers with Untreated Sleep apnea - A Cause of Death and Serious Injury, Arch Intern Med, 1991; 151: 1451-1452
[51] Findley L.J., Unverzagt M., Guchu R., Fabrizio M., Buckner J., Suratt P., Vigilance and automobile accidents in patients with sleep apnea or narcolepsy, Chest, 1995; 108: 619-624
[52] Findley L.J., Suratt P.M., Dinges D.F., Time-on-Task Decrements in "Steer Clear" Performance of Patients With Sleep Apnea and Narcolepsy, Sleep, 1999; 22 (6): 804-809

[53] Findley L.J., Smith C., Hooper J., Dineem M., Suratt P.M., Treatment with nasal CPAP decreases automobile accidents in patients with sleep apnea, Am J Respir Crit Care Med, 2000; 161: 857-859
[54] George C.F.P., Nickerson P., Hanly P., Miller T., Kryger M., Sleep apnea patients have more automobile accidents (letter), Lancet, 1987; 1: 447
[55] George C.F.P., Boudreau A.C., Smiley A., Simulated driving performance in patients with obstructive sleep apnea, Am J Respir Crit Care Med, 1996a; 154: 175-181
[56] George C.F.P., Boudreau A.C., Smiley A., Comparison of simulated driving perfomance in narcolepsy and sleep apnea patients, Sleep, 1996b; 19 (9): 711-717
[57] George C.F.P., Boudreau A.C., Smiley A., Effects of nasal CPAP on simulated driving performance in patients with obstructive sleep apnea, Thorax, 1997; 52: 648-653
[58] George C.F.P., Smiley A., Sleep Apnea, Automobile Crashes, Sleep, 1999; 22 (6): 790-795
[59] George C.F.P., Vigilance Impairment, Assesment by Driving Simulators, Sleep, 2000; 23 (Suppl. 4): 115-118
[60] Gerdesmeyer C., Randerath W., Rühle K.-H., Zeitliche Abhängigkeit der Fehlerzahl bei Messung der Daueraufmerksamkeit mittels Fahrsimulator vor und nach nCPAP-Therapie bei Schlafapnoesyndrom, Somnologie, 1997; 1: 165-170
[61] Greenberg G.D., Watson, R.K., Deptula, D., Neuropsychological Dysfunction in Sleep Apnea, Sleep, 1987; 10 (3): 254-262
[62] Gresele C., Hein H., Eggert F., Beurteilung der Aufmerksamkeitsparameter bei Schlafapnoe-Patienten, Wien Med Wochenschr, 1996; 146 (13-14): 344-345
[63] Guilleminault C., van den Hoed J., Mitler M.M., Clinical overview of the Sleep Apnea Syndromes, in: Guilleminault C., Dement W.C. (Hrsg.), Sleep Apnea Syndromes, New York, Liss., 1978, 1-12
[64] Guilleminault C., Partinen M., Quera-Salva M.A., Hayes B., Dement W.C., Nino-Murcia G., Determinants of Daytime Sleepiness in Obstructive Sleep Apnea, Chest, 1988; 94: 32-37
[65] Guilleminault C., Mignot E., Partinen M., Controversies in the diagnosis of Narcolepsy. Sleep 1994; 17: 1-6
[66] Harnatt J., Kortikale Aktivierung von Daueraufmerksamkeit, Psych Beitr, 1975; 17: 188-210
[67] Hartse K.M., Roth T., Zorick F.J., Daytime sleepiness and daytime wakefulness: The effect of instruction, Sleep, 1982; 5: 107-118
[68] He J., Kryger M.H., Zorick F.J., Conway W., Roth Th., Mortality and apnea index in obstructive sleep apnea. Experience in 385 male patients, Chest, 1988; 94: 9-14
[69] Hennevin E., Hars B., Maho C., Bloch, V., Processing of learned information in paradoxical sleep: Relevanz for memory, Behavioural Brain Research, 1995; 69: 125-135
[70] Hildebrandt G., Rehmert W., Rutenfranz,J., Twelve- and 24-h rhythms in error frequency of locomotive drivers and the influence of tiredness, Int J Chronobiol, 1974; 2: 175-180
[71] Hildebrandt G., Chronobiologische Grundlagen der Leistungsfähigkeit und Chronohygiene, in: Hildebrandt G. (Hrsg.), Biologische Rhythmen und Arbeit, Wien/New York: Springer-Verlag, 1976, 1-19

[72] Hobson J.A., McCarley R.W., The brain as a dream state generator: An activation - synthesis hypothesis of the dream process, American Journal of Psychiatry, 1977; 134: 1335-1348
[73] Hoddes E., Zarcone V., Smythe H., Phillipps R., Dement W.C., Quantification of sleepiness: A new approach, Psychophysiology, 1973; 10: 431-436
[74] Horn J.A., Anderson N.R., Wilkinson R.T., Effects of sleep deprivation on signal detection measures of vigilance. Implications for sleep function, Sleep, 1983; 6: 347-358
[75] Horne J.A., Reyner L.A., Driver sleepiness, J Sleep Res, 1995; 4 (Suppl. 2): 23-29
[76] Horstmann S., Hess C.W., Bassetti C., Gugger M., Mathis J., Sleepiness-related accidents in Sleep Apnea patients, Sleep, 2000; 23: 383-389
[77] Ingram F., Henke K.G., Levin H.S., Ingram P.T., Kuna S.T., Sleep Apnea and Vigilance Performance in a Community-Dwelling Older Sample, Sleep, 1994; 17 (3): 248-252
[78] James W., Principles of Psychology, New York, 1890
[79] Jenkins J.C., Dallenbach K.M., Obliviscence during sleep and waking, American Journal of Psychology, 1924; 35: 605-612
[80] Jennum P., Hein HO., Suadicani P., Gyntelberg F., Cognitive Function and Snoring, Sleep, 1993; 16 (8): 62-64
[81] Johns M.W., A new method of measuring daytime sleepiness: The Epworth Sleepiness Scale, Sleep, 1991; 14: 540-545
[82] Johns M.W., Reliability and factor analysis of Epworth Sleepiness Scale, Sleep, 1992; 15: 376-381
[83] Johns M.W. et al., Daytime Sleepiness, Snoring and Obstructive Sleep Apnea. The Epworth Sleepiness Scale, Chest, 1993; 103: 30-36
[84] Johns M.W., Sleepiness in different situations measured by the Epworth Sleepiness Scale, Sleep, 1994; 17: 703-710
[85] Johns M.W., Hocking B., Daytime sleepiness and sleep habits of Australian workers, Sleep, 1997; 20: 844-849
[86] Johns M.W., Rethinking the assessment of sleepiness, Sleep Medicine Review, 1998; 2: 3-15
[87] Johns M.W., Sensitivity and specificity of the Multiple Sleep Latency Test (MSLT), the Maintenance of Wakefulness Test and the Epworth Sleepiness Scale: Failure of the MSLT as a gold standard, Journal of Sleep Research, 2000; 9: 5-11
[88] Johnson L.C., Sleep Deprivation and Performance, in: Webb W.B. (Hrsg.), Biological Rhythms, Sleep and Performance, New York, Wiley, Sons Ltd, 1982, 111-142
[89] Kales A., Caldwell A.B., Cadieux R.J., Vela-Bueno A., Ruch L.G., Mayes S.D., Severe Obstructive Sleep Apnea - II: Associated Psychopathology and Psychological Consequences, J. Chron Dis, 1985; 38 (5): 427-434
[90] Karni A., Tanne D., Rubenstein B.S., Askenasy J.J.M., Sagi D., Dependence on REM sleep of overnight improvement of a perceptual skill, Science, 1994; 265: 679-681
[91] Keller I., Grömminger O., Aufmerksamkeit, in: v. Cramon D. I., Mai N., Ziegler W. (Hrsg.), Neuropsychologische Diagnostik, Weinheim/Basel/Cambridge /New York/Tokio: VCH-Verlag, 1993, 65-90
[92] Kotterba S., Widdig W., Duscha C., Rasche K., Ereigniskorrelierte Potentiale und neuropsychologische Untersuchungen bei Schlafapnoepatienten. Pneumologie, 1997; 51: 712-715

[93] Kotterba S., Rasche K., Widdig W., Duscha C., Blombach S., Schultze-Werninghaus G., Malin JP., Neuropsychological investigations and event-related potentials in obstructive sleep apnea syndrome before and during CPAP-therapy, Journal of the Neurological Sciences, 1998; 159: 45-50
[94] Kotterba S., Orth M., Happe S., Mayer G., Begutachtung der Tagesschläfrigkeit bei neurologischen Erkrankungen und bei dem Obstruktiven Schlafapnoe-Syndrom, Nervenarzt, 2007; 78: 861-870
[95] Kribbs N.B., Getsy J.E., Dinges D.F., Investigation and management of daytime sleepiness in sleep apnea, in: Saunder N.A., Sullivan C.E. (Hrsg.), Sleeping and Breathing 2, New York: M. Dekker Edition, 1993a, 575-604
[96] Kribbs N.B., Pack A.L., Kline L.R., Getsy J.E., Schuett J.S., Henry J.N., Maislin G., Dinges D.F., Effects of one night without nasal CPAP treatment on sleep and sleepiness in patients with obstructive sleep apnea, Am Rev Despir Dis, 1993b; 147: 1162-1168
[97] Krieger J., Meslier N., Lebrun T., Levy P., Phillip-Joet F., Sailly J.C., Racineux J.J., Accidents in obstructive sleep apnea patients treated with nasal continuous positive airway pressure. A prospective study, Chest, 1997; 112: 1561-1566
[98] Lamphere J., Roehrs T., Wittig R., Zorick F., Conway W.A., Roth T., Recovery of alertness after CPAP in apnea, Chest, 1989; 96: 1364-1367
[99] Langlois P.H., Smolensky M.H., Hsi B.P., Weir F.W., Temporal patterns of reported single-vehicle car and truck accidents in Texas, U.S.A. during 1980-1983, Chronobiol Int, 1985; 2 (2): 131-140
[100] LLoberes P., Levy G., Descals C., Sampol G., Roca A., Sagales T. et al., Self-reported sleepiness while driving as a risk factor for traffic accidents in patients with Obstructive Sleep Apnea Syndrome and in non-apnoeic snorers, Respiratory Medicine, 2000; 94: 971-976
[101] Löwenstein O., Feinberg R., Löwenfeld I.E., Pupillary movements during acute and chronic fatigue, Investigative Ophthalmology & Visual Science, 1963; 2: 138-157
[102] Lund R., Diagnose und Therapie von Atemregulationsstörungen, in: Kemper J., Zulley J. (Hrsg.), Gestörter Schlaf im Alter, München: MMV-Verlag, 1994
[103] Mackworth J.F., Effect of amphetamine on the delectability of signals in a vigilance task, Canad J Psychol, 1956; 19: 104-110
[104] Mackworth N.H., The breakdown of vigilance during prolonged visual search, Quarterly Journal of Experimental Psychology, 1948; 1: 6-21
[105] Mackworth N.H., The breakdown of vigilance during prolonged visual search, Q J Exp Psychol, 1958; 1: 6-21
[106] Martin S.E., Engleman H.M., Deary I.J., Douglas N.J., The effect of sleep fragmentation on daytime function, Am J Respir Crit Care Med, 1996; 153: 1328-1332
[107] McNicholas W.T., Sleep apnoea and driving risk, Eur Respir J, 1999; 13: 1225-1227
[108] Meyer M., Ermüdungsbedingte Fahruntüchtigkeit von Berufskraftfahrern, Archiv für Kriminologie, Vol. 185, 1990, 64-79
[109] Mitler M.M., Gujavarty K.S., Brownman C.P., Maintenance of Wakefulness Test, Sleep, 1982; 28: 113-121
[110] Mitler M.M., Carskadon M., Czeiler C., Dement W., Dinges D., Graeber R., Catastrophes, Sleep and public policy: consensus report, Sleep, 1988; 11: 100-109

[111] Mitler M.M., Two peak 24-hour pattern in sleep, mortality and error, in: Peter J.H., Penzel T., Podszus T., von Wichert P. (Hrsg.), Sleep and health risk, Berlin/Heidelberg/ New York: Springer, 1991, 65-77
[112] Mitler M.M., Walsleben J.A., Sangal R.B., Hirshkowitz M., Sleep latency on the Maintenance of Wakefulness Test (MWT) for 530 patients with Sleep Narcolepsy while free of psychoactive drugs, Electroencephalography and Clinical Neurophysiology, 1998; 107: 33-38
[113] Montplaisir J., Bèdard MA., Richer F., Rouleau I., Neurobehavioral Manifestations in Obstructive Sleep Apnea Syndrome Before and After Treatment with Continuous Positive Airway Pressure, Sleep, 1992; 15 (6): 17-19
[114] Müller T.H., Paterok B., Hoffmann M.R., Becker-Carus C., Auswirkungen chronischer Schlafrestriktion auf Leistungsfähigkeit, Stimmung und Müdigkeit, Somnologie, 1997; 2: 65-73
[115] Naègele B., Thouvard V., Pèpin J.L., Lèvy P., Bonnet C., Perret JE., Pellat J., Feuerstein C., Deficits of cognitive Executive Functions in Patients With Sleep Apnea Syndrome, Sleep, 1995; 18 (1): 43-52
[116] Norman D.A., Aufmerksamkeit und Gedächtnis, Weinheim: Beltz-Verlag, 1973
[117] Oswald W.D., Roth E., Der Zahlen-Verbindungs-Test (ZVT), Göttingen/Toronto/Zürich: Hogrefe-Verlag, 1987
[118] Peter J.H., Obstruktive Schlafapnoe und obstruktives Schnarchen, in: Peter J.H., Köhler D., Knab B., Mayer G., Penzel T., Raschke F., Zulley J. (Hrsg.), Weißbuch Schlafmedizin, Regensburg: S. Roderer-Verlag, 1995, 58-61
[119] Peter J.H., Köhler D., Knab B., Mayer G., Penzel T., Raschke F., Zulley J., Einleitung, in: Peter J.H., Köhler D., Knab B., Mayer G., Penzel T., Raschke F., Zulley J. (Hrsg.), Weißbuch Schlafmedizin, Regensburg: S. Roderer-Verlag, 1995, 1-2
[120] Philip P., Mitler M., Sleepiness at the wheel: Symptom or behavior?, Sleep, 2000; 23 (Suppl. 4): 119-121
[121] Poceta J.St., Timms R.M., Jeong D.U., Swui-Ling H., Erman M.K., Mitler M.M., Maintenance of Wakefulness Test in obstructive sleep apnea syndrome, Chest, 1992; 101: 893-897
[122] Podszus T., Bauer W., Mayer J., Penzel T., Peter J.H., von Wichert P., Sleep apnea and pulmonary hypertension, Klin Wochenschr, 1986; 64: 131-134
[123] Posner M.I., Rafal R., Cognitive theories of attention and the rehabilitation of attentional deficits, in: Meier M., Benton A., Diller L. (Hrsg.), Neuropsychological Rehabilitation, Edinburgh: Churchil Livingstone Press, 1987, 182-201
[124] Posner M.I., Petersen S.E., The attention system of the human brain, Ann Rev Neurosciences, 1990; 13: 25-42
[125] Posner M.I., Attention in Cognitive Neuroscience. An Overview, in: Gazzaniga M.S. (Hrsg.), The Cognitive Neurosciences, Cambridge: A Bradford Book, 1995, 615-625
[126] Prokop O., Prokop L., Ermüdung und Einschlafen am Steuer, Dtsch Z Gerichtl Med, 1955; 44: 343-355
[127] Rahm L., Psychologische Aspekte von Schlafproblemen, Bern/Berlin /Frankfurt a.M./New York/Paris/Wien: P. Lang-Verlag, 1994
[128] Randerath W., Gerdesmeyer C., Ströhlein G., Rühle K.-H., Messung der Vigilanz mittels Fahrsimulator vor und nach nCPAP - Vergleich zweier

Simulationsprogramme mit unterschiedlicher Ereignishäufigkeit, Somnologie, 1997; 1: 110-114
[129] Randerath W., Siller C., Gil G., Rühle K.-H., Fahrsimulatortest zur Erfassung der Daueraufmerksamkeit - Untersuchung bei Normalpersonen und bei Patienten mit obstruktiven Schlafapnoe-Syndrom vor und nach Therapie, Klinik Ambrock Hagen, 1998
[130] Randerath W., Gerdesmeyer C., Siller C., Gil G., Sanner B., Rühle K.-H., A test for the determination of sustained attention in patients with obstructive sleep apnea syndrome, Respiration, 2000; 67: 526-532
[131] Rapp G., Aufmerksamkeit und Konzentration, Erklärungsmodelle - Störungen - Handlungsmöglichkeiten, Bad Heilbrunn/Obb.: Klinkhardt-Verlag, 1982
[132] Rechtschaffen A., Kales A. A manual of standardized terminology, techniques and scoring Institutes system for sleep stages of human subjects. National of Health Publication, No. 204, 1968
[133] Richardson G.S., Carskadon M.A., Orav E.J., Dement W.C., Circadian variation of sleep tendency in elderly and young adult subjects, Sleep, 1982; 5: 82-94
[134] Roehrs T., Zoricks F., Wittig R., Conway W., Roth T., Predictors of objective level of daytime sleepiness in patients with sleep-related breathing disorders, Chest, 1989; 95: 1202-1206
[135] Roehrs T., Merrion M., Pedrosi B., Stepanski E., Zorick F., Roth T., Neuropsychological Function in Obstructive Sleep Apnea Syndrome (OSAS) Compared to Chronic Pulmonary Disease (COPD), Sleep, 1995; 18 (5): 382-388
[136] Rollet B., Die integrativen Leistungen des Gehirns und Konzentration: Theoretische Grundlagen und Interventionsprogramme, in: Klauer K.J. (Hrsg.), Kognitives Training, Göttingen: Hogrefe-Verlag, 1993, 257-272
[137] Rühle K.-H., Feier C., Galetke W., Büttner A., Nilius G., Analyse der 8 Fragen (Items) der Epworth Sleepiness Scale, Somnologie, 2005; 9: 154-158
[138] Rühle K.-H., Nilius G., Mamedova N., Ein Lese-Test zur Erfassung der Tagesschläfrigkeit beim obstruktiven Schlafapnoesyndrom. Eine Pilotuntersuchung, Somnologie, 2007, 11 (2), 132-138
[139] Rützel E., Aufmerksamkeit, in: Hermann T., (Hrsg.), Handbuch psychologischer Grundbegriffe, 1977, 49-58
[140] Sangal R.B., Thomas L., Mitler M.M., Maintenance of Wakefulness Test and Multiple Sleep Latency Test. Measurement of different abilities in patients with sleep disorders, Ches,t 1992; 101: 898-902
[141] Sangal R.B., Mitler M.M., Sangal J.A.M., US modafinil in Narcolepsy multicenter study group. MSLT, MWT and ESS. Indices of sleep in 522 drug-free patients with Narcolepsy, Sleep Research, 1997a; 26: 492
[142] Sangal R.B., Sangal J.M., Belisle C., MWT and ESS measure different abilities in 41 patients with snoring and daytime sleepiness, Sleep Research, 1997b; 26: 493
[143] Sanner B., Sturm A., Konermann M., Koronare Herzkrankheit bei Patienten mit obstruktiver Schlafapnoe, Dtsch Med Wochenschr, 1996; 121 (30): 931-935
[144] Säring W., Aufmerksamkeit, in: v. Cramon D., Zihl J., (Hrsg.), Neuropsychologische Rehabilitation, Berlin: Springer-Verlag, 1988, 157-181
[145] Schmidtke H., Die Ermüdung, Bern/Stuttgart: H. Huber-Verlag, 1965

[146] Schmöttke H., Wiedl K.H., Neuropsychologisches Aufmerksamkeitstraining in der Rehabilitation von Hirnorganikern, in: Klauer K.J. (Hrsg.), Kognitives Training, Göttingen: Hogrefe-Verlag, 1993, 273-298

[147] Schwarzenberger-Kesper F., Becker H., Penzel T., Peter J.H., Weber K., von Wichert P., Die exzessive Einschlafneigung am Tage (EDS) beim Apnoe-Patienten . Diagnostische Bedeutung und Objektivierung mittels Vigilanztest und synchroner EEG-Registrierung am Tage, Prax Klin Pneumol, 1987; 41: 401-405

[148] Sharma H., Sharma S.K., Overview and implications of Obstructive Sleep Apnea, The Indian Journal of Chest Diseases und Allied Sciences, 2008; 50: 137-150

[149] Seko Y., Kataoka S., Senoo T., Analysis of driving behaviour under a state of reduced alertness, Int J Vehicle Design (Spec. Issue on vehicle safety), 1986; 318-330

[150] Sforza E., Lugaresi E., Daytime sleepiness and nasal continuous positive airway pressure therapy in obstructive sleep apnea syndrome patients: effects of chronic treatment and 1-night therapy withdrawal, Sleep, 1995; 18 (3): 195-201

[151] Shreter R., Peled R., Pillar G., The 20-min trial of the Maintenance of Wakefulness Test is profoundly affected by motivation, Sleep Breathing, 2006; 10: 173-179

[152] Smith C., Sleep stages, memory processes and synaptic plasticity, Behavioural Brain Research, 1996; 78: 49-56

[153] Squire L.R., Alvarez P., Retrograde amnesia and memory consolidation: A neurobiological perspektive, Current Opinion in Neurobiology, 1995; 5: 169-177

[154] Stephan S., Cassel W., Schwarzenberger-Kesper F., Fett I., Psychological Problems Correlated with Sleep Apnea, in: Peter J.H., Penzel T., Podszus T., v. Wichert P. (Hrsg.), Sleep and Health Risk, Heidelberg: Springer-Verlag, 1991, 167-173

[155] Steyvers F.J.J.M., Gaillard A.W.K., The effects of sleep deprivation and incentives of human performance, Psychol Res, 1993; 55: 64-70

[156] Stoohs R.A., Guilleminault, C., Itoi, A., Dement W.C., Traffic Accidents in Commercial Long-Haul Truck Drivers: The Influence of Sleep-Disordered Breathing and Obesity, Sleep, 1994; 17 (7): 619-623

[157] Stoohs R.A., Bingha, L.A., Ito, A., Guilleminaul, C., Demen, W.C., Sleep and Sleep Disordered Breathing in Commercial Long-Haul Truck Drivers, Chest, 1995; 107: 1275-1282

[158] Stradling J.R., Obstructive sleep apnoea and driving, BMJ, 1989; 298: 904-905

[159] Sturm W., Zimmerman P., Aufmerksamkeitsstörungen, in: Sturm W., Herrmann M., Wallesch C.-W. (Hrsg.). Lehrbuch der klinischen Neuropsychologie. Lisse (NL): Swets & Zeitlinger, 2000, 345-365

[160] Sturm W., Büssing A., Normierungs- und Reliabilitätsuntersuchungen zum Vigilanzgerät nach Quatember und Maly, Diagnostica 1990; Bd. 36, 1 (1) [zitiert nach Schuhfried 1993]

[161] Telakivi T., Kajaste S., Partinen M., Koskenvuo M., Salmi T., Kaprio J., Cognitive Function in Middle-aged Snorers and Controls: Role of Excessive Daytime Somnolence and Sleep-Related Hypoxic Events, Sleep, 1988; 11 (5): 454-462

[162] Terán-Santos J., Jimenez-Gomez A., Cordero-Guevara J., The association between Sleep Apnea and the risk of traffic accidents, New England Journal of Medicine, 1999; 340: 847-851

[163] Thorpy M.J., The clinical use of the Multiple Sleep Latency Test, Sleep, 1992; 1: 268-276.

[164] van den Hoed J., Kraemer H., Guilleminault C., Zarcone V.P., Miles L.E., Dement W.C., Disorders of excessive somnolence: Polygraphic and clinical date for 100 patients, Sleep, 1981; 4: 23-37
[165] Walsleben J.A., The measurement of daytime wakefulness, Chest, 1992; 101: 890-891
[166] Weeß H.-G., Schläfrigkeit und sozialmedizinisches Risiko. Theorethische Grundlagen, Arbeitspapier des Schlaflabors Pfalzklinik Landeck, 30.01.97
[167] Weeß H.-G., Lund R., Gresele C., Böhning W., Sauter C., Steinberg R., AG Vigilanz der DGSM, Vigilanz, Einschlafneigung, Daueraufmerksamkeit, Müdigkeit, Schläfrigkeit. Die Messung müdigkeitsbezogener Prozesse bei Hypersomnien-Theoretische Grundlage, Somnologie, 1998a; 2: 32-34
[168] Weeß H.-G., Lund R., Gresele C., Böhning W., Sauter C., Steinberg R., Vigilanz, Einschlafneigung, Daueraufmerksamkeit, Müdigkeit, Schläfrigkeit: Die Messung müdigkeitsbezogener Prozesse bei Hypersomnien, Somnologie, 1998b; 2: 32-41
[169] Weeß H.-G., Sauter C., Geißler P., Böhning W., Wilhelm B., Rotte M. et al., Vigilanz, Einschlafneigung, Daueraufmerksamkeit, Müdigkeit, Schläfrigkeit - Diagnostische Instrumentarien zur Messung müdigkeits- und schläfrigkeitsbedingter Prozesse und deren Gütekriterien, Somnologie 2000; 4: 20-38
[170] Weeß, H.-G., Tagesschläfrigkeit, Internet: 2011, http://www.pfalzklinikum.de/fileadmin/pfalzklinikum/Dokumente/Handbuch _Schlafmedizin_Diagnostik_Tagesschl__frigkeit.pdf
[171] Wilhelm B., Rühle K.-H., Widmaier D., Lüdtke H., Wilhelm H., Objektivierung und Schweregrad und Therapieerfolg beim Obstruktiven Schlafapnoesyndrom mit dem Pupillographischen Schläfrigkeitstest, Somnologie, 1998; 2: 51-57
[172] Wilhelm B., Körner A., Heldmaier K., Moll K., Wilhelm H., Lüdtke H., Normwerte des Pupillographischen Schläfrigkeitstests für Frauen und Männer zwischen 20 und 60 Jahren, Somnologie, 2001; 5: 115-120
[173] Wilkinson R.T., Interaction of lack of sleep with knowledge of results, repeatet testing and individual differences, J Exp Psychol, 1961; 62: 263-271
[174] Wilson M.A., McNaughton B.L., Reactivation of hippocampal ensemble memories during sleep episodes, Science, 1994; 265: 676-679
[175] Wu H., Yan-Go F., Self-reported automobile accidents involving patients with Obstructive Sleep Apnea, Neurology, 1996; 46: 1254-1257
[176] Yoss R.E., Moyer N.J., Hollenhorst R.W., Pupil size and spontaneous pupillary waves associated with alertness, drowsiness and sleep, Neurology, 1970; 20: 545-554
[177] Young T., Blustein J., Finn, L., Palta M., Sleepiness, Driving, Accidents: Sleep-Disordered Breathing and Motor Vehicle Accidents in a Population-Based Sample of Employed Adults, Sleep, 1997; 20 (8): 608-613
[178] Zimmermann P., Fimm B., Testbatterie zur Aufmerksamkeitsprüfung (TAP), Herzogenrath: Psytest, 1994
[179] Zulley J., Crönlein T., Hell W., Langwieder K., Einschlafen am Steuer: Hauptursache schwerer Verkehrsunfälle, Wien Med Wochenschr, 1995; 17/18: 473
[180] Zwyghuizen-Doorenbos A., Roehrs T., Schaefer M., Roth T., Test-retest reliability of the MSLT, Sleep, 1988; 16: 562-565

10

Parasomnias

F. Gokben Hizli and Nevzat Tarhan
Uskudar University
Turkey

1. Introduction

Sleep is a vital physiological process with important restorative functions. Parasomnias are characterized by undesirable physical or verbal behaviors, such as walking or talking during sleep and occur in association with sleep, specific stages of sleep or sleep-wake transitions. The category of parasomnias comprises some of the most exceptional behavior disorders because complex and apparently purposeful, goal-directed behavior is associated with a deep sleeping brain. Parasomnias occur during REM sleep, any of the four stages of non-REM sleep, and during transitions between sleep and wakefulness. Sleepwalking, sleep terrors, and confusional arousals are associated with non-REM sleep, nightmares and sleep paralysis are associated with REM sleep, while sleep starts and sleep talking are associated with sleep-wake transitions. Sleep enuresis has been observed with all sleep types.

The International Classification of Sleep Disorders subdivides parasomnias into the following four groups (Table 1): Arousal disorders, sleep-wake transition disorders, rapid eye movement (REM) stage sleep parasomnias, and other parasomnias (American academy of Sleep Medicine, 2004).

When accompanied with excessive motor activity and other complex motor behaviors, these parasomnias may significantly affect the patient's quality of life and that of the bed partner. Motor behaviors may or may not be restricted to bed but can become dangerous when the subject ambulates or is agitated. The behaviors are inappropriate for the time of occurrence but may seem purposeful or goal directed. Therefore, appropriate diagnostic and therapeutic strategies are needed (Young, 2008).

2. Causes of parasomnias

Parasomnias occur due to abnormal transitions between the three primary states of being wake, rapid eye movement (REM) sleep, and non rapid eye movement (NREM) sleep. These different states may overlap or intrude into one another, and it is the overlap of wakefulness and NREM sleep that gives rise to confusional arousals, and the intrusion of REM sleep into waking that produces REM sleep behaviour disorder (Matwiyoff et al, 2010).

Parasomnias may have genetic basis, but occurrence is usually triggered by heavy physical activity, febrile illness, sleep deprivation, excessive caffeine drinks, hypnotics, and emotional stress. Intake of alcohol increased occurrence of confusional arousal, night terror, and sleepwalking, while heavy intake of caffeinated drink increased occurrence of sleep walking in a population study (Oluwole, 2010).

Arousal disorders
Confusional arousals Sleepwalking Sleep terrors
Sleep-wake transition disorders
Rhythmic movement disorder Sleep starts Sleep-talking Nocturnal leg cramps
Parasomnias usually associated with REM sleep
Nightmares Sleep paralysis Impaired sleep-related penile erections Sleep-related painful erections REM sleep sinus arrest REM sleep behavior disorder
Other parasomnias
Sleep bruxism Sleep enuresis Sleep-related abnormal swallowing syndrome Nocturnal paroxysmal dystonia Sudden unexplained nocturnal death syndrome Primary snoring Infant sleep apnea Congenital central hypoventilation syndrome Sudden infant death syndrome Benign neonatal sleep myoclonus

Table 1. The International Classification of Sleep Disorders classification of parasomnias

Heredity was described for many forms of parasomnias but detailed genetic studies are lacking. The composition of non-REM and REM sleep was shown to have genetic roots. Especially the amount of slow-wave sleep was recently shown to be genetically predisposed by a specific gene, the retinoid acid receptor beta encoding gene (Young, 2008; Maret et al., 2005).

3. Diagnosis of parasomnias

All parasomnias more commonly affect persons who have breathing disorders during sleep. Polysomnography is appropriate for any patient with symptoms or signs of obstructive sleep apnea, such as daytime hypersomnolence, nocturnal hypoxia, loud snoring and increased neck circumference. REM behavior disorder often occurs concomitantly with degenerative neurologic illnesses that may require further evaluation. In adults, the onset of arousal disorders such as somnambulism and night terrors may reflect underlying neurologic disease. Thus, neurologic evaluation, including imaging of the central nervous system, may be indicated (Bornemann et al., 2006).

Diagnosis of parasomnias relies on a comprehensive clinical evaluation. Additional testing with polysomnogram and time-synchronized video recording may be indicated for cases that are associated with very frequent episodes, complaints of excessive sleepiness, unusual presentation, or injury to the individual or bed partner. A formal laboratory sleep study or polysomnogram with an expanded electroencephalographic montage can help distinguish among non-REM and REM parasomnias and nocturnal seizures. The latter may manifest clinically as arousals from sleep associated with vocalization and/or complex behaviours (Farid et al., 2004).

4. Epidemiology

Generally parasomnias, particularly those that are associated with non-REM sleep are commoner in childhood, but studies showed that non- REM parasomnias are not uncommon in adults. Parasomnias have been reported in approximately 4% of the adult population (Ohayon et al., 2000).

Prevalence of sleepwalking, which consists of a series of complex behaviours that are initiated during slow wave sleep and result in walking during sleep, varies from 10 per 1,000 to 145 per 1,000. In a population of adults prevalence of sleep walking was 20 per 1,000 (Guilleminault et al., 2003).

Sleep terrors, which are characterized by sudden arousal from slow wave sleep with a piercing scream or cry, accompanied by autonomic and behavioral manifestations of intense fear, are a common parasomnia in childhood. Its prevalence in children varies from 30% to 398 per 1,000, but prevalence of 22 per 1,000 was found in an adult population (Kales et al., 1980).

Nightmares are frightening dreams that usually awaken the sleeper from REM sleep. Between 10 and 20% of children experience nightmares that disturb their parents while 50% of adults have occasional nightmares and 1% have one or more nightmares per week.

Sleep paralysis consists of a period of inability to perform voluntary movements at sleep onset, hypnagogic or predormital form, or upon awakening, either during the night or in the morning, hypnopompic or postdormital. Lifetime prevalence of isolated sleep paralysis in the general population in Germany and Italy was shown to be 62 per 1,000.

Sleep enuresis is characterized by recurrent involuntary micturition that occurs during sleep. In children prevalence of sleep enuresis could be up to 250 per 1,000. In adults prevalence of nocturnal enuresis varies from 2 to 38 per 1,000.

Sleepwalking occurs more frequently in children with an estimated prevalence of up to 40 per cent in this age group. Prevalence among adults is about 4 per cent.
Prevalence of RBD is estimated to be about 0.5 per cent13. REM sleep behaviour disorder tends to affect older adults, with a mean age of onset of 50 to 60 years, predominantly affecting males.

5. Clinical features and symptoms

The disorders that are primarily discussed in this chapter are confusional arousals, sleep terror disorder, sleepwalking disorder, nightmare disorder and REM sleep behavior disorder.

5.1 Confusional arousals

Arousal disorders, including sleepwalking, sleep terrors, and confusional arousals, are the most common forms of parasomnias. They are predominantly associated with arousals from slow-wave sleep, which in turn occur most prominently in the first third of the night. They can present as one disorder or any combination of the three forms mentioned. Awakening the person during the arousal type of parasomnia is difficult; the affected individual usually will not remember the event on awakening in morning. Confusional arousals can occur throughout the night but are seen most commonly during the first half of the major sleep period when NREM density is highest. Confusional arousals are estimated to affect 4 percent of adults. It is characterized by abrupt awakenings with apparent confusion, diminished vigilance, disorientation and occasional violent or inappropriate behaviour (Farid et al, 2004).
Confusional arousal typically appears in young children up to the age of five years. Polysomnographic recordings of affected individual show clear association of confusional arousal episodes with slow-wave sleep mainly in the first part of the night. Confusional arousals usually are not harmful to the patient and are usually self-limited. Usually, there is no indication to intervene during the episodes of confusional arousal (Young, 2008).

5.2 Sleep terror

Sleep terror (pavor nocturnus) is an abrupt, terrifying arousal from sleep, usually in preadolescent boys although it may occur in adults as well. It is distinct from sleep panic attacks. These emerge when normal wake and NREM state boundaries become destabilized and elements of the waking state intrude into NREM sleep. Sleep terrors are believed to be a reaction to a frightening image that results in agitated arousal and sympathetic nervous activation. Polysomnographic recordings of these events have shown that they are associated with 2 abnormalities during the first sleep cycle: abnormally low electroencephalogram (EEG) power and frequent, brief, nonbehavioral EEG-defined arousals.
Symptoms are fear, sweating, tachycardia, and confusion for several minutes, with amnesia for the event. Demystification of these conditions and reassurance, particularly for parents of pediatric patients, is an important aspect of clinical intervention. Patients rarely remember the events in detail, but if actively probed after 4 years of age, they often report vague memories of having to act—run away, escape, or defend themselves—against monsters, animals, snakes, spiders, ants, intruders, or other threats. Children may report

feeling complete isolation and fear. Parents often describe terrified facial expressions, mumbling, shouting, and inability to be consoled.

5.3 Sleepwalking

Among arousal parasomnias, sleepwalking (somnambulism) is the most common. Sleepwalking (somnambulism) includes ambulation or other intricate behaviors while still asleep, with amnesia for the event. Sleepwalking is a complex behavior that ranges from limited and noninjurious activities to dangerous activities associated with injuries to self or others. Up to 40% of normal children have experienced at least one episode of sleepwalking and 2% to 3% of children experience it at least once a month (Klackenberg, 1971).

It affects mostly children aged 6-12 years, and episodes occur during stage 3 or stage 4 sleep in the first third of the night and in REM sleep in the later sleep hours. Despite widespread prevalence of these disorders and the recognition that they may arise from incomplete arousal, their pathophysiology is not well understood. Evidence for a strong genetic background of sleepwalking was shown in epidemiological surveys as in twin studies. Further evidence for heredity of sleepwalking is documented by the 10-fold increased prevalence of sleepwalking in relatives of patients suffering from sleepwalking. Sleepwalking in elderly people may be a feature of dementia. Idiosyncratic reactions to drugs (eg, marijuana, alcohol) and medical conditions (eg, partial complex seizures) may be causative factors in adults. During an episode of sleepwalking, a person may appear agitated or calm and behaviour may range from simple ambulation with a "glassy stare" to more complex activities such as driving. Sleepwalking may be preceded by confusional arousals or sleep terrors.

Depending on the degree of confusion, bedroom location, furniture, and strength of the subject, sleepwalking may lead to accidents and self-injury. Safety precautions should be taken for sleepwalking. These include removing dangerous objects, placing heavy drapes on glass doors and windows, and special locks on doors. Sleepwalking episodes occur in slow-wave sleep, during which time the individual is not easily arousable. Family members may gently guide the person back to the bed; strong stimuli to awaken the patient may cause resistance or aggression and are not recommended. Sleep terror and sleepwalking episodes are disturbing to parents but prepubertal sleepwalking is usually self-limited. Adult-onset sleepwalking with complicated patterns of sleepwalking, however, may contain a psychiatric component. These patients may benefit from psychotherapy, relaxation, or hypnosis (Farid et al, 2004).

5.4 Nightmares

Nightmares are vivid nocturnal events that cause feelings of fear and terror, with or without feeling anxiety. In most cases, a person having a nightmare will be abruptly awakened from REM sleep and is able to give a detailed account of what he dreamt about. Also, the person having a nightmare has difficulty returning to sleep. Episodes typically occur in the latter half of the night. Following the awakening, the individual becomes fully alert and profoundly anxious. There is vivid recall of the preceding dream as well as difficulty returning to sleep. Compared to sleep terrors, there is less autonomic activation, and tachycardia and tachypnea, if present, are not as severe. Episodes can be precipitated by

illness, traumatic experiences, and alcohol and medication use, such as antidepressants and beta-antagonist antihypertensive agents.
Nightmares affect 20 to 39 percent of children between five and 12 years of age. Contrary to popular belief, frequent nightmares in children do not suggest underlying psychopathology. Nightmares and night terrors in children are usually disturbing to parents and family members; therefore, proper diagnosis and education of family members are important components of management. It is essential to control the environment by removing dangerous objects and providing barriers to prevent escape from a safe sleeping environment. Reassurance and support are often the only therapy required because these disorders rarely, if ever, reflect underlying illness and usually disappear with maturity. Pharmacologic intervention is not usually indicated; in fact, it should be discouraged because it may contribute to further sleep disruption. Behavioral methods for treatment of frequent nightmares are effective in older children.

5.5 Rapid Eye Movement (REM) sleep behavior disorder

REM sleep is characterized by a paucity of muscle activity with near complete somatic muscular atonia. REM sleep behaviour disorder is characterized by the intermittent loss of REM atonia due to disinhibition of normally inhibitory mid-brain projections to spinal motor neurons. This, in conjunction with an active dream state, results in behavioural release and the apparent "acting out of dreams". Abnormal behaviours include sleep talking, yelling, limb movement, and complex motor activities. Patients with REM sleep behaviour disorder arouse from sleep to full alertness often with complete recall of fearful dream content, which may involve being chased or attacked. The motor behaviour exhibited tends to correlate with dream content. REM sleep periods typically occur in the latter half of the night. The most common symptom at time of presentation is injury of the patient or bed partner. As a result of the behaviors, bed partners often simply move to another bed or room. Also, patients and families may have a sense of guilt or shame regarding the behaviors, even though the behaviors may not be consistent with patients' personalities. This is particularly true when sexual behaviors are involved. Sleep disruption and daytime sleepiness are often part of the history. REM sleep behaviour disorder tends to be a disease that occurs in older men, although women and people of all ages may be affected. The reason for the strong predominance toward men, with an approximately nine-to-one men-to-women ratio, is not clearly known. The average age of onset is between 52.4 years to 60.9 years. Unlike those who experience sleep terrors, the victim will recall vivid dreams. The frequency of these episodes varies from once every few weeks to several times a night. Episodes tend to occur 90 min or more after sleep onset, when the first REM period typically begins. (Mahowald et al., 2005).
REM sleep behavior disorder has been linked to a number of other neurological conditions; thus, a careful review of systems and a physical examination are crucial. Polysomnographic monitoring in patients with REM sleep behavior disorder reveals increased tonic and/or phasic electromyographic activity, often accompanied by muscle twitching, extremity flailing, or vocalization during REM sleep. REM sleep behavior disorder is often associated with a growing number of underlying neurologic disorders, and may be induced by numerous medications, particularly selective serotonin reuptake inhibitors (Boeve et al., 2004).

REM sleep behavior disorder can be controlled with medication. Clonazepam is the mainstay in the treatment of REM sleep behavior disorder and leads to either a complete or partial response in approximately 90% of cases. Before it is prescribed, the potential benefits of treatment should be weighed against the possible side effects. Other medications have been tried when clonazepam is not effective or is poorly tolerated. Discussions related to safety are very important, because precautionary measures may prevent serious injury to the patient or family members (Schenck et al., 2002).

5.6 Other parasomnias

Ten disorders are classified under this category (Table 1). The most common are sleep bruxism, sleep enuresis, and primary snoring.

Sleep bruxism is the third most common parasomnia and it can be bothersome to the bed partner. Bruxism is not a dangerous disorder. However, it can cause permanent damage to the teeth and uncomfortable jaw pain, headaches, or ear pain. Approximately 8.2% of people experience it at least once a week. Sleep apnea and anxiety disorders are the most prominent risk factors for bruxism. Bruxism could be a reflex to open the airway after an apneic or hypopneic event. Bruxism may improve with treatment of sleep apnea with continuous positive airway pressure. Sleep bruxism does not have a definite cure. The goals of treatment are to reduce pain, prevent permanent damage to the teeth, and reduce clenching as much as possible. Stress reduction, relaxation, biofeedback, hypnosis and improvement of sleep hygiene have been tried with no persistent or significant improvement. To prevent damage to the teeth, mouth guards or appliances (splints) have been used since the 1930s to treat teeth grinding, clenching, and TMJ disorders. A splint may help protect the teeth from the pressure of clenching. Pharmacologic interventions are indicated for short-term management of patients who experience complications of sleep bruxism, including pain in the temporomandibular joint. Benzodiazepines could be effective because of their muscle-relaxing and anti-anxiety properties. Additionally, they increase the arousal threshold that could precede teeth grinding. (Farid et al., 2004)

Sleep enuresis, more commonly known as bedwetting, refers to the lack of ability to maintain urinary control during sleep. This recurrent involuntary urination is also called nocturnal enuresis, which is characterized by at least two occurrences per month in 3 to 6 years old infants and at least one occurrence per month for older children. Sleep enuresis is observed in 10% of children at the age of 6. The prevalence decreases with age. Approximately 77% of children had enuresis when their parents were enuretic, whereas 44% of children with one parent who was enuretic developed enuresis. Simple behavior modifications can be very effective treatments for children with enuretic episodes. For example, intake of liquids and dietary bladder irritants such as citrus products should be discouraged before bedtime. Taking note of when the enuresis actually occurs, and waking and taking the child to toilet before that hour, can also be very helpful Matthias et al., 2002).

Psychological treatments such as encouragement of self-reliance, participation in management, inculcation of self-respect and responsibility are also recommended by many experts. Physical punishments and coercion, on the other hand, are considered to be the most counterproductive measures and should be avoided at all costs.

Using devices such as bedwetting alarms and moisture alarms, combined with bladder muscle exercises, dietary changes, retention control training etc can also be helpful remedies in treating sleep enuresis. Education, encouragement, and patience are prudent approaches for younger children. For older children who may be embarrassed by the occurrences, and who may be affected by the emotional concerns, more aggressive treatment is recommended. Biofeedback, including enuresis alarms, arousal training and desmopressin have been tried with prominent success rates, although they are associated with high relapse rates. Hypnotherapy and imipramine have been somewhat helpful in the management Schenck et al., 1996).

Primary snoring is reported in 40% to 50% of people over the age of 65 and approximately 25% of the middle-age group. Snoring is usually a symptom of sleep disordered breathing. Oral appliances and otolaryngologic procedures, including velopharyngeal surgery, can effectively resolve snoring. Most of the studies on oral appliances are conducted for treatment of obstructive sleep apnea syndrome, with no clear data on primary snoring. They have decreased the frequency of snoring by 50%.

6. Treatment options

The primary therapy for disorders of arousal is reassurance and prevention. For most, the disease course is usually benign and tends to resolve spontaneously with time. It is essential that both the patient and bed partner be educated about safety precautions for the home and bedroom environment, such as reducing or eliminating potential sources of injury (e.g., relocating the bedroom to a room on the ground floor, securing doors, using heavy draperies over the windows, removing mirrors, and keeping the floor free of objects that the sleepwalker might potentially trip over). Bed partners should be counseled not to attempt to stimulate the patient during an episode as this may trigger violent behaviour.

A trial of sleep extension or scheduled awakening may be considered. With scheduled awakening, the patient is awakened just before the typical time of the parasomnia episode and thereafter allowed to return to sleep.

Relaxation training and guided imagery may be helpful strategies for some patients, especially those with disorders of arousal or rhythm movement disorders.

When the events are frequent or particularly dramatic, medication with a long- or medium-acting benzodiazepine, such as clonazepam, at bedtime is effective therapy in most cases of non-REM disorders of arousal and REM sleep behavior disorder. In non-REM disorders, pharmacologic agents that have been used with some success include paroxetine and trazodone and low-dose benzodiazepines. Typically, medication should be used in combination with nonpharmacologic treatments after such techniques have been tried and found to be ineffective and only when the sleep disorder is affecting daytime function.

7. Conclusion

Although parasomnias can be distressing and it is important to recognize that parasomnias are diagnosable and treatable in the vast majority of patients. With recent understanding of the sleep stages and transition of these stages, many of the parasomnias are readily diagnosable and treatable.

8. References

American Academy of Sleep Medicine. The International Classification of Sleep Disorders. (2004). Chicago

Boeve, B. F; Silber, M. H. &, Ferman, T.J. (2004). REM sleep behavior disorder in Parkinson's disease and dementia with Lewy body disease. *J Geriatr Psychiatry Neurol*, No: 17, pp. 146-157

Bornemann, M. A. C.; Mark, W. & Schenck, C. H. (2006). Parasomnias: Clinical Features and Forensic Implications. *Chest*, No: 130, pp. 605-610

Farid, M. & Kushida, C. A. (2004). Non-Rapid Eye Movement Parasomnias. *Current Treatment Options in Neurology*, Vol: 6, pp. 331-337

Guilleminault, C.; Poyares, D.; Aftab; F. A. & Palombini, L. (2001). Sleep and wakefulness in somnambulism: a spectral analysis study. *J Psychosom Res*; No: 51, pp. 411-416

Guilleminault, C., Palombini, L.; Pelayo, R. & Chervin, R. D. (2003). Sleepwalking and Sleep Terrors in Prepubertal Children: What Triggers Them? *Pediatrics*, No: 111; pp. 17, DOI: 10.1542/peds.111.1.e17

Kales, A.; Soldatos, C. R.; Bixler, E. O.; Ladda, R. L.; Charney, D. S.; Weber, G. & Schweitzer, P. K. (1980). Hereditary factors in sleepwalking and night terrors. *Br J Psychiatry*,No: 137, pp. 111-118

Klackenberg, G. (1971). A prospective longitudinal study of children. *Acta Paediatr Scand.* No: 224(suppl), pp.1-239

Mahowald, M. W. & Schenck, C.H. (2005). REM sleep parasomnias. In: *Principles and practice of sleep medicine*, 4th ed. Elsevier Saunders; pp. 906-907, Philadelphia

Maret, S.; Franken, P.; Dauvilliers, Y.; Ghyselinck, N. B.; Chambon, P. & Tafti, M. (2005). Retinoic acid signaling affects cortical synchrony during sleep. *Science, No:* 310, pp. 111-113

Matthias, K.L. & Guilleminault, C. (2002). Rapid Eye Movement Sleep-related Parasomnias. *Current Treatment Options in Neurology*, Vol: 4, pp. 113-120

Matwiyoff, G. & Lee-Chiong, T. (2010). Parasomnias: an overview. *Indian J Med Res*, No:131, (February 2010), pp 333-337

Ohayon, M. M.; Priest, R. G.; Zulley, J. & Smirne, S. (2000). The place of confusional arousals in sleep and mental disorders: findings in a general population sample of 13,057 subjects. *J Nerv Ment Dis*, No: 188, pp. 340-348

Olson, E. J., Boeve, B. F. & Silber, M. H. (2000). Rapid eye movement sleep behaviour disorder: demographic, clinical and laboratory findings in 93 cases. *Brain*, No:123, pp. 331-339

Oluwole, O. S. A. (2010). Lifetime prevalence and incidence of parasomnias in a population of young adult Nigerians. *Journal of Neurology*, No: 257, pp. 1141-1147, DOI 10.1007/s00415-010-5479-6

Schenck, C. H. & Mahowald, M. W. (1996). REM sleep parasomnias. *Neurol Clin*, No: 14, pp. 697-720

Schenck, C. H. & Mahowald, M.W. (2002). REM sleep behavior disorder: clinical, developmental, and neuroscience perspectives 16 years after its formal identification in sleep. *Sleep*, No: 25, pp. 120-130

Young, P. (2008). Genetic aspects of parasomnias. *Somnologie,* Vol:12, pp. 7-13

11

Risk Factors and Treatment of Restless Legs Syndrome in Adults

John A. Gjevre and Regina M. Taylor-Gjevre
Department of Medicine University of Saskatchewan, Canada

1. Introduction

Restless legs syndrome (RLS) is a common clinical entity consisting of an uncomfortable sensation in one's legs and irresistible urge or desire to move them usually occurring in the evening. This syndrome has been sub optimally diagnosed in the past and remains overall misunderstood and under-recognized by many primary health care providers. However, RLS is increasingly recognized to cause significant disease burden and decreased quality of life (Kushida C et al., 2007). The initial modern clinical description was published by Ekbom in 1945 but was largely ignored until the late 1980s when there was a resurgence of interest in RLS (Walters AS & Hening W, 1987). Because of ongoing clinical confusion and the need for more clear epidemiologic assessment, a research group was organized in 1995 and the original IRLSSG criteria were developed (Walters AS, et al., 1995). In 2003, the International Restless Legs Syndrome Study Group (IRLSSG) issued revised guidelines to assist in clinical diagnosis and research of RLS (Allen RP et al., 2003).

2. RLS description and diagnosis

RLS is described by the RLS foundation as a neurological condition that is characterized by the irresistible urge to move the legs. Patients will describe an uncomfortable itching or "creepy-crawling" sensation on the legs in the evenings and report that it feels like "bugs crawling under the skin." The IRLSSG has listed 4 essential criteria to clinically diagnose RLS. Physical examination is usually normal. There is no single test used which will make the diagnosis although many patients suffer from iron deficiency with low ferritin levels. While overnight polysomnography (PSG) in a sleep laboratory is helpful to assess periodic limb movements of sleep (PLMS), a PSG is not necessary to make the clinical diagnosis of RLS. PLMS are defined as a repetitive or periodic bursts of leg (or arm) electromyographic (EMG) activity during sleep associated with discrete, stereotypical movements of the legs or arms. PLMS are felt to be a related but separate disease from RLS. Although most (80%) patients with RLS with have PLMS on PSG testing, approximately 12-20% of RLS patients will not have evidence for PLMS (Montplaisir J et al., 1997). Approximately 30% of patients with PLMS will have RLS symptoms. The revised 2003 IRLSSG essential criteria include 1) An urge to move the legs accompanied or caused by uncomfortable sensations in the legs, 2) The urge to move or unpleasant sensations beginning or worsening during periods or rest or inactivity such as lying or sitting, 3) The urge to move or unpleasant sensations are partially or totally relieved by movements such as walking or stretching, at least as long as the activity continues, 4) The urge to move or unpleasant sensations are worse in the evening or night than during the day or only occur in the evening or night (Allen RP et al., 2003). Despite these revised guidelines, there are still difficulties in excluding mimics such as leg cramps that can confound the diagnosis and the specificity of the 4 diagnostic criteria is 84% (Hening WA et al., 2009). It has been suggested that the validated self-completed Cambridge-Hopkins RLS questionnaire (CH-RLSq) is more useful with a sensitivity of 87.2% and a specificity of 94.4%. (Allen RP et al., 2008). In addition to the diagnostic criteria, the IRLSSG developed a validated, patient-completed 10 item severity rating scale called the IRLS severity scale or IRLSSS (Walters AS et al., 2003).

3. RLS prevalence

RLS has been mainly studied in North America and Europe and appears to have a prevalence of 5 to 15% with up to a 2:1 female ratio (Berger K et al., 2004, Phillips B et al., 2000). Prevalence is markedly higher in certain groups such as Icelandic women where RLS prevalence was found to be 24.4% (Benediktsdottir B et al., 2010). Of interest, the increased risk of RLS in women appears to be linked to parity with an increased risk of RLS directly proportional to the number of children (Berger K et al. 2004). In contrast, nulliparous women have the identical risk of RLS as men the same age. While, most of the epidemiology of RLS has been researched in Europe and North America, there are studies from other areas. Research from Asia appear to yield lower prevalence rates. (Chen NH et al., 2010). Overall, the prevalence of RLS appears to be higher in North American/European populations, especially in women.

4. RLS pathogenesis

The scientific basis of RLS remains unclear but appears to be related in part to the dopaminergic pathways and iron metabolism in the substantia nigra. In 2003, Connor et. al. published an autopsy-based study suggesting that the cause of RLS was related to a defect in the regulation of transferrin receptors in the brain (Connor JR, et al., 2003). In addition, MRI, PET, and SPECT imaging studies have likewise shown alterations in the dopaminergic receptors of the brain (Michaud M et al., 2002). Recently, further evidence has accumulated to support that there is a primary iron insufficiency leading to an overly activated dopaminergic system (Connor JR et al., 2009, Quiroz C et al., 2010). Low iron levels can increase extracellular dopamine and decrease D2 receptors (Earley CJ et al., 2011). Thus, overall the pathophysiologic basis of RLS is not fully understood but there is increasing evidence of iron deficiency related dopaminergic abnormalities. In addition to dopamine and iron physiology, there are clear familial clusterings and genetic linkages. In 2007, researchers in Iceland reported on the first genetic variant associated with a susceptibility to periodic limb movements of sleep (Stefansson H et al., 2007). A total of 4 main genetic variants have since been discovered which account for approximately 80% of primary RLS.

5. Primary RLS

RLS is divided into two main categories which are primary (idiopathic) RLS and secondary RLS. Patients with primary RLS tend to have onset at an earlier age, often under age 45. In addition, there is a significantly higher family history of RLS (Allen RP & Earley CJ, 2000).

6. Clinical associations with RLS or secondary RLS

6.1 RLS and multiple sclerosis

After an initial 2002 meeting presentation where data from 100 multiple sclerosis (MS) patients with a prevalence of RLS of 32%was described, Auger et al reported a prevalence of 37.5% in their 200 French-Canadian MS patients meeting the 2003 IRRLSG criteria. Interestingly, in their patient population, more women than men met RLS criteria and 30% of patients reported that RLS symptoms started or worsened during pregnancy. A positive family history for RLS was reported by 36% of these French-Canadian patients meeting RLS criteria. They speculated whether MS plaque formation and involvement in the basal ganglia may be pathogenic for RLS in these patients. This concept may be supported by the therapeutic effect of dopaminergic therapeutic agents. The concept of potential common susceptibility genes for both MS and RLS is raised by the authors (Auger C et al, 2005). The following year, Kilfoyle et al reported a myelin protein zero (MPZ) mutation which was associated in the individuals studied with various neurological manifestations including RLS and MS (Kifoyle DH, et al, 2006).

In 2007, Manconi et al examined prevalence of RLS in an Italian population of MS patients. In this population of 156 patients, 100 were female and a prevalence of 32.7% was found who met the 2003 IRRLSG diagnostic criteria. However, in contrast to the French-Canadian population, a positive family history for RLS was only reported by 5% of the (total) population. In the majority of these patients (> 90%), RLS symptoms followed or were simultaneous in onset with MS clinical features onset. The authors speculate that the co-existence of MS and RLS may be the result of a particular lesional pattern (Manconi et al, 2007). In a subsequent study of 82 MS patients of whom 30 patients had co-existing RLS, brain and cervical spinal cord MRIs were done. The MS and RLS patients were observed to have a greater degree of cervical cord involvement than those MS patients without RLS. The authors state that cervical cord damage represents a significant risk factor for RLS in MS patients (Manconi et al, 2008).

The Italian REMS Study Group, published the 'REstless legs syndrome in Multiple Sclerosis' or REMS study in 2008 in the journal SLEEP. This group reported a prospective, multicenter case-control epidemiologic survey which involved 20 sleep centers certified by the Italian Association of Sleep Medicine and included 861 MS patients and 649 control patients. They reported a 19% prevalence of RLS, using the IRRLSG criteria, in the MS patients compared to a 4.2% in the control population. This provided a relative risk for RLS in the MS patients of 5.4. Risk factors associated with RLS in the MS patients were identified as older age, longer duration of MS, the primary progressive form of MS, higher global, pyramidal, and sensory disability and the presence of leg jerks before sleep onset. Additionally, RLS symptom severity was reported to be worse in the MS patient group compared to symptoms of control group patients with RLS. The authors comment that their results strengthen the hypothesis that MS inflammatory lesions may induce a secondary form of RLS (The Italian REMS Study Group, 2008).

In a study of French patients with MS by Douay et al, the authors report a prospective evaluation of 242 MS patients and found 18% met the international RLS criteria, consistent with the REMS study report. In this French population, the authors reported RLS symptoms to be more frequent in patients with the relapsing-remitting form of MS (Douay et al. 2009).

A Brazilian study of 44 MS patients reported by Moreira et al, found 27% of their patients met the RLS criteria. The authors did not observe any association of specific patient characteristics associated with the presence of RLS compared to those MS patients not meeting RLS criteria, in this small prevalence study (Moreira et al, 2008).

Deriu et al published a case-control study of Italian MS patients. The authors enrolled 202 MS patients and 212 age and gender matched healthy controls. Interestingly, 45% of the MS patients met the IRRLSG diagnostic criteria for RLS, however, after neurologic review and examination of the each patient who responded positively to the questionnaire instrument, only 14.6% of the MS patients were felt to truly have a diagnosis of RLS. In the control group, 16.03% were positive responders to the questionnaire criteria, but only 2.8% had a final diagnosis of RLS following neurologic review and examination. The authors comment on the high false positive number of questionnaire responders (Deriu et al, 2009).

In summary, there is evidence of an increased prevalence of RLS in the MS population. Several interesting possibilities have been suggested to explain this association. The weight of evidence seems to support the concept of a secondary RLS likely arising from strategic geographic involvement of demyelinating lesions.

6.2 RLS and other neurologic disorders

Peripheral neuropathy has also been associated with RLS. A recent case-control study (Hattan E et al 2009) in a Quebec population examined 245 patients with a diagnosis of peripheral neuropathy and 245 age and gender matched controls. The authors considered a positive response to three of the four essential criteria to be 'screen-positive'. All 'screen-positive' patients were subsequently evaluated by a blinded movement disorders specialist. Of the 245 peripheral neuropathy patients, 26.5% were 'screen-positive', compared to 10.2% of controls. Confirmation by neurologist, however, revealed only 46% of the 'screen-positive' peripheral neuropathy patients were felt to truly have a diagnosis of RLS compared to 80% of the 'screen-positive' control patients. After this diagnostic confirmation, the overall prevalence of RLS did not differ between the peripheral neuropathy patients and the control group.

The prevalence of RLS was evaluated in a cohort of 99 Italian patients with acquired diabetic peripheral neuropathy (Gemignani et al, 2007). Using IRRLSG diagnostic criteria, RLS was found to be present in a third of the patients in this study population (33/99). The authors reported that of the various forms of diabetic neuropathy represented within this population, small fiber sensory neuropathy was more common than other forms. A prominent symptom associated with RLS was 'burning feet'. The authors suggest that RLS may be triggered peripherally by abnormal sensory inputs from small fibers.

A case series of 12 patients with essential mixed cryoglobulinemia and associated peripheral neuropathy reported a frequency of RLS, using pre-2003 diagnostic measures, of one third (4/12) (Gemignani et al, 1997).

A recent report (Bachmann CG et al 2010) suggest response to specific stimuli may be able to distinguish between primary RLS and RLS secondary to small fiber neuropathy. In this study of 21 primary RLS patients and 13 patients with secondary RLS related to small fiber neuropathy, the authors describe thermal hypoesthesia to cold and warm in those with secondary RLS compared to both the primary RLS study patients and controls. They also suggest support for the RLS pathogenesis concept of central disinhibition of nociceptive pathways which might be induced by conditioning afferent input from damaged small fiber neurons in secondary RLS.

Restless legs syndrome has been reported as increased in prevalence in German hereditary spastic paresis patients (Sperfeld AD, et al, 2007) and in Argentinian patients with Fabry's disease (Dominguez RO, et al, 2007). RLS has also been reported to be present in 18.1% of

227 Charcot-Marie Tooth disease patients compared to 234 controls with a 5.6% prevalence. RLS severity was correlated with worse sleep quality and reduced health-related quality of life measures. Variation in prevalence was not observed between subtypes of Charcot-Marie Tooth disease, but women were more severely affected by RLS than male patients (Boentert M, et al 2010). A series of 28 patients with Friedreich's Ataxia were surveyed for prevalence of RLS with 32% meeting diagnostic criteria (Synofzik M et al, 2011). In a population of 28 chronic inflammatory demyelinating polyneuropathy (CIDP), a prevalence of 39.3% for RLS was found, compared to 7.1% prevalence in age and gender matched control patients.

Isolated case reports of RLS symptomatology following development of hyperparathyroidism (Agarwal P et al, 2008), administration of interferon therapy (LaRochelle JS, et al, 2004), development of multifocal motor neuropathy (Lo Coco D, et al, 2009), and Guillain-Barré syndrome have been reported (Marin LF, et al, 2010). Additionally, a case report has been published reporting a patient who experienced remission of severe RLS following excision of multiple foot neuromata (Lettau LA, et al 2010).

The question has also been raised as to whether RLS in seen in a higher prevalence in patients with Parkinson's Disease. This has been addressed in an Italian population of 118 Parkinson's Disease outpatients using a case-control study design. The authors report a failure to demonstrate increased prevalence of RLS in the Parkinson's patients in comparison to age and gender matched control patients. They further acknowledge the RLS prevalence assessment may be impeded by the concurrent treatment of Parkinson's Disease with dopaminomimetic drugs, which may also be expected to impact on RLS symptomatology (Calzetti et al, 2009). Another study from the Netherlands in 269 non-demented Parkinson's Disease patients, found RLS to be present in 11% of patients. RLS severity was noted to correlate positively with Parkinson's Disease severity. RLS was also significantly more common in male patients than female. The authors note the similar prevalence of RLS in their study population to the general population and submit that this could potentially relate to concurrent dopaminergic therapy. They also suggest that in view of the relationship of severity of RLS to severity of Parkinson's Disease related primarily non-dopaminergic symptoms, that non-dopaminergic systems may play a role in any potential relationship between RLS and Parkinson's Disease (Verbaan D, et al, 2010).

In a reverse style of assessment, 23,119 participants in the Health Professional Follow-up study who were free of diabetes and arthritis were surveyed. The IRRLSG diagnostic criteria were applied and concurrent diagnoses of Parkinson's Disease were investigated. The adjusted odds ratios for Parkinson's Disease in men with RLS symptoms with frequency from 5-14 times per month was 1.1, and in those with a frequency of RLS of 15 or more times per month the odds ratio was higher at 3.09. The authors concluded that men with RLS symptomatology were more likely to have concurrent Parkinson's Disease (Gao X, et al, 2010).

6.3 RLS and pregnancy

Lower extremity symptoms consistent with RLS have been reported in pregnancy. In a study of 642 pregnant Italian women, data was collected around the time of delivery and at follow-up evaluation up to six month post-delivery. Patients were screened with the IRRLSG diagnostic criteria. The authors reported that 26% of women acknowledged symptoms of RLS during their pregnancy. It was most strongly related to the last trimester of the pregnancy and tended to disappear around the time of delivery. The authors concluded that pregnancy was associated with transient RLS. They did also observe that women with RLS symptoms had lower hemoglobin levels and MCV compared to healthy subjects. (Manconi M et al, 2004). An American study of 189 nulliparous women who were enrolled between six and 20 weeks of gestation and were followed up in the third trimester, reported an increase in patients meeting RLS criteria from 17.5% at enrollment up to 31.2% in the third trimester (Facco FL, et al, 2010).

In a questionnaire study of female members of the French Association of Patients with RLS, Ghorayeb et al applied both the International RLS Severity Scale (IRLSSS) and a questionnaire addressing reproductive behaviour and RLS history. Interestingly, women who had had a pregnancy showed a higher mean IRLSSS score than women who had never had a child. Worsening of symptoms during pregnancy were reported by 23% of patients, 29% of non-menopausal women reported increased severity of RLS symptoms during menses, and 69% of women reported worsening of symptoms following menopause (Ghorayeb I, et al, 2008). An Australian case-control study of pregnant women demonstrated a RLS prevalence of 22.5% of 211 women. A positive family history of RLS and of 'growing pains', as well as a personal childhood history of 'growing pains' were associated with meeting RLS criteria in this study population (Balendran et al 2011).

In a Turkish study of 146 pregnant women, 38 were diagnosed with RLS. The authors report lower hemoglobin levels to be a risk factor for RLS in pregnancy (Tunc et al 2007). In a study of pregnant women in Pakistan, 81 of 271 women met diagnostic criteria for RLS. The authors reported anemia and a positive family history of RLS to be predictive for development of de novo RLS, whereas, a positive family history for RLS and multiparity were predictors for pre-existing RLS with odds ratios of 12.39 and 6.84 respectively (Sikandar R, et al, 2009). A previous pregnancy was also identified by Pantaleo NP et al as a significant risk factor for RLS in a re-analysis of data from a prior RLS study. They observed that in family members of RLS probands, the prevalence of RLS was significantly higher for parous women (49.5%) than for nulliparous women (33.7%) or for men (30%). These differences were not observed in control proband family members. The authors suggest that in patients with a positive family history of RLS, pregnancy has a major influence on the risk of developing RLS (Pantaleo NP, et al, 2010).

Examining hormonal influences on RLS, Dzaja et al, studied 10 pregnant German women with RLS and nine healthy pregnant controls. Blood hormone levels of estradiol were higher in patients with RLS than in control patients. The authors suggest estrogens may contribute via a pathophysiological mechanism to triggering of RLS symptoms during pregnancy (Dzaja A, et al, 2009).

Neau et al, in a cross-sectional questionnaire study of 1.022 pregnant French women from a single town, screened for RLS using IRRLSG criteria. They found 24% of these women to be affected by RLS during their pregnancy. The symptoms of RLS were strongly related to the third trimester of the pregnancy. In a follow-up study of a smaller number of patients, the authors report resolution of RLS symptoms within a short time interval following delivery in the majority of women (Neau JP et al, 2010a, Neau JP et al, 2010b). A follow-up study of RLS in pregnant Italian women performed after a mean lapse of 6.5 years, reported on 74 women with pregnancy associated RLS and 133 women who did not have RLS symptoms during their pregnancy. During the time between the original study and this follow-up investigation, the prevalence of RLS had increased to 56% person/year in women who had experienced RLS symptoms transiently during their pregnancy and 12.6% person/year in subjects who had not been troubled with RLS symptoms during pregnancy. The authors conclude the transient pregnancy RLS form to be a significant risk factor for development of a future chronic form of RLS (Cesnick et al, 2010).

6.4 RLS and renal disease

Renal disease has been associated with RLS symptomatology. A recent hospital based study of 301 patients, revealed a prevalence for meeting RLS criteria of 18.3%. Multivariate analysis identified iron deficiency and chronic renal disease to be independent predictors for RLS in this population (Quinn C et al, 2011). In a Japanese study of 490 uremic patients on hemodialysis (HD), 12.2% were found to meet criteria for RLS. The authors found a relationship between RLS, anxiety, anemia and high serum phosphorus level. They failed to find evidence of previously identified risk factors including relationship to gender, longer duration of HD therapy, frequency of HD sessions, and smoking (Takaki J et al, 2003). The significance of an elevated serum phosphorus in RLS is unclear.

A lower frequency of RLS was observed in an Indian study of 121 HD patients and 99 controls, where only 6.6% of HD patients and 0% of controls met RLS criteria. Nerve conduction studies conducted on RLS patients found the majority to have evidence of sensori-motor neuropathy (Bhowmik D, et al, 2003). Another prevalence study in Brazil in 176 HD patients observed a prevalence of RLS of 14.8% (Goffredo et al, 2003). A similar prevalence was established in 894 dialysis patients participating in the CHOICES (Choices for Healthy Outcomes In Caring for End Stage renal disease) study, where a prevalence of 15% for 'severe' RLS was observed. Age and diabetes were positive predictors for RLS in this population. The authors also report an increase in the adjusted mortality hazard ratio of 1.39 in patients with severe RLS. Reduced quality of life measures in these patients was also observed (Unruh ML, et al, 2004). In a small study from the Netherlands, 48 patients with renal disease and RLS were studied by polysomnogram (PSG) and questionnaire. A prevalence of 58.3% for meeting RLS criteria was observed. In addition the authors report nearly all RLS patients had evidence of severe periodic limb movement disorder on PSG (Riisman RM, et al, 2004). Examining a population who were not yet dialysis dependent, Merlino et al enrolled 138 chronic renal failure patients and 151 controls. RLS criteria were met by 10.9% of the chronic renal failure group and 3.3% of the control population. An association with iron deficiency and female gender was observed (Merlino et al, 2005).

6.5 RLS and rheumatic diseases

In the rheumatoid arthritis (RA) patient population, increased prevalence of RLS has been reported by several investigators. Reynolds et al studied hospitalized RA patients employing a 'control' group of osteoarthritis (OA) patients, and found a 30% prevalence of RLS in RA compared to 3% in OA (Reynolds G et al, 1986). A subsequent study again comparing RA and OA found comparable prevalence rates for RLS of 25% in RA and 4% in OA (Salih AM, et al, 2004). Auger et al in their study of MS patients employed a RA patient group for contrast, finding a prevalence rate for RLS of 31% in their RA group (Auger C, et al, 2005). A more recent study employing the 2003 IRRLSG criteria for RLS found a prevalence of RLS of 27.7% in RA and a prevalence of 24.4% in OA patients (Taylor-Gjevre, et al, 2009). Increased frequency of RLS has also been reported in other rheumatic disease populations, including Sjogren's Syndrome, scleroderma and fibromyalgia patients (Taylor-Gjevre, et al, 2011). A recent study of RLS in Systemic Lupus Erythematosus patients has also suggested an increased prevalence in that population (Hassan N, et al, 2011).

6.6 RLS and Iron deficiency

An increased prevalence of anemia or iron deficiency has been observed in many RLS patient populations. Treatment with iron supplementation has been efficacious in many cases of RLS in patients with low serum ferritin levels. This is discussed in greater depth in the treatment section of this chapter. Consistent with these observations, there has been an increased prevalence of RLS in patients with celiac disease, a disorder with associated abnormal iron absorption (Moccia M, et al, 2010) and as mentioned previously in this chapter, many instances of secondary RLS appear to be also associated with anemia or low iron status.

There have been several studies assessing prevalence of RLS in regular blood donors. A large Swedish study of 946 consecutive blood donors, aged 18-64, who were evaluated for RLS, found a gender difference in prevalence. In male blood donors 14.7% met RLS criteria, in female donors the frequency increased to 24.7%. Further, in patients with laboratory evidence consistent with iron-deficiency, the frequency of RLS increased to 37.5%. The authors conclude RLS to be common amongst female blood donors (Ulfberg J, et al, 2004). Conversely, in an American study of 144 blood donors, only a 4% prevalence of definite RLS was appreciated. The authors comment that their relatively small sample size may influence their results (Arunthari V, et al, 2010).

From a pathologic viewpoint, decreased iron content has been observed in the substantia nigra which is felt to contribute to the pathophysiology of RLS (Synder AM, et al, 2009). In a recent study, Connor et al examined expression of iron management proteins in proximity to the blood-brain interface in brains from eleven RLS patients and in 14 control brains. The authors report a significant decrease in heavy chain ferritin, transferrin and it's receptor in the microvessels in RLS patients compared to controls. Additionally, activity of an iron regulatory protein was observed to be diminished in the RLS patients compared to controls. These relative differences between brains from RLS patients and control patients suggest fundamental differences in brain iron acquisition in RLS patients (Connor JR, et al, 2011)

7. Treatment options for RLS

Historically, there were a variety of treatments for RLS ranging from bloodletting to opiates. Indeed, Sir Thomas Willis over 325 years ago described the first probable case of RLS and used opium to alleviate the symptoms. When RLS was "rediscovered" by researchers in the 1980s, once again opioid narcotics were the treatment of choice (Hening WA, et al. 1986). In that study, five patients with RLS were given opioid drugs which relieved their awake RLS symptoms as well as PLMs and sleep disturbance. When counteracted with intravenous naloxone, the RLS symptoms and findings returned leading the authors to speculate on the endogenous opiate system playing a role in RLS pathogenesis. However, with increasing research in the last two decades, it has become clear that the underlying pathology of RLS is largely due to alternations in dopaminergic pathways. This has lead to the use of both non-specific and specific dopamine receptor agents.

7.1 Pharmacological treatments for RLS

7.1.1 Iron replacement therapy

While Ekbom did recognize the possible role of iron therapy in RLS, it was not until 1994 when O'Keeffe in Dublin did the first clinical trial of iron replacement therapy. In that study of 18 elderly patients with 18 matched controls, iron status and RLS response to iron therapy was observed. The researchers found that serum ferritin levels were reduced in RLS subjects compared to the control group and that levels were inversely correlated to the severity of RLS symptomatology. In the 15 RLS patients treated with iron replacement therapy for 2 months, there was a significant improvement in RLS symptoms (O'Keeffe ST, 1994). In a recent double-blinded, placebo-controlled study, Wang and colleagues showed the benefit of iron replacement in RLS patients with low serum ferritin. In this study, 373 patients were screened and 157 (42%) met the 2003 IRLSSG criteria for RLS. Of these, there were only 18 patients who consented to participate and met the inclusion criteria (which included having a low-normal serum ferritin between 15-75 ng/ml). Eleven patients were randomized to iron replacement (ferrous sulfate 325mg po bid) and 7 to placebo for 12 weeks and IRLS scores were obtained at the start and end of the study. The researchers found a clinically significant ($p = 0.01$) improvement in IRLS scores in the iron therapy group and a non-significant ($p = 0.07$) trend towards improvement in quality of life (Wang J, 2009).

7.1.2 Dopamine precursors

Dopamine is a catecholamine which acts as a neurotransmitter but cannot cross the blood-brain barrier. Levodopa (L-DOPA) is a precursor to dopamine (as well as norepinephrine and epinephrine) and can cross the blood-brain barrier. Once in the brain, L-DOPA is converted by DOPA decarboxylase to dopamine which can act on the dopamine receptors to treat RLS. However, because peripheral L-DOPA is also converted to dopamine leading to adverse effects, L-DOPA is usually given with a peripheral DOPA decarboxylase inhibitor (usually carbidopa). There is a large body of evidence supporting the effectiveness of L-DOPA in RLS. One of earliest randomized trials was done in the USA and published in 1993. This study was a randomized, double-blind, placebo-controlled, cross-over design trial evaluating carbidopa/levodopa with proproxyphene and placebo. The primary outcome was PSG measurements and sleep latency tests. The researchers found that carbidopa/levodopa normalized the PLMs and improved sleep, especially in the first 3 hours of sleep (Kaplan PW et al., 1993). However, it soon became apparent that carbidopa/levodopa had a serious drawback in regards to augmentation or rebound of RLS symptoms the following morning and/or early afternoon. In a report from 1996, Allen and colleagues prospectively evaluated 46 consecutive patients being treated with carbidopa/levodopa. They found that 82% of RLS patients and 31% of PLMS patients experienced augmentation problems and this was severe enough to lead to medication changes in 50% of the RLS patients (Allen RP, Earley CJ, 1996). Because of augmentation issues, other researchers have evaluated using sustained-release L-DOPA preparations. Trenkwalder and colleagues did an open-label extension trial of an earlier double-blinded, cross-over study evaluating standard and sustained-release L-DOPA. In this 1 year trial they found that 60% of patients discontinued therapy due to aggravating daytime symptoms (Trenkwalder C et al., 2003). In a 2006 review, Paulus & Trenkwalder examined the world literature and concluded that augmentation is a result of severely increased dopamine concentration in the CNS and that overstimulation of the D1 receptors compared to the D2 receptors in the spinal cord may cause discomfort and PLMS. Also, iron deficiency may be a significant predisposing factor for the development of augmentation. The researchers concluded that therapy with L-DOPA or dopamine agonist should endeavour to be low-dose and that iron replacement and/or opiates are the therapies of choice to use with augmentation (Paulus W & Trenkwalder C, 2006). In summary, L-DOPA is a widely available and inexpensive therapy for RLS which has been shown in numerous studies to be beneficial in improving objective PSG findings as well as subjective measures of sleep and RLS symptoms. Unfortunately, there are problems particularly linked to L-DOPA with next morning augmentation of RLS symptoms. This does impair the usefulness of L-DOPA especially when there are newer effective dopamine agonists with a better side effect profile.

7.1.3 Ergot-derived dopamine agonists

Ergotamine is related to ergot alkaloids and is structurally similar to several neurotransmitters including dopamine. Ergotamine derivatives include bromocriptine, pergolide, and cabergoline. It most be noted that all ergot derivatives have been associated with cardiac valve disease. In a recent Italian study, researchers found that patients taking pergolide or cabergoline had a relative risk of 4.2 to 6.3 for valve regurgitation compared to patients using non-ergot dopamine agonists and controls (Zanettini R, 2007). Thus it is recommended to conduct close cardiac monitoring in patients on ergot-derived dopamine agonists.

Bromocriptine is an ergot-derivative dopamine agonist that preferentially acts on the D2 dopamine receptor. It has traditionally been used in the treatment of pituitary tumors and Parkinson Disease but has been tried for RLS with some efficacy. In a small, double-blinded, randomized crossover study, researchers found that 83% of patients had partial subjective improvement in RLS symptoms but no significant change in PLMD by PSG (Walters AS, 1988). A more recent study from Europe compared bromocriptine to pramipexole (a preferential D3 receptor agonist) showing that while both helped to improve RLS symptoms, pramipexole was superior. In addition, pramipexole improved PSG parameters including PLM frequency (Manconi M, 2011). Thus, bromocriptine is not commonly used as a therapy for RLS at this time.

Pergolide is a semi-synthetic ergot-derivative that acts as a dopamine agonist at both the D2 and D1 receptors. In a major study, Trenkwalder and colleagues found pergolide significantly improved RLS symptom severity and PLMD (Trenkwalder et al. 2004). The researchers conducted a double-blinded, placebo-controlled, randomized study of pergolide therapy; the Pergolide European Australian RLS (PEARLS) study. In this study, 100 patients with primary (idiopathic) RLS were randomized to either pergolide or placebo for 6 weeks. In addition, there was a 12 month follow-up phase with open-label pergolide for placebo non-responders. PLMS were assessed by PSG and RLS symptoms by the IRLS severity scale (IRLSSS) questionnaire. They found that pergolide significantly improved IRLSSS results at 6 weeks. In addition, the pergolide treated patients had substantial improvements in the 6 week and 12 month PLM index. The authors concluded that pergolide significantly improves PLM findings as well as subjective RLS sleep disturbance.

Cabergoline is a newer, semi-synthetic, long-acting, ergot-derivative dopamine agonist that particularly acts on the D2 receptors but also has some affinity for the D1 and D3 receptors. One of the earliest studies examining cabergoline in RLS was from Germany in 2000. In that study, researchers conducted a 12 week open label trial assessing efficacy with baseline and 12 week PSG and RLS subjective questionnaires. The research team found improvements in PLMs and subjective relief of symptoms and concluded that cabergoline was effective and well-tolerated (Stiasny K et al., 2000). A more recent randomized, double-blinded, placebo-controlled, multicenter PSG study examined the efficacy of cabergoline in RLS (the CATOR study). In this study, 40 patients with moderate to severe RLS were randomized to either cabergoline or placebo for 5 weeks. Baseline and end of study PSGs were obtained as well as IRLSSS and quality of life questionnaires. The researchers found the cabergoline group had significant improvements in PSG parameters, IRLSSS severity scores, and the RLS quality of life scores. They concluded that cabergoline is an efficacious and well-tolerated therapy for RLS symptoms and associated sleep abnormalities (Oertel WH et al., 2006). Unfortunately, like pergolide, cabergoline has been implicated in cardiac valvular heart disease and patients treated with this agent need close cardiac monitoring.

7.1.4 Nonergot-derived dopamine agonists

There are three newer fully-synthetic dopamine agonists that are not derived from ergot. The three drugs include ropinirole, pramipexole, and rotigotine. As of July 2011, rotigotine is not approved by the FDA for use for RLS in the USA. These nonergot agents are not associated with valvular heart disease but have been associated with impulse control disorders including pathological gambling, compulsive overeating, hypersexuality, and pyschosis. There is increasing recognition that patients treated with these agents should be monitored for impulse control disorders.

Ropinirole acts as a dopamine agonist primarily on the D3 as well as D2 & D4 receptors. It was originally studied in the early 1990s for Parkinson's Disease and later found to be beneficial for RLS. Ondo studied 16 RLS patients in an open-label trial of ropinirole. Three patients discontinued ropinirole use. Of the remaining 13 patients, the average duration of use was 3.9 months and there was a 58.7% improvement in symptoms (Ondo W, 1999). Further studies reinforced the safety and efficacy of ropinirole in RLS. The TREAT RLS 1 study (Therapy with ropinirole; efficacy and tolerability in RLS 1) was a randomized, double-blinded, placebo-controlled trial of 12 weeks duration. 146 subjects were randomized to the ropinirole group and 138 to the placebo group. The key endpoint was the IRLS severity score which showed significant improvement in the ropinirole group over the placebo group at week 12 ($p=0.0036$). The researchers concluded that ropinirole improves RLS compared with placebo and was generally well-tolerated (Trenkwalder C et al. 2004). More recent similar studies from the USA and Canada confirm the efficacy and safety of ropinirole, including long-term duration in the Canadian study. In the USA study, Bogan and colleagues studied 331 subjects in a multicenter, double-blinded, placebo-controlled, flexible dose trial of 12 weeks duration. The primary endpoint was the IRLS score at week 12 which showed a significant improvement in the ropinirole group ($p<0.001$). In addition, the treatment group showed improvements in subjective measures of sleep disturbance and quantity and quality of life scores also improve. The authors concluded that ropinirole improves RLS symptoms and was generally well-tolerated over a 12 week study period (Bogan RK et al. 2006). In the Canadian study, researchers studied the long-term efficacy (36 weeks) of ropinirole and also evaluated for the potential of symptom relapse after drug discontinuation. They identified 202 patients and found significantly fewer subjects relapsed in the ropinirole arm compared to placebo (32.6% versus 57.8%, $p=0.0156$). In addition, the time to relapse symptoms was longer in the ropinirole group and less patients withdrew from lack of efficacy in that group. The authors concluded that ropinirole was highly efficacious and well-tolerated over a 36 week period (Montplaisir J et al. 2006). In 2008, Allen and colleagues reviewed RLS age-of-onset and the response to treatment. They observed no relationship between the RLS symptoms age-of-onset and baseline IRLS score, and between dose administered at week 12 and age-of-onset. The authors concluded that ropinirole provides effective RLS symptom relief that is not affected by age of symptom onset (Allen RP, Ritchie SY, 2008). In 2009, a large meta-analysis was conducted to evaluate the effect of ropinirole versus placebo on sleep outcomes as measured by the Medical Outcomes Study (MOS) sleep scale. The validated MOS sleep scale is a 12 question scale which evaluates sleep disturbance, sleep adequacy, snoring, somnolence, quantity of sleep, and other measures. In this review, the authors found that ropinirole improved sleep quality and decreased daytime somnolence in patients with primary RLS (Hansen RA, et al., 2009). Finally, researchers assessed the efficacy of ropinirole on depressive symptoms and RLS. In a multicenter, randomized, double-blinded, placebo-controlled trial, 231 patients with moderate to severe primary RLS and at least mild depression were studied. Ropinirole versus placebo was given for 12 weeks with measurements obtained at baseline and 12 weeks for the Montgomery-Asberg Depression Rating Scale, the Hamilton Scale for Depression and Beck Depression Inventory-II score, and the Medical Outcomes Study sleep scale. There were significant improvements in the Montgomery and Hamilton scores as well as 3 of the 4 domains of the MOS sleep scale. The authors concluded that in patients with RLS and mild to moderate depression, appropriate therapy for RLS should first be tried and antidepressant medication may be needed later if the depression symptoms still persist (Benes H et al., 2011). In summary, ropinirole is a newer nonergot-derived dopamine agonist with a particular affinity for the D3 dopamine receptors. It has been shown to be beneficial in RLS symptom improvement both short and long-term with improvement in daytime somnolence and quality of life indicators.

Pramipexole is a nonergot-derived dopamine agonist that acts on the D3 as well as D2 and D4 receptors. One of the earliest RLS studies was conducted by Lin at the Mayo Clinic in 1998. In that research, 16 patients were studied who had failed other dopaminergic therapies for symptomatic RLS. An open-label trial showed that after 2 to 3 months usage, there was clinically significant improvements in nocturnal leg restlessness and involuntary leg movements. The authors proposed that pramipexole was an effective therapy for the treatment of RLS (Lin SC et al., 1998). Following that encouraging initial report, a small randomized trial was conducted in Quebec. Researchers studied 10 RLS subjects with PSG and RLS symptom questionnaire using a double-blinded crossover study. They found a significant reduction in PLMs and RLS symptoms of bedtime/nocturnal leg discomfort (Montplaisir J et al., 1999). A larger randomized trial from Finland evaluated the efficacy and safety of pramipexole in 2006. In this study (the PRELUDE study), 109 patients with moderate to severe RLS (based on the IRSS severity score) were randomized in a 3 week, double-blinded, placebo-controlled, dose-finding study. PSG measures and IRLS severity scores were assessed. At all doses, the PLM index was reduced and IRLS severity scores reduced. The authors concluded that pramipexole was an effective and safe therapy for treatment of both the objective (PSG measures) and subjective (IRLS severity) aspects of RLS (Partinen M et al., 2006) In a long-term 52 week open-label study, Japanese researchers found that pramipexole was both effective and safe (with no RLS augmentation), especially in patients with an IRLS score less than 20 (Inoue Y, et al., 2010). In a more recent, multicenter trial, pramipexole was evaluated for efficacy and augmentation problems over a 6 month period. This was a 6 month, randomized, double-blinded, placebo-controlled trial in which 321 patients were recruited. Primary endpoint for efficacy was the change in the IRLS severity score. In addition, patients maintained a symptom diary and cases that met pre-defined criteria for suspected augmentation were reviewed by a blinded panel. The study showed that pramipexole was significantly more effective than placebo in improvements of IRLS severity ($p=0.0077$). Over 6 months, the incidence of confirmed augmentation was 9.2% in the pramipexole group versus 6.0% in placebo and the rate increased with treatment in the intervention group but not placebo. Overall, the authors felt that pramipexole was effective and safe but did suggest it should be studied over a longer duration for further assess augmentation issues (Hogl B, et al., 2011). More recent trials evaluating pramipexole has focused on comparison with other dopaminergic agonist. In a recent study by Manconi, pramipexole (mainly a D3 receptor agonist) was compared with bromocriptine (largely a D2 receptor agent) and researchers found that pramipexole was more effective than bromocriptine in reduction of PLMs and that while both drugs reduced RLS symptoms, the pramipexole group had greater symptom improvements (Manconi M et al., Neurology 2011). The same Italian group also did a recent comparison of pramipexole to ropinirole. Researchers found that both treatment groups improved RLS symptoms and reduced PLMs on PSG compared to the placebo group and that there was no significant differences between the pramipexole and ropinirole treatment arms (Manconi M et al. Mov Disorders 2011). In summary, pramipexole is a newer nonergot-derived dopamine agonist with preferential action on the D3 dopamine receptor site. It has been shown to be beneficial for both objective PSG PLM findings as well as subjective improvements in RLS clinical symptoms. It is generally well-tolerated although there may be an issue with augmentation long-term.

Rotigotine is another newer nonergot-derived dopamine agonist. It is formulated as a once daily transdermal patch and approved to treat RLS in Europe but not FDA-approved for the USA. It appears to mainly work on the D2, D3, and D4 receptor sites. In one of the earliest pilot studies to show benefit for RLS patients, German researchers in 2004 evaluated 63 patients. In this randomized, multicentre, double-blind, parallel-group trial, 63 subjects were studied using the IRLS severity score as the primary endpoint. Researchers found a significant improvement in the treatment group and concluded that transdermal rotigotine was efficacious and well-tolerated (Stiasny-Kolster K et al., 2004). More recently in a multicenter, randomized, double-blind, placebo-controlled 6 month trial, 505 patients with moderate to severe RLS were placed on placebo or rotigotine with the primary endpoints being the IRLS severity score and the CGI-1 score. The treatment group had significantly improved IRLS and CFI-1 outcomes. There was an overall 27% incidence of skin reactions to the transdermal patch. Overall, the authors concluded that rotigotine significantly reduced the severity of RLS symptoms and that treatment effectiveness was maintained throughout the 6 month study period (Hening WA et al., 2010). Rotigotine was also recently assessed in an overnight PSG study evaluating objective PLM measurements. This study was a multicenter, randomized, double-blind, placebo-controlled trial that evaluated 67 subjects over a 4 week period. Baseline and 4 week PSG and subjective questionnaires (IRLS, CGI-1, MOS-S) were obtained. The authors found significant improvements in both the subjective questionnaires but also the objective PSG PLM data. The researchers concluded that rotigotine was effective and well tolerated in the 4 week treatment of both motor symptoms and subjective sleep disturbances caused by RLS (Oertel WH et al., 2010). Finally, in a long term follow-up study, rotigotine was shown to provide sustained effectiveness in treating moderate to severe RLS symptoms for up to 5 years and was generally well-tolerated (Oertel W et al., 2011).

7.1.5 Other pharmacological treatments for RLS

A number of other therapies have be evaluated for RLS including opioids, gabapentin and pregabalin, clonazepam, and case reports of melatonin, buproprion, and other agents. Overall, there is a long experience with opioids and those drugs have been especially useful in dopaminergic resistant RLS with augmentation problems. Clonazepam has also been widely used but is not particularly efficacious and now has been largely replaced by dopaminergic agents. In April 2011, the FDA approved extended release gabapentin for use in moderate to severe RLS. This anticonvulsant agent has recently been shown to be beneficial in RLS and may be especially useful when dopamine agents provide incomplete resolution of RLS symptoms and/or augmentation issues arise. Please remember that the extended release form of gabapentin gives different concentrations of drug than the shorter acting form. Finally, it is important to note that all epilepsy drugs carry a suicide warning label including gabapentin.

7.2 Non-pharmacological treatments for RLS

7.2.1 Exercise

Traditionally, one of the basic clinical recommendations in treating RLS symptoms involves exercise and stretching maneuvers. This has been endorsed by the RLS Foundation (www.rls.org) in their latest patient brochure although the data supporting this is limited. There have been earlier studies by suggesting that exercise close to bedtime is counterproductive for RLS. In a large study, Ohayon assessed the prevalence of RLS and PLMD in the general population. During the multivariate analysis of the secondary results, the researchers (Ohayon, 2002) found that physical exercise close to bedtime (within 2 hours for at least 15 minutes exercise 3 or more times per week) was associated with an increased risk of RLS (OR 1.34, $p<0.05$) and PLMD (OR 1.43, $p<0.05$). However, in a conflicting study from 2000, Phillips et al. found that a lack of exercise was significantly associated with RLS. In a telephone survey of over 1800 participants, a single question (modified from the 1995 IRLSSG criteria) was used to screen for RLS. In this study, there was an age-adjusted prevalence of RLS of 10.0% and a lack of exercise (less than 3 hours/month) was significantly associated with RLS (OR 3.32). In 1996, a Brazilian study evaluated 11 volunteers with to study the effect of acute physical activity on RLS and PLMD. In this report using a baseline PSG followed the next day by exercise and then a repeat PSG, there was a reduction in PLMD noted on the second night PSG (de Mello, 1996). In the only randomized-controlled trial of exercise in RLS, Aukerman studied 28 individuals in a 12 week exercise trial. The average age was 53.7 years and 39% of study subjects were male. Subjects were randomized to either a control group with usual activities or to an exercise group. The exercise program consisted of 3 days a week aerobic and lower extremity resistance/conditioning training. The IRLSSG severity scale and an RLS ordinal severity scale were checked at 0, 3, 6, 9, and 12 weeks. Of the 28 subjects, most (23) completed the trial with 11 in the exercise training group. The researchers found that the exercise group had a significant improvement in RLS symptoms compared to the control group with a $p = 0.001$ for the IRLSSG severity score and $p < 0.001$ for the RLS ordinal scale. The research team concluded that a prescribed exercise program is effective in improving RLS symptoms (Aukerman MM 2006).

7.2.2 Sequential compression devices

There is a hypothesis that reduced blood flow to the extremities may play a role in RLS symptoms. Research has been undertaken to ascertain whether sequential (pneumatic) compression devices may alleviate RLS symptomatology. In a small preliminary study from 2005, researchers from New Jersey evaluated 6 patients using enhanced external counter pulsation (EECP) devices on the legs for one hour daily Monday to Friday for 7 weeks (Rajaram SS, 2004). All 6 patients met the 2003 IRLSSG criteria and were assessed with the IRLS rating scale (IRLSSS) before and after the intervention. It should be noted that 3 subjects did not complete the IRLSSS until 4-5 months after EECP treatment. Further complicating the results, 4 of the 6 patients suffered from diabetic peripheral neuropathy and no electromyography or nerve conduction studies were done before or after EECP treatment to assess any potential neuropathy changes. Nevertheless, the research team found that the IRLS rating scale was significantly improved after EECP intervention and suggested that decreases in vascular flow may affect the nervous system (peripheral or central) causing the sensory symptoms of RLS. In a more rigorous prospective, randomized, double-blinded sham-controlled trial, Lettieri and Eliasson studied 35 subjects in 2009. Consecutive patients attending a sleep clinic for RLS for approached for recruitment. 41 RLS patients were assessed for eligibility with 6 excluded (4 not meeting inclusion criteria and 2 refused to participate). The remaining 35 patients were randomized into either therapeutic or sham treatment with a sequential compression device for 1 hour daily for 4 weeks. Validated questionnaires were administrated at the start and end of the intervention. These forms included the International Restless Legs Syndrome Study Group Severity Scale (IRLSSS), the Johns Hopkins Restless Legs Severity Scale (JHRLSS), and the restless legs syndrome quality of life instrument (RLS-QLI). Iron therapy and RLS pharmacological use was similar between the sham control and intervention groups. The researchers found significant improvements in the IRLSSS, JHRLSS, and the RLS-QLI for the intervention group and suggest that pneumatic compression devices are a useful adjunctive or alternative therapy for RLS (Lettieri CJ, 2009).

7.2.3 Massage therapy

Massage therapy has been long recommended as an additional therapy for RLS symptoms. However, there is a dearth of scientific evidence to support this claim. In a case report from 2006, Russell presented a 35 year old women with RLS type symptoms. There was no indication whether the patient actually met the 2003 IRLSSG criteria. It was noted that the patient had previously tried ropinirole without benefit. In this case report, the patient was treated with twice weekly massage therapy of 45 minute duration to the lower extremities for a 3 week period and reported improvements on a subjective symptom intensity scale from 40% at baseline to 10% at the end of therapy (Russell M, 2006). Interestingly, 2 weeks following the end of the massage intervention, the patient reported a return of her symptoms. Overall, there is a lack of scientific evidence to routinely support the use of massage therapy in RLS.

7.2.4 Acupuncture

Acupuncture has also been recommended by some as a therapy for RLS. Nonetheless, similar to massage therapy, there is minimal evidence to recommend acupuncture for RLS symptoms. In a Cochrane review, the authors found out of 14 potential studies only 2 met the inclusion criteria to be valid and both trials had methodological and/or reporting issues. Overall, the Cochrane reviewers felt that there was no significant data to support the use of acupuncture in RLS (Cui Y, 2008).

7.2.5 Endovenous laser ablation & sclerotherapy

Recently, Hayes and colleagues have reported on the use of endovenous laser ablation and sclerotherapy for the treatment of RLS. They screened 89 patients for RLS using the 2003 IRLSSG criteria. A total of 35 patients met inclusion criteria with 16 assigned to the control group and 19 to the interventional group. IRLS scores were obtained at baseline and 6 weeks later and showed a significant symptom improvement of 80% in the interventional group. The authors suggest that endovenous laser ablation therapy improves symptoms in RLS patients with superficial venous insufficiency (Hayes CA, 2008). The only other study assessing the efficacy of sclerotherapy in RLS was published by Kanter in 1995. In that paper, 1397 patients presenting to a varicose vein clinic were screened for RLS using an interview and a questionnaire (pre-1995 IRLSSG). Of these, 312 patients (22%) were felt to have RLS with 113 patients receiving treatment with sclerotherapy. The vast majority of patients (98%) reported subjective initial improvement in RLS symptoms although a substantial minority reported recurrent symptoms at 2 year follow-up (Kanter AH, 1995).

8. Conclusion

RLS is a common medical disorder which remains underdiagnosed. The underlying etiology is still not fully elucidated but there is increasing understanding of some mechanisms of disease especially in secondary RLS. Many treatment options are available although issues of augmentation and rebound continue to cause problems with RLS control. It is highly recommended that health care providers be aware of RLS symptoms and recognize the disease in their patients.

9. References

Agarwal P, Griffith A. (2008) Restless legs syndrome: a unique case and essentials of diagnosis and treatment. *Medscape J Med.* 2008;10(12):296.

Allen RP, Earley CJ. (1996) Augmentation of the restless legs syndrome with carbidopa/levodopa. *Sleep.* 1996 Apr;19(3):205-13.

Allen RP, Earley CJ. (2000) Defining the phenotype of the restless legs syndrome (RLS) using age-of-symptom-onset. *Sleep Med* 2000; 1: 11–9.

Allen RP, Picchietti D, Hening W, Trenkwalder C, Walters A, Montplaisi J. (2003) Restless legs syndrome: diagnostic criteria, special considerations, and epidemiology. A report from the restless legs syndrome diagnosis and epidemiology workshop at the National Institutes of Health. *Sleep Med.* 2003 Mar;4(2):101-19.

Allen RP, Ritchie SY. (2008) Clinical efficacy of ropinirole for restless legs syndrome is not affected by age at symptom onset. *Sleep Med.* 2008 Dec;9(8):899-902.

Auger C, Montplaisir J, Duquette P. (2005) Increased frequency of restless legs syndrome in a French-Canadian population with multiple sclerosis. *Neurology* 2005;65:1652-53.

Arunthari V, Kaplan J, Fredrickson PA, Lin SC, Castillo PR, Heckman MG. (2010) Prevalence of Restless Legs Syndrome in Blood Donors. *Mov Disord.* 2010 Jul 30;25(10):1451-5.

Bachmann CG, Rolke R, Scheidt U, Stadelmann C, Sommer M, Pavlakovic G, Happe S, Treede RD, Paulus W. (2010) Thermal hypoesthesia differentiates secondary restless legs syndrome associated with small fiber neuropathy from primary restless legs syndrome. *Brain.* 2010 Mar;133(Pt 3):762-70.

Balendran J, Champion D, Jaaniste T, Welsh A. (2011). A common sleep disorder in pregnancy: Restless legs syndrome and its predictors. *Aust N Z J Obstet Gynaecol.* 2011 Jun;51

Benes H, Mattern W, Peglau I, Dreykluft T, Bergmann L, Hansen C, Kohnen R, Banik N, Schoen SW, Hornyak M. (2011) Ropinirole improves depressive symptoms and restless legs syndrome severity in RLS patients: a multicentre, randomized, placebo- controlled study. *J Neurol.* 2011 Jun;258(6):1046-54.

Benediktsdottir B, Janson C, Lindberg E, Arnardóttir E, Olafsson I, Cook E, Thorarinsdottir EH, Gislason T. (2010) Prevalence of restless legs syndrome among adults in Iceland and Sweden: Lung function, comorbidity, ferritin, biomarkers and quality of life. *Sleep Med.* 2010 Dec;11(10):1043-8.

Berger K, Luedemann J, Trenkwalder C, John U, Kessler C. (2004) Sex and the risk of restless legs syndrome in the general population. *Arch Intern Med.* 2004 Jan 26;164(2):196-202.

Bhowmik D, Bhatia M, Tiwari S, Mahajan S, Gupta S, Agarwal SK, Dash SC. (2004) Low prevalence of restless legs syndrome in advanced chronic renal failure in the Indian population: a case-control study. *Ren Fail.* 2004 Jan;26(1):69-72.

Boentert M, Dziewas R, Heidbreder A, Happe S, Kleffner I, Evers S, Young P. (2010) Fatigue, reduced sleep quality and restless legs syndrome in Charcot-Marie-Tooth disease: a web-based survey. *J Neurol.* 2010 Apr;257(4):646-52.

Bogan RK, Fry JM, Schmidt MH, Carson SW, Ritchie SY; TREAT RLS US Study Group. (2006) Ropinirole in the treatment of patients with restless legs syndrome: a US-based randomized, double-blind, placebo-controlled clinical trial. *Mayo Clin Proc.* 2006 Jan;81(1):17- 27.

Calzetti S, Negrotti A, Bonavina G, Angelini M, Marchesi E. (2009) Absence of co-morbidity of Parkinson's Disease and restless legs syndrome: a case-control study of patients attending a movement disorder clinic. *Neurol Sci.* 2009 Apr;30(2):119-22.

Cesnik E, Casetta I, Turri M, Govoni V, Granieri E, Strambi LF, Manconi M. (2010) Transient RLS during pregnancy is a risk factor for the chronic idiopathic form. *Neurology* 2010; 75(23):2117-20.

Chen NH, Chuang LP, Yang CT, Kushida CA, Hsu SC, Wang PC, Lin SW, Chou YT, Chen RS, Li HY, Lai SC. (2010) The prevalence of restless legs syndrome in Taiwanese adults. *Psychiatry Clin Neurosci.* 2010 Apr;64(2):170-8.

Connor, JR; Boyer, PJ; Menzies, SL, Dellinger B, Allen RP, Ondo WG, Earley CJ. (2003) Neuropathological examination suggests impaired brain iron acquisition in restless legs syndrome. *Neurology* 2003;61(3): 304–9.

Connor JR, Wang XS, Allen RP, Beard JL, Wiesinger JA, Felt BT, Earley CJ. (2009) Altered dopaminergic profile in the putamen and substantia nigra in restless leg syndrome. *Brain* 2009 Sep;132(Pt 9):2403-12.

Connor JR, Ponnuru P, Wang XS, Patton SM, Allen RP, Earley CJ. (2011) Profile of altered brain iron acquisition in restless legs syndrome. *Brain.* 2011 Apr;134(Pt 4):959-68.

Cui Y, Wang Y, Liu Z. (2008) Acupuncture for restless legs syndrome. *Cochrane Database Syst Rev.* 2008 Oct 8;(4):CD006457.

de Mello MT, Lauro FA, Silva AC, Tufik S. (1996) Incidence of periodic leg movements and of the restless legs syndrome during sleep following acute physical activity in spinal cord injury subjects. *Spinal Cord* (1996) 34:294-296.

Deriu M, Cossu G, Molari A, Murgia D, Mereu A, Ferrigno P, Manca D, Contu P, Melis M. (2009) Restless legs syndrome in multiple sclerosis: a case control study. *Mov Disord.* 2009 Apr 15;24(5):697- 701.

Domínguez RO, Michref A, Tanus E, Amartino H. (2007) Restless legs syndrome in Fabry disease: clinical feature associated to neuropathic pain is overlooked. *Rev Neurol.* 2007 Oct 16- 31;45(8):474-8.

Douay X, Waucquier N, Hautecoeur P, Vermersch P; G-SEP (Groupe Septentrional d'Etudes et de Recherche sur la Sclérose en Plaques). (2009) High prevalence of restless legs syndrome in multiple sclerosis. *Rev Neurol (Paris)* 2009 Feb;165(2):194-6.

Dzaja A, Wehrle R, Lancel M, Pollmächer T. (2009) Elevated estradiol plasma levels in women with restless legs during pregnancy. *Sleep.* 2009 Feb;32(2):169-74.

Earley CJ, Kuwabara H, Wong DF, Gamaldo C, Salas R, Brasic J, Ravert HT, Dannals RF, Allen RP. (2011) The dopamine transporter is decreased in the striatum of subjects with restless legs syndrome. *Sleep* 2011 Mar 1;34(3):341-7.

Ekbom K. (1945) Restless legs: a clinical study. *Acta Med Scand Suppl* 1945;158:1–123.

Facco FL, Kramer J, Ho KH, Zee PC, Grobman WA. (2010) Sleep disturbances in pregnancy. *Obstet Gynecol*. 2010;115(1):77-83.

Gao X, Schwarzschild MA, O'Reilly EJ, Wang H, Ascherio A. (2010) Restless legs syndrome and Parkinson's Disease in men. *Mov Disord*. 2010 Nov 15;25(15):2654-7.

Gemignani F, Marbini A, Di Giovanni G, Salih S, Margarito FP, Pavesi G, Terzano MG.(1997) Cryoglobulinaemic neuropathy manifesting with restless legs syndrome. *J Neurol Sci*. 1997 Nov 25;152(2):218- 23.

Gemignani F, Brindani F, Vitetta F, Marbini A, Calzetti S. (2007) Restless legs syndrome in diabetic neuropathy: a frequent manifestation of small fiber neuropathy. *J Peripher Nerv Syst*. 2007 Mar;12(1):50-3.

Ghorayeb I, Bioulac B, Scribans C, Tison F. (2008) Perceived severity of restless legs syndrome across the female life cycle. *Sleep Med*. 2008 Oct;9(7):799-802.

Goffredo Filho GS, Gorini CC, Purysko AS, Silva HC, Elias IE. (2003) Restless legs syndrome in patients on chronic hemodialysis in a Brazilian city: frequency, biochemical findings and co-morbidities. *Arq Neuropsiquiatr*. 2003 Sep;61(3B):723-7.

Hansen RA, Song L, Moore CG, Gilsenan AW, Kim MM, Calloway MO, Murray MD. (2009) Effect of ropinirole on sleep outcomes in patients with restless legs syndrome: meta-analysis of pooled individual patient data from randomized controlled trials. *Pharmacotherapy*. 2009 Mar;29(3):255-62.

Hassan N, Pineau CA, Clarke AE, Vinet E, Ng R, Bernatsky S. (2011) Systemic lupus and risk of restless legs syndrome. *J Rheumatol* 2011; 38(5):874-6.

Hattan E, Chalk C, Postuma RB. (2009) Is there a higher risk of restless legs syndrome in peripheral neuropathy? *Neurology* 2009 Mar 17;72(11):955-60.

Hayes CA, Kingsley JR, Hamby KR, Carlow J. (2008) The effect of endovenous laser ablation on restless legs syndrome. *Phlebology* 2008;23:112–117.

Hening WA, Walters A, Kavey N, Gidro-Frank S, Côté L, Fahn S. (1986) Dyskinesias while awake and periodic movements in sleep in restless legs syndrome: treatment with opioids. *Neurology*. 1986 Oct;36(10):1363-6.

Hening WA, Allen RP, Ondo WG, Walters AS, Winkelman JW, Becker P, Bogan R, Fry JM, Kudrow DB, Lesh KW, Fichtner A, Schollmayer E; SP792 Study Group. (2010) Rotigotine improves restless legs syndrome: a 6-month randomized, double-blind, placebo- controlled trial in the United States. *Mov Disord*. 2010 Aug 15;25(11):1675-83.

Högl B, Garcia-Borreguero D, Trenkwalder C, Ferini-Strambi L, Hening W, Poewe W, Brenner SS, Fraessdorf M, Busse M, Albrecht S, Allen RP. (2011) Efficacy and augmentation during 6 months of double- blind pramipexole for restless legs syndrome. *Sleep Med*. 2011 Apr;12(4):351-60.

Inoue Y, Kuroda K, Hirata K, Uchimura N, Kagimura T, Shimizu T. (2010) Long-term open-label study of pramipexole in patients with primary restless legs syndrome. *J Neurol Sci*. 2010 Jul 15;294(1- 2):62-6.

Italian REMS Study Group, Manconi M, Ferini-Strambi L, Filippi M, Bonanni E, Iudice A, Murri L. (2008) Multicenter case-control study on restless legs syndrome in multiple sclerosis: the REMS study. *Sleep*. 2008 Jul;31(7):944-52.

Kaplan PW, Allen RP, Buchholz DW, Walters JK. (1993) A double-blind, placebo-controlled study of the treatment of periodic limb movements in sleep using carbidopa/levodopa and propoxyphene. *Sleep*. 1993 Dec;16(8):717-23.

Kanter AH. (1995) The effect of sclerotherapy on restless legs syndrome. *Dermatol Surg*. 1995 Apr;21(4):328-32.

Kilfoyle DH, Dyck PJ, Wu Y, Litchy WJ, Klein DM, Dyck PJ, Kumar N, Cunningham JM, Klein CJ. (2006) Myelin protein zero mutation His39Pro: hereditary motor and sensory neuropathy with variable onset, hearing loss, restless legs and multiple sclerosis. *J Neurol Neurosurg Psychiatry*. 2006 Aug;77(8):963-6.

Kushida C, Martin M, Nikam P, Blaisdell B, Wallenstein G, Ferini-Strambi L, Ware JE Jr. (2007) Burden of restless legs syndrome on health related quality of life. *Qual Life Res*. 2007;16:617-624.

LaRochelle JS, Karp BI. (2004) Restless legs syndrome due to interferon- alpha. *Mov Disord*. 2004 Jun;19(6):730-1.

Lettau LA, Gudas CJ, Kaelin TD. (2010) Remission of restless legs syndrome and periodic limb movements in sleep after bilateral excision of multiple foot neuromas: a case report. *J Med Case Reports*. 2010 Sep 17;4:306.

Lettieri CJ, Eliasson AH. (2009) Pneumatic compression devices are an effective therapy for restless legs syndrome: a prospective, randomized, double-blinded, sham-controlled trial. *Chest*. 2009 Jan;135(1):74-80.

Lin SC, Kaplan J, Burger CD, Fredrickson PA. (1998) Effect of pramipexole in treatment of resistant restless legs syndrome. *Mayo Clin Proc*. 1998 Jun;73(6):497-500.

Lo Coco D, Cannizzaro E, Lopez G. (2009) Restless legs syndrome in a patient with multifocal motor neuropathy. *Neurol Sci*. 2009 Oct;30(5):401-3.

Manconi M, Govoni V, De Vito A, Economou NT, Cesnik E, Casetta I, Mollica G, Ferini-Strambi L, Granieri E. (2004) Restless legs syndrome and pregnancy. *Neurology*. 2004 Sep 28;63(6):1065-9.

Manconi M, Fabbrini M, Bonanni E, Filippi M, Rocca M, Murri L, Ferini- Strambi L. (2007) High prevalence of restless legs syndrome in multiple sclerosis. *Eur J Neurol*. 2007 May;14(5):534-9.

Manconi M, Rocca MA, Ferini-Strambi L, Tortorella P, Agosta F, Comi G, Filippi M. (2008) Restless legs syndrome is a common finding in multiple sclerosis and correlates with cervical cord damage. *Mult Scler*. 2008 Jan;14(1):86-93.

Manconi M, Ferri R, Zucconi M, Oldani A, Giarolli L, Bottasini V, Ferini- Strambi L. (2011). Pramipexole versus ropinirole: polysomnographic acute effects in restless legs syndrome. *Mov Disord*. 2011 Apr;26(5):892-5.

Manconi M, Ferri R, Zucconi M, Clemens S, Giarolli L, Bottasini V, Ferini- Strambi L. (2011) Preferential D2 or preferential D3 dopamine agonists in restless legs syndrome. *Neurology*. 2011 12;77(2):110-7.

Marin LF, dos Santos WA, Pedroso JL, Ferraz HB, de Carvalho LB, do Prado GF. (2010) Restless legs syndrome associated with Guillain- Barré syndrome: a report of two cases. *Parkinsonism Relat Disord*. 2010 Jul;16(6):418-9.

Merlino G, Lorenzut S, Gigli GL, Romano G, Montanaro D, Moro A, Valente M. (2010) A case-control study on restless legs syndrome in nondialyzed patients with chronic renal failure. *Mov Disord*. 2010 Jun 15;25(8):1019-25.

Michaud M, Soucy JP, Chabli A, Lavigne G, Montplaisir J. (2002) SPECT imaging of striatal pre- and postsynaptic dopaminergic status in restless legs syndrome with periodic leg movements in sleep. *J Neurol*. 2002;249:164–70.

Moccia M, Pellecchia MT, Erro R, Zingone F, Marelli S, Barone DG, Ciacci C, Strambi LF, Barone P. (2010) Restless legs syndrome is a common feature of adult celiac disease. *Mov Disord.* 2010 May 15;25(7):877-81.

Montplaisir J, Boucher S, Poirier G, Lavigne G, Lapierre O, Lesperance P. (1997) Clinical,vpolysomnographic, and genetic characteristics of restless legs syndrome: a study of 133 patients diagnosed with new standard criteria. *Mov Disord* 1997;12(1):61–5.

Montplaisir J, Nicolas A, Denesle R, Gomez-Mancilla B. (1999) Restless legs syndrome improved by pramipexole: a double-blind randomized trial. *Neurology.* 1999 Mar 23;52(5):938-43.

Montplaisir J, Karrasch J, Haan J, Volc D. (2006) Ropinirole is effective in the long-term management of restless legs syndrome: a randomized controlled trial. *Mov Disord.* 2006 Oct;21(10):1627-35.

Moreira NC, Damasceno RS, Medeiros CA, Bruin PF, Teixeira CA, Horta WG, Bruin VM. (2008) Restless legs syndrome, sleep quality and fatigue in multiple sclerosis patients. *Braz J Med Biol Res.* 2008 Oct;41(10):932-937.

Neau JP, Porcheron A, Mathis S, Julian A, Meurice JC, Paquereau J, Godeneche G, Ciron J, Bouche G. (2010) Restless legs syndrome and pregnancy: a questionnaire study in the Poitiers district, France. *Eur Neurol.* 2010; 64(5):268-74.

Neau JP, Marion P, Mathis S, Julian A, Godeneche G, Larrieu D, Meurice JC, Paquereau J, Ingrand P. (2010) Restless legs syndrome and pregnancy: follow-up of pregnant women before and after delivery. *Eur Neurol.* 2010;64(6):361-6.

Oertel WH, Benes H, Bodenschatz R, Peglau I, Warmuth R, Happe S, Geisler P, Cassel W, Leroux M, Kohnen R, Stiasny-Kolster K. (2006) Efficacy of cabergoline in restless legs syndrome: a placebo- controlled study with polysomnography (CATOR). *Neurology.* 2006 Sep 26;67(6):1040-6.

Oertel WH, Benes H, Garcia-Borreguero D, Högl B, Poewe W, Montagna P, Ferini-Strambi L, Sixel-Döring F, Trenkwalder C, Partinen M, Saletu B, Polo O, Fichtner A, Schollmayer E, Kohnen R, Cassel W, Penzel T, Stiasny-Kolster K. (2010) Rotigotine transdermal patch in moderate to severe idiopathic restless legs syndrome: a randomized, placebo-controlled polysomnographic study. *Sleep Med.* 2010 Oct;11(9):848-56.

Oertel W, Trenkwalder C, Beneš H, Ferini-Strambi L, Högl B, Poewe W, Stiasny-Kolster K, Fichtner A, Schollmayer E, Kohnen R, García- Borreguero D; on behalf of the SP710 study group. (2011) Long- term safety and efficacy of rotigotine transdermal patch for moderate-to-severe idiopathic restless legs syndrome: a 5-year open-label extension study. *Lancet Neurol.* 2011 Jun 24. [Epub ahead of print]

O'Keeffe ST, Gavin K, Lavan JN. (1994) Iron status and restless legs syndrome in the elderly. *Age Ageing* 1994;23(3):200–3.

Ondo W. (1999) Ropinirole for restless legs syndrome. *Mov Disord.* 1999 Jan;14(1):138-40.

Ohayon MM, Roth, T. (2002) Prevalence of restless legs syndrome and periodic limb movement disorder in the general population. *J Psychosom Res* 2002 Jul;53(1):547–554.

Phillips B, Young T, Finn L, Asher K, Hening W, Purvis C. (2000), Epidemiology of Restless Legs Symptoms in Adults. *Arch Intern Med.* 2000;160:2137-2141

Pantaleo NP, Hening WA, Allen RP, Earley CJ. (2009) Pregnancy accounts for most of the gender difference in prevalence of familial RLS. *Sleep Med.* 2010 Mar;11(3):310-3.

Partinen M, Hirvonen K, Jama L, Alakuijala A, Hublin C, Tamminen I, Koester J, Reess J. (2006) Efficacy and safety of pramipexole in idiopathic restless legs syndrome: a polysomnographic dose- finding study--the PRELUDE study. *Sleep Med.* 2006 Aug;7(5):407-17.

Paulus W, Trenkwalder C. (2006) Less is more: pathophysiology of dopaminergic-therapy-related augmentation in restless legs syndrome. *Lancet Neurol.* 2006 Oct;5(10):878-86.

Quinn C, Uzbeck M, Saleem I, Cotter P, Ali J, O'Malley G, Gilmartin JJ, O'Keeffe ST. (2011) Iron status and chronic kidney disease predict restless legs syndrome in an older hospital population. *Sleep Med.* 2011 Mar;12(3):295-301.

Quiroz C, Pearson V, Gulyani S, Allen R, Earley C, Ferré S. (2010) Up-regulation of striatal adenosine A(2A) receptors with iron deficiency in rats: effects on locomotion and cortico-striatal neurotransmission. *Exp Neurol.* 2010 Jul;224(1):292-8.

Reynolds G, Blake DR, Pall HS, Williams A. (1986) Restless leg syndrome and rheumatoid arthritis. *BMJ* 1986;292:659-60.

Rijsman RM, de Weerd AW, Stam CJ, Kerkhof GA, Rosman JB. (2004) Periodic limb movement disorder and restless legs in dialysis patients. *Nephrology (Carlton).* 2004 Dec;9(6):353-61.

Russell, M. (2007) Massage therapy and restless legs syndrome. *J Bodywork Movement Ther* 2007 11(2):146–150.

Salih AM, Gray RES, Mills KR, Webley M. (1994) A clinical, serological and neurophysiological study of restless legs syndrome in rheumatoid arthritis. *Br. J Rheumatol* 1994;33:60-3.

Sikandar R, Khealani BA, Wasay M. (2009) Predictors of restless legs syndrome in pregnancy: a hospital based cross sectional survey from Pakistan. *Sleep Med.* 2009 Jun;10(6):676-8.

Snyder AM, Wang X, Patton SM, Arosio P, Levi S, Earley CJ, Allen RP, Connor JR. (2009) Mitochondrial ferritin in the substantia nigra in restless legs syndrome. *J Neuropathol Exp Neurol.* 2009 Nov;68(11):1193-9.

Sperfeld AD, Unrath A, Kassubek J. (2007) Restless legs syndrome in hereditary spastic paraparesis. *Eur Neurol.* 2007;57(1):31-5.

Stiasny K, Röbbecke J, Schüler P, Oertel WH. (2000) Treatment of idiopathic restless legs syndrome (RLS) with the D2-agonist cabergoline--an open clinical trial. *Sleep.* 2000 May 1;23(3):349-54.

Stiasny-Kolster K, Kohnen R, Schollmayer E, Möller JC, Oertel WH; Rotigotine Sp 666 Study Group. (2004) Patch application of the dopamine agonist rotigotine to patients with moderate to advanced stages of restless legs syndrome: a double-blind, placebo-controlled pilot study. *Mov Disord.* 2004 19(12):1432-8.

Synofzik M, Godau J, Lindig T, Schöls L, Berg D. (2011) Restless legs and substantia nigra hypoechogenicity are common features in Friedreich's ataxia. *Cerebellum.* 2011 Mar;10(1):9-13.

Takaki J, Nishi T, Nangaku M, Shimoyama H, Inada T, Matsuyama N, Kumano H, Kuboki T. (2003) Clinical and psychological aspects of restless legs syndrome in uremic patients on hemodialysis. *Am J Kidney Dis.* 2003 Apr;41(4):833-9.

Taylor-Gjevre RM, Gjevre JA, Skomro R, Nair B. (2009) Restless legs syndrome in a rheumatoid arthritis patient cohort. *J Clin Rheumatol* 2009;15:12-15.

Taylor-Gjevre RM, Gjevre JA, Skomro RP, Nair BV. (2011) Assessment of sleep health in patients with rheumatic disease. *International Journal of Clinical Rheumatology* 2011; 6(2):207-218.

Trenkwalder C, Collado Seidel V, Kazenwadel J, Wetter TC, Oertel W, Selzer R, Kohnen R. (2003) One-year treatment with standard and sustained-release levodopa: appropriate long-term treatment of restless legs syndrome? *Mov Disord.* 2003 Oct;18(10):1184-9.

Trenkwalder C, Hundemer HP, Lledo A, Swieca J, Polo O, Wetter TC, Ferini-Strambi L, de Groen H, Quail D, Brandenburg U; PEARLS Study Group. (2004) Efficacy of pergolide in treatment of restless legs syndrome: the PEARLS Study. *Neurology.* 2004 Apr 27;62(8):1391-7.

Trenkwalder C, Garcia-Borreguero D, Montagna P, Lainey E, de Weerd AW, Tidswell P, Saletu-Zyhlarz G, Telstad W, Ferini-Strambi L; Therapy with Ropiunirole; Efficacy and Tolerability in RLS 1 Study Group. (2004) Ropinirole in the treatment of restless legs syndrome: results from the TREAT RLS 1 study, a 12 week, randomised, placebo controlled study in 10 European countries. *J Neurol Neurosurg Psychiatry.* 2004 Jan;75(1):92-7.

Tunç T, Karadağ YS, Doğulu F, Inan LE. (2007) Predisposing factors of restless legs syndrome in pregnancy. *Mov Disord.* 2007 Apr 15;22(5):627-31.

Ulfberg J, Nyström B. (2004) Restless legs syndrome in blood donors. *Sleep Med* 2004;5(2):115-8.

Unruh ML, Levey AS, D'Ambrosio C, Fink NE, Powe NR, Meyer KB; Choices for Healthy Outcomes in Caring for End-Stage Renal Disease (CHOICE) Study. (2004) Restless legs symptoms among incident dialysis patients: association with lower quality of life and shorter survival. *Am J Kidney Dis.* 2004 May;43(5):900-9

Verbaan D, van Rooden SM, van Hilten JJ, Rijsman RM. (2010) Prevalence and clinical profile of restless legs syndrome in Parkinson's Disease. *Mov Disord.* 2010 Oct 15;25(13):2142-7.

Walters AS, Hening WA, Kavey N, Chokroverty S, Gidro-Frank S. (1988) A double-blind randomized crossover trial of bromocriptine and placebo in restless legs syndrome. *Ann Neurol.* 1988 24(3):455-8.

Walters AS, Hening W. (1987) Clinical presentation and neuropharmacology of restless legs syndrome. *Clin Neuropharmacol.* 1987 Jun;10(3):225-237.

Walters AS. The International Restless Legs Syndrome Study Group. (1995) Toward a better definition of the restless legs syndrome. *Mov Disord* 1995;10:634–42.

Walters AS and the International Restless Legs Syndrome Study Group. (2003) Validation of the International Restless Legs Syndrome Study Group rating scale for restless legs syndrome. *Sleep Med* 2003; 4: 121–32.

Wang J, O'Reilly B, Venkataraman R, Mysliwiec V, Mysliwiec A. (2009) Efficacy of oral iron in patients with restless legs syndrome and a low-normal ferritin: A randomized, double-blind, placebo- controlled study. *Sleep Med.* 2009 Oct;10(9):973-5.

Zanettini R, Antonini A, Gatto G, Gentile R, Tesei S, Pezzoli G. (2007) Valvular heart disease and the use of dopamine agonists for Parkinson's disease. *N Engl J Med.* 2007 Jan 4;356(1):39-46.

12

Screening Methods for REM Sleep Behavior Disorder

Masayuki Miyamoto[1], Tomoyuki Miyamoto[2],
Keisuke Suzuki[1], Masaoki Iwanami[2] and Koichi Hirata[1]
[1]*Department of Neurology, Center of Sleep Medicine,*
Dokkyo Medical University School of Medicine
[2]*Department of Neurology Dokkyo Medical University Koshigaya Hospital*
Japan

1. Introduction

REM sleep behavior disorder (RBD) is a parasomnia characterized by dream-enacting behavior and vivid, action-filled or unpleasant dreams and presents a risk for self-injury and harm to others (e.g., a bed partner) due to abnormal REM sleep during which control of muscle tonus is lacking. Polysomnography is required to establish the diagnosis and represents the diagnostic gold standard for revealing loss of REM-related muscle atonia with excessive sustained or intermittent elevation of submental EMG tone or excessive phasic submental or limb EMG twitching. Idiopathic RBD (iRBD) has a male preponderance and usually emerges after the age of 50 and has a known association with neurodegenerative diseases, in particular the α-synucleinopathies such as Parkinson's disease (PD), dementia with Lewy body disease and multiple system atrophy (Schenck & Mahowald, 2002). Even more important, evidence is growing that iRBD precedes parkinsonism by years or even decades, and that iRBD might present an early stage in the development of neurodegenerative disorders (Schenck et al., 1996). Thus, to identify clinical RBD as early as possible appears to be useful for early diagnosis, a clinical trial with a potentially neuroprotective substance, and also for epidemiological studies. To meet the need for an easily applicable diagnostic screening tool, Stiasny-Kolster et al. developed and validated a specific screening scale for assessment of RBD, the RBD screening questionnaire (RBDSQ) (Stiasny-Kolster et al., 2007). Subsequently we developed a Japanese version of the RBDSQ (RBDSQ-J) after obtaining approval from the patent owner and investigated its validity and reliability (Miyamoto et al., 2009). We found that detection of RBD using the RBDSQ-J would be useful in the stepwise diagnostic process. We will discuss screening methods for RBD and describe RBD screening questionnaires, including the RBDSQ-J.

2. Prevalence of REM sleep behavior disorder

The overall prevalence of RBD remains largely unknown. A large telephone survey using the Sleep-EVAL system for assessing violent behaviors during sleep in the general population (4972 individuals aged 15-100 years) in the United Kingdom suggested an estimated prevalence of RBD of about 0.5% (Ohayon et al., 1997). A study of 1034 elderly subjects aged 70 years or above in the Hong Kong area found an estimated prevalence of polysomnography (PSG)-confirmed RBD of 0.38% (Chiu et al., 2000). There is a male predominance (87%) with primarily men over the age of 50 being affected (Schenck & Mahowald, 2002). Boeve summarized the demographics and clinical phenomenology of RBD (Table 1) (Boeve, 2010a).

Male gender predilection
Age of onset typically 40-70 years (range 15-80 years)
Abnormal vocalizations –orating, yelling, swearing, screaming
Abnormal motor behavior- limb flailing, punching, kicking, lurching out of bed
Altered dream mentation - typically involves a chasing/attacking theme with insects, animals or other humans being the aggressors and the patient being the defender
Exhibited behaviors mirror dream content
Behaviors tend to occur in the latter half of the sleep period

Table 1. Demographics and clinical phenomenology of RBD (Modified from Boeve, 2010a)

3. Diagnosis for REM sleep behavior disorder

Until recently, the diagnosis of RBD was based on clinical manifestations, namely the presence of limb or body movements associated with dream mentation and at least one of the following: (1) harmful or potentially harmful sleep behaviors during sleep; (2) dreams that appear to be acted out; and (3) sleep behaviors that disrupt sleep continuity. Polysomnographic observations of patients were not necessary for diagnosis according to the International Classification of Sleep Disorders-1 (ICSD-1).

Eisensehr et al. and Gagnon et al. pointed out the limitations of these criteria because one half of the cases of RBD with PD would have been undetected based clinical interviews alone (Eisensehr et al., 2001; Gagnon et al., 2002). RBD-like features can occur with other sleep conditions such as obstructive sleep apnea syndrome (OSAS), sleepwalking, night terrors, and sleep-related seizures (see below 4). In the second version of the ICSD (ICSD-2), PSG findings were required to establish the diagnosis. The first essential criterion is the presence of REM sleep without atonia. The second criterion is the presence of either sleep-related injurious or disruptive behaviors revealed by history or abnormal REM sleep behaviors documented during PSG recording. Time-synchronized video recording is essential for helping to establish the diagnosis of RBD during PSG. The last two criteria are exclusion criteria, which are the absence of epileptiform activity during sleep and the presence of other sleep disorders or medical or neurological disorders that could better explain the sleep disturbance. The diagnostic criteria are listed in Table 2.

A. Presence of REM sleep without atonia: EMG finding of excessive amounts of sustained or intermittent elevation of submental EMG tone or excessive phasic submental or (upper or lower) limb EMG twitching.

B. At least one of the following is present:

i. Sleep related injurious, potentially injurious, or disruptive behaviors by history

ii. Abnormal REM sleep behaviors documented during polysomnographic monitoring

C. Absence of EEG epileptiform activity during REM sleep unless RBD can be clearly distinguished from any concurrent REM sleep related seizure disorder.

D. The sleep disturbance is not better explained by another sleep disorder, medical or neurological disorder, mental disorder, medication use, or substance use disorder.

Table 2. Diagnostic criteria for REM sleep behavior disorder in ICSD-2

4. Differential diagnosis of REM sleep behavior disorder

RBD is a relatively rare condition and is largely unknown to most physicians (see above 2), therefore it is often misdiagnosed and mistreated.
The differential diagnosis of recurrent dream enactment behavior includes NREM parasomnia, nocturnal panic attacks, nocturnal seizures, nightmares, nocturnal wandering associated with dementia, and OSAS (Boeve, 2010a). A complaint of nocturnal disruptive behaviors is the major clinical feature of several other conditions, such as primary and secondary disorders of arousal, dreaming, and panic disorders (Table 3).

Primary disorders of arousal (from NREM sleep)
Confusional arousals
Sleepwalking
Sleep terrors
Secondary arousal disorders
Obstructive sleep apnea syndrome (pseudo RBD)
Sleep-related epilepsy
Psychiatric diseases
Sleep-related dissociative disorder
Panic disorder
Posttraumatic stress syndrome

Table 3. Differential diagnosis of RBD

Primary arousal disorders from NREM sleep include confusional arousals, sleepwalking, and sleep terrors. In contrast to RBD, sleepwalking and sleep terrors are more frequent in children and rarely appear *de novo* in middle-aged or elderly individuals. They are also characterized by confusion and retrograde amnesia upon awakening at the time of nocturnal episodes; these phenomena are not seen in patients with RBD. In general, RBD involves attempted enactment of altered dreams and rapid awakening from an episode that usually occurs two or more hours after sleep onset. In contrast, sleepwalking and sleep terror episodes often emerge within two hours after sleep onset, are not usually associated with rapid alertness, and are rarely associated with dreaming in children. Adults can have associated dreaming, but it is usually more fragmentary and more limited than RBD dreams.

Severe OSAS and nocturnal epilepsy may mimic the symptoms of RBD. Patients with severe OSAS may present with unpleasant dreams and dream-enacting behaviors (Iranzo & Santamaria, 2005). Continuous positive airway pressure (CPAP) therapy can eliminate abnormal nocturnal behaviors. Sleep-related seizures usually present with repetitive stereotypical behaviors.

When a diagnostic clarification is necessary, particularly when the risk for injury is high, the behaviors occur at any time of the night, other features suggesting an evolving neurodegenerative are present, or loud snoring and observed apnea suggestive of OSA are present, PSG with simultaneous video monitoring is warranted (Boeve, 2010a).

5. The need for screening and screening methods for RBD

PSG is clearly necessary for establishing the diagnosis of RBD, but the procedure requires appropriate monitoring equipment, including time synchronized video recordings, specially trained technologists, bed availability in a sleep laboratory, and clinicians who can interpret the data. The procedure is costly, especially for patients with limited insurance coverage.

Subjects must be willing and able to sleep in a sleep laboratory and undergo monitoring. Some patients with coexisting neurologic disorders are too cognitively or physically impaired to tolerate and undergo an adequate study, are too uncooperative to permit all of the monitoring equipment to remain in place, are at risk for falls during the night, or are institutionalized. RBD cannot be accurately assessed in the home. Due to the limited number of sleep disorder centers in many countries, PSG is not possible even when clearly medically warranted. As it is impractical to perform PSG in large numbers of subjects in epidemiologic studies of sleep disorders, the availability of a simple, short, reliable, and accurate measure to screen for the presence of various sleep disorders would be highly valuable (Boeve, 2010a).

A recent study suggested that a clinical interview by expert clinicians could provide good sensitivity (100%) and specificity (99.6%) in diagnosing RBD in non-PD patients (Eisensehr et al, 2001). The interobserver reliability of ICSD-R criteria for RBD was also found to be substantial (Bologna, Genova, Parma and Pisa Universities group for the study of REM sleep Behaviour Disorder (RBD) in Parkinson's Disease, 2003). Nevertheless, conducting a useful clinical interview may require considerable expertise, training, time and resources. In addition, waiting times might be long for and access limited to clinical and PSG assessments in some medical settings. Hence, an easily applicable questionnaire may be considered as a supplemental assessment tool in clinical practice to provide a quick and accurate appraisal of RBD symptoms in order to prioritize assessment and intervention.

We describe RBD screening questionnaires such as the Mayo Sleep Questionnaire (MSQ), RBDSQ (English/German version and Japanese version) and RBDQ-HK.

5.1 Mayo sleep questionnaire

RBD is a parasomnia that can develop in otherwise neurologically-normal adults as well as in those with a neurodegenerative disease. Confirmation of RBD requires PSG. A simple screening measure for RBD is desirable for clinical and research purposes. Boeve et al.

developed the Mayo Sleep Questionnaire (MSQ), a 16-item measure to screen for the presence of RBD, periodic legs movement disorder (PLMD), restless legs syndrome (RLS), sleepwalking, OSAS and sleep-related leg cramps (Boeve, 2010a; Boeve et al., 2002a, 2002b, 2010b, 2011). The data presented herein refer to the primary question on RBD (Question 1); if the primary question is answered affirmatively, subquestions are asked (subquestions 1b-e) as shown in Table 4.

1. Have you ever seen the patient appear to "act out his/her dreams"while sleeping?
(punched or flailed arms in the air, shouted or screamed).

If yes,

(a) How many months or years has this been going on? (data on this subquestion were not analyzed in this analysis)

(b) Has the patient ever been injured from these behaviors (bruises, cuts, broken bones)?

(c) Has a bed partner ever been injured from these behaviors (bruises, blows, pulled hair)?

(d) Has the patient told you about dreams of being chased, attacked or that involve defending himself/herself?

(e) If the patient woke up and told you about a dream, did the details of the dream match the movements made while sleeping?

Table 4. Primary question on RBD in the Mayo Sleep Questionnaire (MSQ)
(from the website: http://www.mayoclinic.org/pdfs/MSQ-copyrightfinal.pdf.)

Among the community-dwelling elderly, the MSQ has high sensitivity (100%) and specificity (95%) for diagnosis of RBD and was particularly specific for RBD in the absence of an OSA feature (Boeve, 2010b).
Boeve et al. also assessed the validity of the MSQ by comparing the responses of patients' bed partners with the findings (REM sleep without atonia) on PSG. The study subjects were 176 individuals (150 males; median age 71 years (range 39-90)) with the following clinical diagnoses: normal (n=8), mild cognitive impairment (n=44), Alzheimer's disease (n=23), dementia with Lewy bodies (n=74), and other dementia and/or parkinsonian syndromes (n=27). Sensitivity and specificity for question 1 on the MSQ for PSG-proven RBD were 98% and 74%, respectively. They concluded that the MSQ has adequate sensitivity and specificity for the diagnosis of RBD among aged subjects with cognitive impairment and/or parkinsonism (Boeve et al, 2011).

5.2 RBDSQ

Stiasny-Kolster et al. in 2007 developed the original German/English RBD Screening Questionnaire (RBDSQ) (Stiasny-Kolster et al., 2007). The RBDSQ is a 10-item patient self-rating instrument that assesses sleep behavior with short questions that have to be answered by either "yes" or "no" by the patient. Since patients do not always have a long-time companion, the bed partner's input was encouraged but not required. Items 1 to 4 address the frequency and content of dreams and their relationship to nocturnal movements and behavior. Item 5 asks about self-injuries and injuries of the bed partner. Item 6 consists of four subitems that assess nocturnal motor behavior more specifically, e.g., questions about nocturnal vocalization, sudden limb movements, complex movements, or items around the bed that fell down. Items 7 and 8 deal with nocturnal awakenings. Item 9 focuses on disturbed sleep in general and item 10 on the presence of any neurological disorder. The maximum total score for the RBDSQ is 13 points. The RBDSQ was applied to 54 RBD patients (mean age 53.7 years, range 19-79) who had been clinically diagnosed with iRBD (n=19), narcolepsy (n=33), early PD (n=2)) and 160 patients without RBD (age 50.8 years, range 20-83) who had been diagnosed as having RLS (n=73), narcolepsy (n=27), OSAS (n=21), hypersomnia (n=10), PLMD (n=8), insomnia (n=4), sleepwalking (n=4), epilepsy (n=3), nightmares (n=1), sleep bruxisum (n=1), or depression. (n=1). Also studied were 133 healthy subjects (mean age 46.9 years, range 20-72). Using a cut-off value of five points on the RBDSQ as a discriminatory variable, the questionnaire revealed a sensitivity of 96% and a specificity of 56%, correctly diagnosing 66% of subjects with sleep disorders. They mentioned that the lower specificity might be due to the fact that most of their control patients had sleep disturbances or neurological disorders that are known to be associated with periodic leg movements, e.g., RLS, PLMD, narcolepsy, and OSAS. This selection bias predisposed to positive answers for items that are related either to limb movements such as items 4, 5, 6.2, and 7 or to the presence of sleep and/or neurologic disorders such as for items 9 and 10, leading to higher RBDSQ total scores and thus to a lower specificity. Considering its high sensitivity, the RBDSQ represents an adequate tool to detect subjects with RBD. In subjects without additional neurologic or sleep disorders, the specificity was high, but in patients with either neurologic diseases or sleep disorders, the specificity is poorer but acceptable. The authors demonstrated the RBDSQ might be applied within a stepwise diagnostic process (questionnaire, interview, PSG).

5.3 RBDSQ-J

We developed a Japanese version of the RBDSQ (RBDSQ-J) after obtaining approval from the patent owner and investigated its validity and reliability (Miyamoto et al., 2009). The RBDSQ-J was administered to 52 consecutive patients with iRBD diagnosed according to criteria in the ICSD-2 (mean age 66.4 years; 36 males, 16 females), 55 consecutive OSAS patients who had responded well to CPAP therapy (mean age 63.1 years; 44 males, 11 females) after a diagnosis of RBD was ruled out by history and PSG and 65 apparently healthy subjects (mean age 64.6 years; 37 males, 28 females).

The mean RBDSQ-J scores for the iRBD group, the OSAS group and the healthy subjects were 7.5, 1.9, and 1.6 points, respectively. Sensitivity and specificity using a cut-off of 4.5 were high in differentiating the iRBD group from healthy subjects or the OSAS group. An RBDSQ-J score cut-off of 5.0 was considered useful for differentiating the iRBD group from the healthy subjects or the OSAS group. Cronbach's alpha for the entire RBDSQ-J was 0.866. The RBDSQ-J score had no correlation with the duration of RBD (mean disease duration in the iRBD group from symptom onset was 4.6 years, range 0.2 to 18 years). Answers to some items varied or had lower sensitivity. For example, for items 5, 6.2, and 6.3 a bed partner would be needed to provide answers, and the situations referred to in items 6.4 and 8 were often obscure. In evaluation of reliability, items that enlarged the kappa coefficient were 1, 2, 5 and 6.1 for iRBD. It can be proposed that future evaluations should use weighted scores for RBDSQ-J items, which may improve the accuracy of the questionnaire. The RBDSQ-J has high sensitivity, specificity, and reliability and would be applicable as a screening method for iRBD in an elderly Japanese population. Early-onset patients (≦50 years) were reported to have significantly more past and present psychiatric diagnoses and antidepressant usage than late-onset patients (>50 years) (Teman et al., 2009). It may be necessary to validate the RBDSQ-J in early-onset patients.

Nomura et al. evaluated the usefulness of the RBDSQ-J among patients with PD (Nomura et al., 2011). A total score of 6 points on the RBDSQ-J represented the best cut-off value for detecting RBD. This cut-off value for RBD secondary to PD was approximately 1 point higher than that reported for iRBD in studies performed by Stiasny-Kolster et al. and Miyamoto et al. However, the cut-off value with the RBDSQ-J for PD patients would become equal to the above-indicated value for iRBD patients if item 10 were removed. Nomura et al. showed that the RBDSQ-J may be useful for detecting RBD among a PD population regardless of the RBD symptoms. In addition, positivity for item 6.1 might represent a key criterion for analyzing populations with non-violent RBD.

5.4 RBDQ-HK

The existing RBD questionnaires may overlook the prevalence, frequency and severity of the clinical symptoms. There remains an obstacle for physicians to quantitatively observe and monitor treatment progress in clinical settings without the availability of timely PSG. Screening instruments for diagnosis of RBD are limited and there are none for quantifying the severity of the disease. Li et al. developed and validated a 13-item self-reported RBD questionnaire for diagnostic and monitoring purposes (Li et al., 2010). The patient always answered and the bed partner sometimes also answered in addition to the patient. Items 1-5 (Q1-Q5) were pertinent to patients' dreams and nightmares and the last eight items (Q6-Q13) elicited information on the typical behavioral consequences as a result of patients' dream enactments. Each item assesses two scales: lifetime occurrence and recent 1-yr frequency (5 point scale: 3 times or above per week; 1-2 times per week; once or a few times per month; once or few times per year; none). Scores are weighted in 7/13 questions according to the clinical importance of the behavioral manifestations of RBD. Scores range from 0-100. In a study to validate the instrument, 107 PSG-confirmed RBD patients (mean age 62.5 y) with the diagnosis of cryptogenic RBD, symptomatic RBD (PD, dementia, PD with dementia, narcolepsy), RBD-like disorder) and 107 controls (mean age 55.3 y) participated. The best RBDQ-HK cut-off score for RBD detection was 18-19, with 82% sensitivity, 87% specificity, and 86% positive predictive value; there was high test-retest reliability. Among the RBD cases, the scores of RBDQ-HK based on patients' self-reports were slightly lower compared to those provided by both patients and their relatives (e.g., bed partner)[self-report: 40.56(21.26) vs. self and relatives: 54.89(17.34), p=0.05]. The RBDQ-HK can be completed by patients with or without other informants such as a bed partner. However, abnormal nocturnal behaviors can go unnoticed in some RBD cases (e.g., when there is no assault or injury to self or bed partner), making the sensitivity of the RBDQ-HK different between those living and sleeping on their own and those living and sleeping with others. Hence, input on RBDQ-HK from relatives of patients is encouraged as it may enhance accuracy of the diagnosis and provide a better appraisal of treatment progress.

6. Conclusion

We have described screening methods for RBD as well as some of the available RBD screening questionnaires. All of the questionnaires had high sensitivity in screening for RBD, but lower specificity. There were some problems and limitations related to these instruments. These validation studies were mainly performed in middle aged and elderly subjects. Therefore, validation of RBD screening questionnaires should be done in younger people. In the case of self-reported questionnaires, information from a bed partner is useful in achieving higher sensitivity and specificity for the instrument. Boeve suggested that the MSQ likely to be more appropriate for use in those with cognitive impairment/dementia since the responses are provided by bed partners (Boeve, 2010a). In any of the instruments that might be applied but are unable or unwilling to undergo PSG, or who have little or no apparent REM sleep during PSG, then a diagnosis of probable RBD would be justified (Boeve, 2010a). OSAS may represent a confounding factor in the clinical diagnosis of RBD (Comella et al., 2002). To differentiate RBD from OSAS, simultaneously screening for OSAS by pulse oxymetry may be useful. It is impractical to frequently perform PSG and the availability of PSG is often limited. Therefore, it is important to evaluate and follow up the severity of RBD through instruments such as RBDQ-HK. It is also necessary to develop a severity index for RBD. Tachibana recently developed an RBD severity index (RBDSI) in Japanese (Tachibana, 2009).

In conclusion, RBD questionnaires may be applied within a stepwise diagnostic process (questionnaire, interview, polysomnography) for RBD (Table 5).

1st step	Screening	Questionnaire
2nd step	Interview	Sleep specialist, Neurologist
3rd step	Final diagnosis	Video PSG

Table 5. Diagnostic process for RBD

7. APPENDIX

RBD Screening Questionnaire (RBDSQ-J) (from Miyamoto T, et al., 2009)
（RBD スクリーニング問診票）

English (Japanese)	Questions（質問）	Answer（答え）	
1.	**I sometimes have very vivid dreams.** とてもはっきりした夢をときどき見る。	Yes （はい）	No （いいえ）
2.	**My dreams frequently have an aggressive or action-packed contents.** 攻撃的だったり、動きが盛りだくさんだったりする夢をよく見る。	Yes （はい）	No （いいえ）
3.	**The dream contents mostly match my nocturnal behavior.** 夢を見ているときに、夢の中と同じ動作をすることが多い。	Yes （はい）	No （いいえ）
4.	**I know that my arms or legs move when I sleep.** 寝ている時にうでや足を動かしていることがある。	Yes （はい）	No （いいえ）
5.	**It thereby happened that I (almost) hurt my bed partner or myself.** 寝ている時にうでや足を動かすので、隣で寝ている人にケガを負わせたり、自分がケガをしたりすることもある。	Yes （はい）	No （いいえ）

6. **I have or had the following phenomena during my dreams.** 夢を見ているときに以下のできごとが以前にあったり、今もある。		
6.1- **speaking, shouting, sweating, laughing, loudly** 誰かとしゃべる、大声でどなる、大声でののしる、大声で笑う。	Yes (はい)	No (いいえ)
6.2- **sudden limb movements, "fights"** うでと足を突如動かす/ けんかをしているように。	Yes (はい)	No (いいえ)
6.3- **gesture, complex movements, that are useless during sleep, e.g. to wave, to salute, to frighten mosquitoes, falls off the bed** 寝ている間に、身振りや複雑な動作をする。(例:手を振る、挨拶をする、何かを手で追い払う、ベッドから落ちる)	Yes (はい)	No (いいえ)
6.4 - **things that fell down around the bed, e.g. bedside lamp, book glasses.** ベッドの周りの物を落とす。(例:電気スタンド、本、メガネ)	Yes (はい)	No (いいえ)
7. **It happens that my movements awake me.** 寝ている時に自分の動作で目が覚めることがある。	Yes (はい)	No (いいえ)
8. **After awakening I mostly remember the content of my dreams well.** 目が覚めた後、夢の内容をだいたい覚えている。	Yes (はい)	No (いいえ)
9. **My sleep is frequently disturbed.** 眠りがよく妨げられる。	Yes (はい)	No (いいえ)
10. **I have/had a disease of the nervous system (e.g. stroke, head trauma, parkinsonism, RLS, narcolepsy, depression, epilepsy, inflammatory disease of the brain), which?** 以下のいずれかの神経系の病気を、以前患っていた、または現在患ってますか。(例:脳卒中、頭部外傷、パーキンソン病、むずむず脚症候群、ナルコレプシー、うつ病、てんかん、脳の炎症性疾患)	Yes (はい)	No (いいえ)

8. References

American Sleep Disorders Association, Diagnostic Classification Steering Committee. (1997). The International Classification of Sleep Disorders, Revised: Diagnostic and Coding Manual. American Sleep Disorders Association, Rochester, MN.

American Academy of Sleep Medicine. (2005) . The International Classification of Sleep Disorders: Diagnostic and Coding Manual. 2nd ed. American Academy of Sleep Medicine, Westchester, IL.

Boeve,BF., Ferman, TJ., Silber,MH., Smith, GE.(2002a). Validation of a Questionnaire for the Diagnosis of REM Sleep Behavior Disorder. *Neurology* 58 (Suppl 3): A509.

Boeve,BF., Silber ,MH., Ferman, TJ., Smith, GE.(2002b). Validation of a questionnaire for the diagnosis of REM sleep behavior disorder. *Sleep* (Abstract Suppl): A 486.

Boeve ,BF. (2010a). REM sleep behavior disorder: Updated review of the core features, the REM sleep behavior disorder-neurodegenerative disease association, evolving concepts, controversies,and future directions. *Ann. N.Y. Acad. Sci.* 1184: 15-54.

Boeve ,BF., Molano, J., Ferman ,T., Smith ,G., Bieniek, KF., Tippmann-Peikert ,M., Knopman ,D., Pankratz ,VS., Geda ,Y., Roberts ,R., Tangalos,E., Silber ,M., Petersen ,R. (2010b). Screening for REM Sleep Behavior Disorder in the Community-Dwelling Elderly: Validation of the Mayo Sleep Questionnaire in the Mayo Clinic Study of Aging. *Neurology* 74 (Suppl 2): A432.

Boeve, BF., Molano, JR., Ferman, TJ., Smith, GE., Lin, SC., Bieniek, K., Haidar, W., Tippmann-Peikert, M., Knopman, DS., Graff-Radford, NR., Lucas, JA., Petersen, RC,. Silber, MH. (2011). Validation of the Mayo Sleep Questionnaire to screen for REM sleep behavior disorder in aging and dementia cohort. *Sleep Med* ,doi: 10.1016/j.sleep.2010.12.009.

Bologna, Genova, Parma and Pisa Universities group for the study of REM sleep Behaviour Disorder (RBD) in Parkinson's Disease. (2003). Interobserver reliability of ICSD-R criteria for REM sleep behavior disorder. *J Sleep Res* 12: 255-257.

Chiu,HFK., Wing,YK., Lam,LCW., Li,SW., Lum,CM., Leung,T., Ho,CKW. (2000). Sleep-related injyury in the elderly- An epidemiological study in Hong Kong. *Sleep* 23(4): 513-517.

Comella, CL., Stevens, S., Stepanski, E., Leurgans (2002). Sensitivity analysis of the clinical diagnostic criteria for REM behavior disorder (RBD) in Parkinson's disease. *Neurology* 58 (Suppl 3):A434.

Eisensehr, I., Lindeiner, HV., Jäger, M., Noachtar, S.(2001). REM sleep behavior disorder in sleep-disordered patients with versus without Parkinson's disease: is there a need for polysomnography? *J Neurol Sci* 186: 7-11.

Gagnon, JF., Bēdard, MA., Fantini, ML., Petit, D., Panisset, M., Romprē, S., Carrier, J., Montplaisir, J. (2002). REM sleep behavior disorder and REM sleep without atonia in Parkinson's disease. *Neurology* 59: 585-589.

Iranzo, A., Santamaria, J.(2005). Severe obstructive sleep apnea/hypopnea mimicking REM sleep behavior disorder. *Sleep* 28: 203-206.

Iranzo, A., Molinuevo, JL., Santamaria, J., Serradell, M., Marti, MJ., Valldeoriola, F., Tolosa, E. (2006). Rapid-eye-movement sleep behavior disorder as an early marker for a neurodegenerative disorder: a descriotive study. *Lancet Neurol* 5 (7): 572-577

Li,SX., Wing ,YK., Lam, SP., Zhang, J., Yu, MWM,. Ho, CKW., Tsoh, J., Mok, V. (2010).Validation of a new REM sleep behavior disorder questionnaire (RBDQ-HK). *Sleep Med* 11:43-48.

Miyamoto, T., Miyamoto, M., Iwanami, M., Kobayashi, M., Nakanura, M., Inoue, Y., Ando, C., Hirata, K. (2009). The REM sleep behavior disorder screening questionnaire: Validation study of a Japanese version. *Sleep Med* 10 :1151-1154.

Nomura, T., Inoue, Y., Kagimura, T., Uemura, Y., Nakajima, K. (2011). Utility of the REM sleep behavior disorder screening questionnaire (RBDSQ) in Parkinson's disease patients. *Sleep Med,* doi:10.1016/j.sleep.2011.01.015.

Ohayon, MM., Caulet, M., Priest, RG. (1997). Violent Behavior During Sleep. *J Clin Psychiatry* 58: 369-376.

Postuma, RB., Gagnon, JF., Vendette, M., Fantini, ML., Massicotte-Marquez, J., Montplaisir, J. (2009). Quantifying the risk of neurodegenerative disease in idiopathic REM sleep behavior disorder. *Neurology* 72(15): 1296-1300.

Schenck, CH., Bundlie, SR., Mahowald, MW. (1996). Delayed emergence of a parkinsonian disorder in 38% of 29 older men initially diagnosed with idiopathic rapid eye movement sleep behavior disorder. *Neurology* 46: 388-393.

Schenck, CH, Mahowald, MW. (2002). REM sleep behavior disorder: Clinical developmental, and neuroscience perspectives 16 years after its formal identification in SLEEP. *Sleep* 25(2): 120-138.

Stiasny-Kolster, K., Mayer, G., Schäfer, S., Möller, JC., Heinzel-Gutenbrunner, M., Oertel,WH.(2007). The REM Sleep Behavior Disorder Screening Questionnaire- A New Diagnostic Instrument. *Mov Disord* 22(16): 2386-2393.

Tachibana, N. (2009). Historical overview of REM sleep behavior disorder in relation to its pathophysiology. *BRAIN and NERVE* 61(5): 558-568.

Teman, PT., Tippmann-Peikert, M., Silber, MH., Slocub, NL., Auger, RR.(2009). Idiopathic rapid-eye-movement sleep disorder: Associations with antidepressants, psychiatric diagnoses, and other factors, in relation to age of onset. *Sleep Med* 10: 60-65.